Medical Decision Making

Medical Decision Making

Second Edition

Harold C. Sox, M.D.
Geisel School of Medicine at Dartmouth, Hanover, New Hampshire

Michael C. Higgins, Ph.D.
Stanford University, Stanford, California

Douglas K. Owens, M.D., M.S.
Department of Veterans Affairs Palo Alto Health Care System, Palo Alto, California
Stanford University, Stanford, California

WILEY-BLACKWELL
A John Wiley & Sons, Ltd., Publication

Library of Congress Cataloging-in-Publication Data

Sox, Harold C.
  Medical decision making / Harold C. Sox, Michael C. Higgins, Douglas K. Owens. -- 2nd ed.
    p. ; cm.
  Rev. ed. of: Medical decision making / Harold C. Sox, Jr. . . . [et al.]. c1998.
  Includes bibliographical references and index.
  Summary: "This title provides a thorough understanding of the key decision making infrastructure of clinical practice and retains its emphasis on practice and principles of individualized medical decision making" – Provided by publisher.
    ISBN 978-0-470-65866-6 (paper)
  I. Higgins, Michael C. (Michael Clark), 1950- II. Owens, Douglas K. III. Medical decision making. IV. Title.
  [DNLM: 1. Diagnosis, Differential. 2. Cost-Benefit Analysis. 3. Decision Making. 4. Probability. WB 141.5]
  616.07'5 – dc23

                                                    2012047951

A catalogue record for this book is available from the British Library.

Wiley also publishes its books in a variety of electronic formats. Some content that appears in print may not be available in electronic books.

Cover design by Rob Sawkins for Opta Design Ltd.

Set in 9.5/12pt Palatino by Laserwords Private Limited, Chennai, India
Printed and bound in Malaysia by Vivar Printing Sdn Bhd

1 2013

To Jean and Kathleen
To Sara, Rachel, and Christopher
To Carol, Colin, and Lara
Their support has meant everything.

Contents

Foreword

The maturation of medical science during the last half of the twentieth century was most impressive. Clinical trials displaced observational studies that typically consisted of a dozen or fewer patients; the pathophysiology and genetics of many diseases were discovered; and diagnostic and therapeutic methods advanced. Crude diagnostic tests such as cholecystography and barium enemas and risky tests such as air encephalograms, needle biopsies, and exploratory laparotomies were made obsolete by technology. Flexible tubes, some outfitted with lights and cameras, CT, MRI, and PET scanners, and sophisticated immuno-analyses of blood and other body fluids gained immediate acceptance. Many therapies that were formulated by grinding up organs, desiccating them, and hoping that they would correct a deficit were replaced by new, potent chemicals.

Clinical reasoning, the processes behind both diagnosis and medical decision making, including the complex tradeoffs between the risks and benefits of tests and treatments, lagged behind advances in medical science. In the run-up to the last quarter of the century, students learned how to reason about patient problems by observing expert clinicians at work, and (if they dared) by asking them why they ordered this test or that, why they gave one drug or another. Because this apprenticeship approach was not codified, objectified, or quantified, medical texts struggled to explain clinical reasoning, and students struggled to learn it. And when the evidence of confusion about the use of tests and treatments first emerged, alarm bells clanged. Researchers had discovered extreme variations in the use of tests and treatments from one community to another and in regions across the country without a corresponding benefit for patients. Irrational testing and treating had begun to contribute substantially to an impossible escalation in the cost of care.

During the last three decades of the twentieth century, clinician–scientists began to examine the processes of diagnosis and decision making with tools from other disciplines, including cognitive science, decision science, probability, and utility theory. From these diverse sources the clinical science of medical decision making was hatched. Elements of the diagnostic process were identified and a language for explaining and teaching diagnosis was formulated. Cognitive errors in diagnosis were sought and methods developed to avoid them. The critical importance of a probabilistic representation of diagnosis, in terms of prior probabilities, conditional probabilities, and likelihood ratios, was recognized and put to use in the form of a centuries-old formulation of Bayes' Rule. Decision analysis, a discipline formerly used by the military, was applied first to individual clinical problems, later to classes of problems, and eventually to issues of cost and efficacy of tests and treatments. Before the end of the twentieth century, a science of medical decision making and a language for teaching it had been born.

Implementing the new science, however, proved more difficult than developing it. Skeptics averred that physicians' estimates of probabilities were often flawed, that applying Bayes' Rule was not easy, and that decision trees were either too simple (and thus did not represent a clinical problem sufficiently) or too complex (and thus could not be understood). Many wondered whether medicine could be convinced to adopt these new approaches and whether the average physician could be expected to use them in their day-to-day practices.

As the field has evolved, some of these questions have been answered. Now, in the second decade of the twenty-first century, Bayes' Rule is used to design clinical trials, to develop decision rules that help physicians judge whether to admit patients suspected of having an acute myocardial infarction, and to develop compiled strategies for diagnosing and treating pulmonary emboli, to name a few applications. Decision analysis has been used to formulate answers for individual patients' dilemmas, but this use is time consuming, expensive, and requires special expertise. Nonetheless, decision analysis has found extensive application in clinical practice guideline development, cost-effective analyses, and comparative effectiveness studies. A cadre of physicians has become sufficiently skilled in the methods to apply them in active clinical teaching environments and to integrate them into medical student and residency curricula.

It is legitimate to ask why a student or resident should spend the intellectual capital to learn these methods. The answer is compelling. First, they help in learning and teaching the process of diagnosis. Second, the principles of screening and diagnostic and management decision making become transparent from an understanding of Bayes' Rule, diagnostic and therapeutic thresholds, decisional toss-ups, and decision analysis. Subjecting such issues to rational examination improves decision making and, consequently, patient care. Moreover, because these methods are the basis for so many analyses of health practices, appreciation of their limitations provides a healthy skepticism of their applications. Lastly, the approaches are powerful tools to pass on the concepts to others, as well as critical templates to understand honest differences of opinion on controversial medical practices.

For the past 25 years, *Medical Decision Making* has been an ideal venue for developing a rich comprehension of these methods and for understanding how to approach diagnosis; the new second edition is even better. Its chapter on Bayes' Rule, for example, is exemplary, explaining the method in multiple different formats. The chapters on selection of diagnostic tests and decision analysis are meticulously crafted so as to leave little uncertainty about the methods. A new chapter on modeling methods is richly illustrated by actual analyses; the chapters on expected value decision making, utility assessment, and Markov modeling have been extensively revised.

In short, this book has been a standard of the field, and the new edition will continue its dominance. There is little doubt that in the future many clinical analyses will be based on the methods described in *Medical Decision Making,* and the book provides a basis for a critical appraisal of such policies. Teachers of medical decision making will require it; medical students will dig into it repeatedly as they learn clinical medicine; residents will go back to it again and again to refresh their diagnostic and therapeutic skills. And from its lucid pages, practicing physicians will attain a richer understanding of the principles underlying their work.

Jerome P. Kassirer, M.D.
Distinguished Professor, Tufts University School of Medicine, US
Visiting Professor, Stanford Medical School, US

Preface

The first edition of *Medical Decision Making* was a small project that took on a life of its own. The chapters began as sketches for a course on medical decision making that the authors undertook as part of a foundation grant to study methods for teaching medical decision making. Thanks to the enthusiasm of co-authors Keith Marton and Michael Higgins, the project took off and turned into a book published by Butterworths in 1988. A Stanford medical student, Marshal Blatt, read the chapters and gave us invaluable advice about making the book more understandable to beginning students. We must have listened to him because many students have thanked us for writing a book that they could understand.

Twenty-five years have elapsed since publication. *Medical Decision Making* has sold steadily through a succession of publishers. Physicians and decision analysts from every corner of the globe have approached me to say that the book was pivotal in their engagement with the field of medical decision making. People have called for a second edition, but the authors, having moved on in disparate careers, were never ready until the past year. I have been an advocate for medical decision analysis as a teacher, practicing internist, medical journal editor, and participant in the emergence of comparative effectiveness research as a new discipline. Michael Higgins worked for companies that developed medical software, while teaching courses at Stanford University. Douglas Owens, an internist and a leader in the application of medical decision analysis to clinical policy, has become the third author.

How has the book changed? Hopefully, the writing has benefited from my experience of eight years as a full-time medical journal editor. I updated Chapters 1 through 5, 9, and 11 and served as the editor for my co-authors. I rewrote my chapters, updated the examples, and added new developments (particularly a stronger emphasis on likelihood ratios (Chapter 4), systematic reviews and meta-analysis of diagnostic test sensitivity and specificity (Chapter 5), and cost–benefit analysis (Chapter 11)).

Michael Higgins wrote new chapters (Chapters 6 through 8) that covered expected value decision making, utility assessment, Markov models, and mathematical models of life expectancy. The treatment of these topics reflects his long teaching experience, in which he relied on mathematical models that simplify the process of assessing utilities. Any reader who can recall the concepts of high school algebra will be able to understand these chapters.

Dr. Owens' chapter on decision modeling reflects the growing influence of decision analysis to support clinical and public health policy making (and the waning influence of decision models created to solve a specific patient's decision problem). The chapter describes different types of models and provides extended examples, but it is not a tutorial in how to create a decision model. The reader who wants to learn decision modeling should take the short courses offered at the annual meeting of the Society for Medical Decision Making and spend some time apprenticing with an expert in the field.

From the simple (likelihood ratios) to the complex (microsimulation modeling), what is the future of medical decision analysis? In two words, both hand-held computer applications ("apps" in current usage) and shared decision making. Hand-held devices will bring decision models – simple and complex – to the office and the bedside, where clinicians and patients will use them to individualize their discussions of the big decisions.

What can textbooks like *Medical Decision Making* contribute to this world of shared, informed decision making using computer-based decision analysis? As in the past, textbooks will shape the way that future decision analysts learn and later practice the discipline of their life's work. We think that clinicians-in-training should master the material in Chapters 3, 4, and 5. They should be able to use the time-tradeoff method to assess a patient's utilities for a health state. They should have a cultural understanding of decision modeling. Finally, we hope that aspiring master clinicians will read a book like ours to gain a greater understanding of their daily work and the limitations of the imperfect information that they rely upon.

H.C.S.

CHAPTER 1

Introduction

"Proof," I said, "is always a relative thing. It's an overwhelming balance of probabilities. And that's a matter of how they strike you."

(*Raymond Chandler*, Farewell, My Lovely, 1940)

Probability is the rule of life – especially under the skin. Never make a positive diagnosis.

(*Sir William Osler*)

Thoughtful clinicians ask themselves many difficult questions during the course of taking care of patients. Some of these questions are as follows:

- How may I be thorough yet efficient when considering the possible causes of my patient's problem?
- How do I characterize the information I have gathered during the medical interview and physical examination?
- How should I interpret new diagnostic information?
- How do I select the appropriate diagnostic test?
- How do I choose among several risky treatments?

The goal of this book is to help clinicians answer these important questions.

The first question is addressed with observations from expert clinicians "thinking out loud" as they work their way through a clinical problem. The last four are addressed from the perspective of medical decision analysis, a quantitative approach to medical decision making.

The goal of this introductory chapter is to preview the contents of the book by sketching out preliminary answers to these five questions.

1.1 How may I be thorough yet efficient when considering the possible causes of my patient's problems?

Trying to be efficient in thinking about the possible causes of a patient's problem often conflicts with being thorough. This conflict has no single solution. However, much may be learned about medical problem solving

Medical Decision Making, Second Edition. Harold C. Sox, Michael C. Higgins and Douglas K. Owens.
© 2013 John Wiley & Sons, Ltd. Published 2013 by John Wiley & Sons, Ltd.

by listening to expert diagnosticians discuss how they reasoned their way through a case. Because the single most powerful predictor of skill in diagnosis is exposure to patients, the best advice is "see lots of patients and learn from your mistakes." How to be thorough, yet efficient, when thinking about the possible causes of a patient's problem is the topic of Chapter 2.

1.2 How do I characterize the information I have gathered during the medical interview and physical examination?

The first step toward understanding how to characterize the information one gathers from the medical interview and physical examination is to realize that information provided by the patient and by diagnostic tests usually does not reveal the patient's true state. A patient's signs, symptoms, and diagnostic test results are usually representative of more than one disease. Therefore, distinguishing among the possibilities with absolute certainty is not possible. A 60-year-old man's history of chest pain illustrates this point:

> Mr. Costin, a 60-year-old bank executive, walks into the emergency room complaining of intermittent substernal chest pain that is "squeezing" in character. The chest pain is occasionally brought on by exertion but usually occurs without provocation. When it occurs, the patient lies down for a few minutes, and the pain usually subsides in about 5 minutes. It never lasts more than 10 minutes. Until these episodes of chest pain began 3 weeks ago, the patient had been in good health, except for intermittent problems with heartburn after a heavy meal.

Although there are at least 60 causes of chest pain, Mr. Costin's medical history narrows down the diagnostic possibilities considerably. Based on his history, the two most likely causes of Mr. Costin's chest pain are coronary artery disease or esophageal disease.

However, the cause of Mr. Costin's illness is uncertain. This uncertainty is not a shortcoming of the clinician who gathered the information; rather, it reflects the uncertainty inherent in the information provided by Mr. Costin. Like most patients, his true disease state is hidden within his body and must be inferred from imperfect external clues.

How do clinicians usually characterize the uncertainty inherent in medical information? Most clinicians use words such as "probably" or "possibly" to characterize this uncertainty. However, most of these words are imprecise, as illustrated as we hear more about Mr. Costin's story:

> The clinician who sees Mr. Costin in the emergency room tells Mr. Costin, "I cannot rule out coronary artery disease. The next step in the diagnostic process is to examine the results of a stress ECG." She also says, "I cannot rule out esophageal disease either. If the stress ECG is negative, we will work you up for esophageal disease."
>
> Mr. Costin is very concerned about his condition and seeks a second opinion. The second clinician who sees Mr. Costin agrees that coronary artery

disease and esophageal disease are the most likely diagnoses. He tells Mr. Costin, "Coronary artery disease is a likely diagnosis, but to know for certain we'll have to see the results of a stress ECG." Concerning esophageal disease, he says, "We cannot rule out esophageal disease at this point. If the stress ECG is normal, and you don't begin to feel better, we'll work you up for esophageal disease."

Mr. Costin feels reassured that both clinicians seem to agree on the possibility of esophageal disease, since both have said that they cannot rule it out. However, Mr. Costin cannot reconcile the different statements concerning the likelihood that he has coronary artery disease. Recall that the first clinician said "coronary artery disease cannot be ruled out," whereas the second clinician stated, "coronary artery disease is a likely diagnosis." Mr. Costin wants to know the difference between these two different opinions. He explains his confusion to the second clinician and asks him to speak to the first clinician:

> The two clinicians confer by telephone. Although the clinicians expressed the likelihood of coronary artery disease differently when they talked with Mr. Costin, it turns out that they had similar ideas about the likelihood that he has coronary artery disease. Both clinicians believe that about one patient out of three with Mr. Costin's history has coronary artery disease.

From this episode, Mr. Costin learns that clinicians may choose different words to express the same judgment about the likelihood of an uncertain event:

> To Mr. Costin's surprise, the clinicians have different opinions about the likelihood of esophageal disease, despite the fact that both clinicians described its likelihood with the same phrase, "esophageal disease cannot be ruled out." The first clinician believes that among patients with Mr. Costin's symptoms, only one patient in ten would have esophageal disease. However, the second clinician thinks that as many as one patient in two would have esophageal disease.

Mr. Costin is chagrined that both clinicians used the same phrase, "cannot be ruled out," to describe two different likelihoods. He learns that clinicians commonly use the same words to express different judgments about the likelihood of an event.

The solution to the confusion that can occur when using words to characterize uncertainty with words is to use a number: probability. Probability expresses uncertainty precisely because it is the likelihood that a condition is present or will occur in the future. When one clinician believes the probability that a patient has coronary artery disease is 1 in 10, and the other clinician thinks that it is 1 in 2, the two clinicians know that they disagree and that they must talk about why their interpretations are so disparate. The precision of numbers to express uncertainty is illustrated graphically by the scale in Figure 1.1. On this scale, uncertain events are expressed with numbers between 0 and 1.

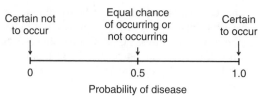

Figure 1.1 A scale for expressing uncertainty.

To understand the meaning of probability in medicine, think of it as a fraction. For example, the fraction "one-third" means 33 out of a group of 100. In medicine, if a clinician states that the probability that a disease is present is 33%, it means that the clinician believes that if she sees 100 patients with the same findings, 33 of them will have the disease in question (Figure 1.2).

Although probability has a precise mathematical meaning, a probability estimate need not correspond to a physical reality, such as the prevalence of disease in a defined group of patients. We define probability in medicine as a number between 0 and 1 that expresses a clinician's opinion about the likelihood of a condition being present or occurring in the future. The probability of an event a clinician believes is certain to occur is equal to 1. The probability of an event a clinician believes is certain not to occur is equal to 0.

A probability may apply to the present state of the patient (e.g., that he has coronary artery disease), or it may be used to express the likelihood that an event will occur in the future (e.g., that he will experience a myocardial infarction within one year).

Any degree of uncertainty may be expressed on this scale. Note that uncertain events are expressed with numbers between 0 and 1. Both ends of the scale correspond to absolute certainly. An event that is certain to occur is expressed with a probability equal to 1. An event that is certain not to occur is expressed with a probability equal to 0.

When should a clinician use probability in the diagnostic process? The first time that probability is useful in the diagnostic process is when the clinician feels she needs to synthesize the medical information she has obtained in the medical interview and physical examination into an opinion. At this juncture the clinician wants to be precise about the uncertainty because she is poised

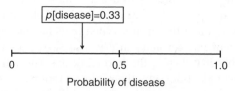

Figure 1.2 A clinician can visualize the level of certainty about a disease hypothesis on a probability scale. Thirty-three is marked on this certainty scale to correspond to the clinician's initial probability estimate concerning the likelihood that Mr. Costin had coronary artery disease.

to make decisions about the patient. The clinician may decide to act as if the patient is not diseased. She may decide that she needs more information and will order a diagnostic test. She may decide that she knows enough to start the patient on a specific treatment. To decide between these options, she does not need to know the diagnosis. She does need to estimate the patient's probability that he has, as in the case of Mr. Costin, coronary artery disease as the cause of his chest pain.

A clinician arrives at a probability estimate for a disease hypothesis by using personal experience and the published literature. Advice on how to estimate probability is found in Chapter 3.

1.3   How do I interpret new diagnostic information?

New diagnostic information often does not reveal the patient's true state, and the best a clinician can do is to estimate how much the new information has changed her uncertainty about it. This task is difficult if one is describing uncertainty with words. However, if the clinician is expressing uncertainty with probability, she can use Bayes' theorem to estimate how much her uncertainty about a patient's true state should have changed. To use Bayes' theorem a clinician must estimate the probability of disease before the new information was gathered (the *prior probability* or pre-test probability) and know the accuracy of the new diagnostic information. The probability of disease that results from interpreting new diagnostic information is called the *posterior probability* (or post-test probability). These two probabilities are illustrated in Figure 1.3.

Chapter 4 describes how to use Bayes' theorem to estimate the post-test probability of a disease.

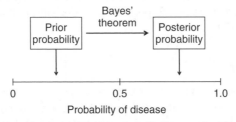

Figure 1.3 The pre-test probability and the post-test probability of disease.

1.4   How do I select the appropriate diagnostic test?

Although the selection of a diagnostic test is ostensibly straightforward, the reasoning must take into account several factors. In the language of medical decision analysis, the selection of diagnostic tests depends on the patient's feelings about states of disease and health, the clinician's estimate of the prior probability of disease, and the accuracy of the diagnostic tests that the clinician is trying to choose between.

A logical approach to selecting diagnostic tests depends on three principles:

- Diagnostic tests are imperfect and therefore seldom reveal a patient's true state with certainty.
- Tests should be chosen if the results could change the clinician's mind about what to do for the patient.
- Clinicians often start treatment when they are uncertain about the true state of the patient.

These three principles lead to an important concept: The selection of diagnostic tests depends on the level of certainty at which a clinician is willing to start treatment. This level of certainty is known as the treatment-threshold probability. How to use the treatment-threshold probability to make decisions is a topic of Chapter 9.

A clinician must take two steps to assess the treatment-threshold probability of disease. The first step is to list the harms and benefits of treatment. The second step is to assess the patient's feelings about these harms and benefits. A decision analyst assesses a patient's attitudes toward the risks and benefits of treatment using a unit of measure called *utility*. Measuring a patient's utilities is covered in Chapter 8 of this text.

1.5 How do I choose among several risky treatment alternatives?

Choosing among risky treatment alternatives is difficult because the outcome of most treatments is uncertain: some people respond to treatment but others do not. If the outcome of a treatment is governed by chance, a clinician cannot know in advance which outcome of the treatment will result. Under these circumstances, the best way to achieve a good outcome is to choose the treatment alternative whose average outcome is best. This concept is called *expected value decision making*. Expected value decision making is the topic of Chapters 6, 7, and 11.

1.6 Summary

The care of patients is difficult in part because of the uncertainty inherent in the nature of medical information: tests are imperfect, and treatments have unpredictable consequences. The application of probability, utility, and expected value decision making provides a framework for making the right decision despite the uncertainty of medical practice. Medical decision analysis helps clinicians and patients to cope with uncertainty.

CHAPTER 2

Differential diagnosis

This chapter is about differential diagnosis, a systematic process for narrowing the range of possible explanations for a patient's problem. The goal of this chapter is to describe a thorough, yet efficient, approach to this process. The chapter has four parts:

2.1 Introduction

Differential diagnosis is the process of considering the possible causes of a patient's symptom or physical finding and making a diagnosis. Differential diagnosis is a safeguard against premature conclusions as well as a time-proven method for attacking what can be a supremely difficult intellectual challenge. All clinicians, regardless of their specialty, use differential diagnosis and strive to master it. For many clinicians, to be called a superb diagnostician is the highest form of praise.

The Challenge of Differential Diagnosis: A patient visits your office on a busy afternoon because of a symptom. She wants you to discover the reason for the symptom and then cure it quickly and painlessly. You must discover its cause or at least assure yourself that it is not due to a serious, treatable disease. This task can be difficult, especially when the symptom has many possible causes. It is hard to recall a long list of possible causes or the key features of even one cause of the symptom. Moreover, these key features typically occur in more than one disease. Time pressure often adds to the intellectual difficulties.

The Purposes of the Interview: The medical interview has many purposes. The first goal is to establish a relationship of mutual trust with the patient. Another goal is to observe the patient closely for clues that may help to focus your investigation. A third goal is to narrow the list of diseases that could be causing the patient's problem and focus the physical examination on a few possible diagnoses. Later on comes the physical examination and decisions about whether to perform diagnostic tests.

Medical Decision Making, Second Edition. Harold C. Sox, Michael C. Higgins and Douglas K. Owens.
© 2013 John Wiley & Sons, Ltd. Published 2013 by John Wiley & Sons, Ltd.

2.2 How clinicians make a diagnosis

We know more about how clinicians *should* reason than about how they *do* reason. This book is about how physicians should reason in specific situations, such as selecting and interpreting diagnostic tests or making a decision between two treatments. These normative methods are based on first principles of logical reasoning and take full advantage of all sources of information. This chapter is about how physicians *do* reason as they strive to narrow the list of possible causes of a patient's symptom.

This chapter describes a logical framework for diagnosis, but we cannot claim that it is based on first principles of logical reasoning. We can claim that expert clinicians use the process. However, the path to expertise only begins with a good process. Research shows that expert clinicians got that way by seeing lots of patients. Moreover, they are skillful at applying what they learned from past experience to solve the problem of the moment.

The process that we will describe is based upon listening to expert diagnosticians think aloud as they solve a diagnostic problem. Diagnosticians, expert or not, use a similar process. The expert has a larger, more accessible fund of knowledge than the average clinician. Some of this knowledge comes from textbooks and articles, but most of it comes from having seen similar patients and remembering their diagnosis (pattern recognition).

The message for beginning students is two-fold. First, they will learn a process that is the foundation of excellence in diagnosis. Second, the pathway to excellence is open to those who constantly strive to enlarge their experience by immersing themselves in clinical medicine and the important details of individual patients and their ultimate fate. The more you challenge yourself, the more you will learn and the more expert you will become. You do not get better by playing it safe and avoiding exposure to the possibility of being wrong. In fact, experts will tell you that they learn more from being wrong than from being right.

The central mystery of medical education is how students acquire skill in differential diagnosis. This topic is seldom taught as a formal discipline. Most learn it while discussing specific patients with a clinical teacher. This gap in the medical curriculum is easily understood: our understanding of the methods used by skilled diagnosticians would scarcely sustain an hour's lecture. What we do know about differential diagnosis is the result of research in which clinicians "think out loud" as they work their way through a diagnostic problem. These observations may be summarized in five conclusions:

1. Hypotheses are generated early in the interview.
2. Only a few hypotheses are being actively considered at any moment.
3. Newly acquired information is often used incorrectly.
4. Clinicians often fail to take full advantage of past experience with similar patients.
5. A clinician's skill in differential diagnosis varies from topic to topic; more experience usually means greater expertise.

Each one of these conclusions requires additional comment:

1. *Hypotheses are generated early:* Beginning students are often instructed to obtain all relevant data before starting to exclude diseases from the list of possible causes of the patient's complaint. They soon outgrow this mistaken teaching. Experienced clinicians observe the patient closely while introducing themselves and often begin to draw tentative conclusions before the patient has spoken. As soon as they identify the patient's main complaint, they use the patient's age and gender to help identify the main diagnostic possibilities. Good diagnosticians will ask the patient to tell the story of the main complaint while they listen, observe, and formulate hypotheses. These hypotheses determine their first specific questions, and the answers bring other hypotheses to mind.

Conclusion: data collection is hypothesis-driven.

2. *Only a few hypotheses are considered simultaneously:* Research about cognition shows that the human mind has a limited working memory. Just as a juggler can keep only a few objects in the air at once, so the clinician can consider only a few hypotheses simultaneously.

The clinician begins evaluating a hypothesis by matching the patient's findings with the clinician's internal representation, or model, of the disease. Sometimes this internal representation is the pathophysiology of the condition. One pathophysiological derangement causes another, as inferred by logical deduction, which leads to another and eventually to the expected clinical manifestations. Reasoning backward along this chain of logical deductions may lead to the cause of the patient's problem. One way to remember the differential diagnosis of a low serum sodium is to reason deductively from the pathophysiology of the condition. Research indicates that expert diagnosticians use pathophysiological reasoning mainly for difficult, atypical cases. Expert diagnosticians typically have an excellent understanding of pathophysiology.

More often, the clinician uses an associative model of disease, also known as pattern recognition. Associative models consist of clinical findings, illness progression, predisposing characteristics, and complications that are associated with a disease. The clinician asks about the typical features of a disease and is often able to eliminate hypotheses solely from the patient's responses. Hypotheses that cannot be readily discarded are further tested during the physical examination. Another mark of an expert diagnostician is the ability to quickly match the patient's findings to a pattern of disease manifestations. Often, the patient's findings remind the clinician of a similar patient seen many years earlier. Expert clinicians retain these experiences and can recall specific patients from many decades earlier.

The supreme mystery of clinical reasoning is the cognitive process that clinicians use to discard or confirm a hypothesis. Several models of this process have been proposed. These models are based on analyzing what clinicians say about how they test hypotheses:

- *Additive model*: In a linear model, clinicians assign a positive weight to findings that tend to confirm a diagnosis and negative weights to findings that disconfirm the diagnosis. In some unknown cognitive process, the clinician decides to discard or accept a hypothesis based on the sum of the diagnostic weights. Clinical prediction rules use this model (see Chapter 3). Physicians probably assign weights subjectively and subconsciously. In the context of this chapter, the analog of the diagnostic weight of a finding might be the likelihood ratio of the finding. The likelihood ratio indicates whether the odds of the target condition go up or down and by how much. It is, therefore, an empirical, quantitative measure of the changes in the odds of the target condition (see Chapters 4 and 5).
- *Bayesian model*: Bayes' theorem is the method to calculate the post-test probability of the target condition. Bayes' theorem tells the clinician how much new information should change the probability. By analogy, clinicians may change their belief in a hypothesis with each new item of information and conclude at some point that the probability is low enough to discard the hypothesis.
- *Algorithmic model*: Algorithms are commonly used to represent the logic of diagnosis. Do clinicians follow an internal flow sheet with branching logic as they test a hypothesis? Does a series of "no" branches eventually lead to discarding a hypothesis? We do not know.

Undoubtedly, clinicians use features of these admittedly speculative models as they consider a diagnostic hypothesis, but the essence of diagnostic reasoning eludes understanding.

3. *Newly acquired information is often used inappropriately:* Mistakes happen when a clinician begins to believe in a diagnostic hypothesis. The clinician may ignore conflicting information or misinterpret it as confirming an existing hypothesis when the correct action is to disregard it, use it to reject the hypothesis, or use it as a clue to a new hypothesis. The clinician may exaggerate the importance of findings that fit with a preconceived idea or accommodate inconsistent data by reformulating a hypothesis to the point where it is too general to be tested parsimoniously.

Example: These errors are illustrated by the story of the medical student who offered a diagnosis of leishmaniasis in a patient with diffuse lymphadenopathy. The patient had taken a steamship cruise to a South American port years before. When the attending physician asked him to justify this arcane diagnosis, the student replied, "what else causes lymphadenopathy?" Unable to remember any other causes of lymphadenopathy, the student exaggerated the importance of a rather dubious travel history in order to support a far-out hypothesis.

Conclusion: placing too much weight on data to support a low-probability hypothesis leads to mistakes.

4. *Past experience can be used inappropriately:* Clinicians use rules of thumb (heuristics) for using experience to estimate probability from the match between the patient's case history and past experience. These heuristics include representativeness (the goodness of fit between the patient's case and past cases) and availability (how easily past cases come to mind). Thoughtless use of these heuristics can lead to mistakes (discussed at length in Chapter 3).

5. *Skill in clinical reasoning varies from topic to topic:* Students of cognitive psychology have assumed that individuals who are able to reason well about one topic should be equally proficient with other topics. In fact, clinicians' reasoning skills vary from topic to topic. Associations between hypotheses and clinical findings are learned by experience. Therefore, mastery of a topic requires experience with a wide variety of cases. A good memory and cognitive facility are not enough.

Conclusion: expertise requires a deep clinical experience.

Summary: Descriptive studies of clinical reasoning provide helpful insights for the beginning clinician. However, despite dogged efforts by researchers, we do not understand many aspects of clinical reasoning.

2.3 The principles of hypothesis-driven differential diagnosis

The most important conclusion from research on how experts make a diagnosis is that the questions they are asking at any moment are intended to test the small number of diagnostic hypotheses that they are considering at that moment. In other words, the main function of the interview and physical examination is to test diagnostic hypotheses. Thinking of this principle may help the clinician to steer the interview back on topic when it threatens to get sidetracked.

While reading this chapter, imagine that you are evaluating a patient with a chief complaint of "nocturnal chest pain for one month." The pain is a substernal tightness that begins an hour or so after lying down. A complete evaluation of this complaint will include the following steps:

1. Taking the history.
2. Doing a physical examination.
3. Selecting and interpreting diagnostic tests.
4. Choosing a treatment.

This book will cover the principles underlying each of these steps in considerable detail. The purpose of this chapter is to describe the thinking processes that guide the history and physical examination. Subsequent chapters prepare the reader to choose diagnostic tests and therapy.

Differential diagnosis is a cyclic process consisting of three steps which ultimately lead to a fourth step, taking action (Figure 2.1).

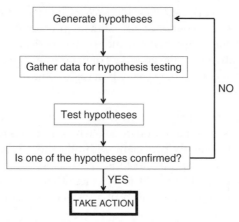

Figure 2.1 The cyclic process of differential diagnosis.

The three steps are repeated many times as hypotheses are considered and rejected, confirmed, or set aside for further testing. Steps 2 and 3 are repeated during the physical examination. The following four sections follow the cyclic process shown in Figure 2.1.

2.3.1 The first step in differential diagnosis: listening and generating hypotheses

This process begins as the patient voices the chief complaint. Most clinicians ask the patient to provide a chronologic account of his illness from its beginning. This approach provides valuable information and perspective on the patient's illness. It also respects the patient. As the patient tells his story, the clinician has time to think, write down some diagnoses to consider, and observe the patient for diagnostic clues.

Hypothesis generation begins at the start of the interview. The first catalyst for hypothesis generation is usually the chief complaint, although the patient's appearance and agility as he take his seat in the examining room also provide a context for interpreting the history. As shown in Figure 2.2, the

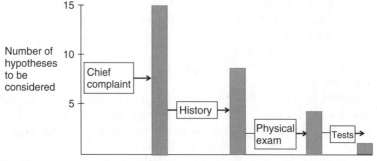

Figure 2.2 Number of diagnostic hypotheses remaining during the steps of evaluating a symptom.

patient's history generates the most hypotheses. The physical examination is usually a time to gather objective clues to confirm or discard a hypothesis. For example, a patient complaining of shortness of breath usually evokes the hypothesis of heart failure. If the patient does not have pulmonary rales, elevated neck veins, cardiac enlargement, or a third heart sound, heart failure is a much less likely diagnosis.

After the physical examination, a skilled clinician will have only a few remaining hypotheses to evaluate. The next step may be to start treatment, do a diagnostic test (see Chapter 9), or simply wait a few days to see if the complaint is resolving spontaneously.

Recall that our patient's complaint is "nocturnal substernal chest pain for one month." This complaint might elicit several of the following hypotheses:

Lung:
- pneumonia
- pulmonary embolus
- tuberculosis
- tumor
- pneumothorax

Bony thorax:
- rib fracture
- muscle strain
- costochondritis

Esophageal:
- reflux esophagitis
- esophageal spasm
- esophageal rupture
- esophageal cancer

Pericardial or pleural:
- pericarditis
- pleuritis

Great vessels:
- dissecting aneurysm

Cardiac:
- coronary artery disease
- aortic stenosis

Mediastinal:
- mediastinitis
- tumor

Referred pain:
- cholecystitis
- peptic ulcer
- pancreatitis
- cervical arthritis

As you generate the first few hypotheses, you may ask these questions:
1. Which hypothesis should I test first?
2. What should I do when I cannot think of possible diagnoses?

1. *Which hypothesis should I test first?* Start with *common* diseases that are *important to treat*:
- Common diseases: Think of them first. These hypotheses are more likely to be true – when supported by confirmatory evidence – than hypotheses about rare diseases. However, hypotheses about common diseases are harder to disconfirm (rule out) than hypotheses about rare diseases. (If this point puzzles you, go to Chapter 5, which explains how new information changes probability.)

   Example: Because coronary artery disease is a common disease, consider it before pericarditis and pulmonary embolus, which are less common.

- Importance of treatment: Consider diagnoses for which delay in starting treatment could lead to death or serious disability. These are "the diseases that you cannot afford to miss."

Example: Be sure to consider two relatively uncommon but treatable causes of our patient's chest pain, pneumonia and pneumothorax (a pocket of air within the thorax and outside the lung). You can safely delay testing hypotheses about diseases that benefit relatively little from treatment, such as muscular strain.

This example is a reminder that always adhering to the usual sequence of history taking followed by physical examination can endanger the patient. Some diagnoses, such as pneumothorax, are very important to treat promptly, do not have a characteristic history, but do have characteristic physical findings. If the patient is in severe distress, you should do a targeted physical examination first in order to rule out diseases, like pneumothorax. Likewise, gently palpating the abdomen of someone complaining of severe abdominal pain can provide clues about serious diseases that can progress quickly, like peritonitis or abdominal aneurysm. The physical examination in such patients provides a context for taking the history.

2. *What should I do when I cannot think of possible diagnoses?* Beginning students are the main victims of this problem. Even experienced clinicians have trouble when the patient's complaint is vague.

- *Vague, non-specific complaints*: Hypotheses can be slow in coming to mind when the patient's chief complaint is non-specific, such as weakness or fever, which can be caused by many different illnesses. While most clinicians have difficulty remembering long lists of possible diagnoses, reliance on memory is unnecessary in the era of hand-held computers.

  When the chief complaint is non-specific, ask the patient about other symptoms that started about the same time as his main complaint. One of these may have a much smaller list of possible causes of the patient's illness. For example, a patient with low-grade fever may volunteer that his right knee has been bothering him since the fever began. Localized joint pain, especially with fever, suggests a relatively small number of diagnoses.

  If this approach fails, many clinicians fall back on a time-honored technique: doing the review of systems immediately, rather than at the end of the interview. Several findings may merge into a pattern that suggests a syndrome or disease. Another, more specific, complaint may emerge. This technique has an inherent risk: you may forget the original complaint as you focus on more easily solved problems.

Example: If our patient with chest pain instead presented with a chief complaint of excessive intestinal gas, an experienced clinician might do the review of systems rather than try to think of causes of this very non-specific main complaint. This strategy might elicit the patient's chest pain, which would become the starting point for the differential diagnosis.

- *Memory failure*: To overcome a temporary lapse of memory, think of categories of disease rather than trying to recall specific diseases. First, think of anatomy. Try to identify the organ system that is the probable source of the patient's symptoms. Then, focus on diseases of that organ system. This strategy usually reduces the number of diseases to consider. Once you have identified a body system, think of categories of etiology. Most diseases are in one of the following categories: congenital, infectious, neoplastic, degenerative, or metabolic.

Example: In our patient, first evaluate the hypothesis that the patient's chest pain is caused by chest wall disease rather than considering the many possible musculoskeletal causes of chest pain individually. If the pain has the characteristics of chest wall pain (pain on deep breathing or movement; pain on palpating the thorax), think of the anatomic components of the chest wall and the diseases that affect them (bone, nerve, cartilage, and muscle).

In the era before hand-held computers, one coat pocket held a notebook listing common chief complaints and their causes. The other pocket held a stethoscope. Now the stethoscope is draped around the neck, and the coat pocket holds a hand-held computer. The principle has not changed: relying on memory is poor practice.

2.3.2 The second step in differential diagnosis: gathering data to test hypotheses

After accumulating a few hypotheses, ask specific questions to test each hypothesis. This phase of history taking is sometimes called the cross-examination. The cross-examination is the most active part of history taking because several diagnostic hypotheses are being considered in rapid succession. The answers to several hypothesis-testing questions may exclude one diagnosis while elevating another to the "active list." Some diagnostic hypotheses are under active consideration only briefly, while others survive the cross-examination and are retested during the physical examination and beyond.

Data gathering can be quite time consuming. Here are several efficient strategies for history taking and the physical examination:
1. Screen and branch.
2. Use pathognomonic findings.
3. Consider the cost of additional information.
4. Avoid getting information simply to reassure yourself.

In the remainder of this section, we will discuss each of these strategies in detail.

1. *Screen and branch*: In screening and branching, the clinician moves from one hypothesis to another with one or two screening questions, rather than exploring each hypothesis in depth. The clinician asks about a clinical finding that is nearly always present in patients with a disease (*screening*). If the finding is not present, the clinician eliminates the diagnostic hypothesis and moves on to other hypotheses (*branching*).

Example: If our patient with chest pain denies having fever or cough, the clinician rapidly excludes pneumonia and moves on to screening questions for other hypotheses. If the clinician can press on the chest without eliciting pain, she decides that the patient does not have musculoskeletal chest pain.

Screening and branching is efficient but risky. If a finding is truly present in all patients with a disease, screening is a reliable method for excluding a hypothesis. However, effective screening questions are the exception rather the rule. Few findings are always present in a disease. Clinicians seldom know exactly how often a finding is absent in patients with a disease, because the information is unknown or easily forgotten.

Errors in screening may be avoided by using the following principle: *do not try to eliminate a common disease with a single screening question*. If you believe that a hypothesis is likely to be true, a negative response to a screening question should not eliminate the hypothesis. On the other hand, you can eliminate a "long shot," low-probability hypothesis if the patient answers no to a screening question. This reasoning is based on principles to be described in Chapter 4.

Screening and branching is also a basic strategy in the physical examination. Clinicians typically begin with a "screening physical examination." If the screening examination of an organ shows an abnormality, the clinician performs a much more detailed examination of the organ (branching) and then moves on to the next part of the screening physical exam.

When to avoid the screening and branching strategy:
- The hypothesized diagnosis has serious consequences if untreated ("the disease you cannot afford to miss").
- The disease is very common and therefore difficult to exclude with a single finding.
- Effective screening questions may not exist.
- The patient's may be unreliable as a source of information.

2. *Pathognomonic findings*: A good screening question excludes disease; a pathognomonic finding establishes a diagnosis. A pathognomonic finding occurs in only one disease. Pathognomonic findings improve diagnostic efficiency, but very few such findings exist. Verifying a claim that a finding is pathognomonic is very difficult because the claimant must show that all patients with the finding have one and only one disease. Unquestioning belief in pathognomonic findings can lead the clinician to prematurely terminate a diagnostic search. A so-called pathognomonic finding is strong evidence in favor of a hypothesis, but supporting evidence should be sought, depending on whether the disease is uncommon (supporting information more necessary) or common (less necessary).

Example: If our patient with chest pain had an easily audible pericardial friction rub, you should conclude that he has pericarditis. A pericardial friction rub is one of the few examples of a pathognomonic finding (this claim is, of course, subject to dispute!).

3. *Consider the cost of information*: As information becomes difficult to obtain, weigh the harms and costs of getting the information against its potential benefits. This principle does not apply to the history and physical examination, which is inexpensive and safe to obtain, except when an excessively thorough history and physical exam delays efforts to treat a critically ill person.

Example: Performing a coronary arteriogram on asymptomatic middle-aged men will occasionally identify someone whose life might be prolonged by coronary bypass surgery. Most clinicians think that testing several hundred men to detect one person who might benefit is not worth the cost.

4. *Avoid getting information simply to reassure yourself*: To improve efficiency, avoid obtaining more data than are necessary to make a decision. Most clinicians frequently start treatment without being absolutely certain of the diagnosis. In Chapter 9, we will argue that the diagnostic search should stop when further information would not change the decision.

2.3.3 Hypothesis testing

Hypothesis testing is the most important but least understood part of differential diagnosis. In this section, we consider principles for evaluating hypotheses. These include:

1. Principles for comparing two hypotheses.
2. Principles for reducing the list of active hypotheses.
3. The final step: testing the adequacy of the proposed explanation for the patient's complaint.

1. *Principles for comparing two hypotheses*: Hypotheses are often evaluated in pairs. In this direct comparison, the less likely hypothesis is discarded. The remaining hypothesis is retained on the list of active hypotheses and then matched against another hypothesis. The rules in schoolyard pick-up basketball games are similar: the winner of a game plays the next challenger and keeps playing until finally losing. Then the players sit and wait their turn to be a challenger.

Typically, clinicians compare hypotheses on the basis of how each one matches up with the features of the patient's history. Whether they also take into account the relative prevalence of the hypothesized diagnoses is not known.

Several principles apply when deciding which hypothesis to discard:

- When deciding between evenly matched hypotheses, favor the diagnosis that is most prevalent in the population. This principle is a direct consequence of Bayes' theorem, which is the subject of Chapter 4. Clinicians typically do not know the exact prevalence and rely on impressions from personal experience and textbooks.

  Example: In patients with chest pain, coronary artery disease is common, and pericarditis is very uncommon. When the patient's findings match up equally well with the typical features of both of these two diagnoses, favor coronary artery disease. Perhaps the patient has some features of coronary artery disease and some features of pericarditis. In that case, favor coronary artery disease.

- If the patient's pattern of findings is more likely to occur in diagnosis A than diagnosis B, favor diagnosis A.

  Example: In a patient with chest pain that is aggravated by breathing, signs of pulmonary consolidation are more common in pneumonia than in a fractured rib. When deciding between pneumonia and fractured rib, we should favor pneumonia if consolidation is present. This statement is equivalent to saying that the patient's findings are more representative of pneumonia than of a fractured rib. It is an example of the *representativeness heuristic*, which we will discuss in Chapter 3. This principle also follows from the definition of the likelihood ratio, which is the single number that best characterizes the value of the information contained in a pattern of clinical findings (see Chapters 4 and 5).

- Strong evidence against one hypothesis increases the probability that another hypothesis is correct. This principle follows from the requirement that the sum of the probabilities of a set of mutually exclusive findings must add up to 1. Therefore, if the patient does not have a finding that is usually present in diagnosis A, diagnosis A becomes less likely and diagnosis B more likely. This principle underlies the "diagnosis of exclusion," in which we assume that a disease is present because we have excluded all other diseases.

After taking the history, several hypotheses often remain. By using the principles just described, the clinician can reduce this list still further during the physical examination. Often, however, more than one hypothesis may remain after performing the physical examination. Diagnostic tests or re-evaluation a short time later may resolve a diagnostic impasse, but one should first try to reduce the number of active hypotheses, if only to reduce the number of tests to choose between.

2. *Principles for reducing the list of active hypotheses*:
(a) Rank the remaining hypotheses and list the evidence for each and against each.
(b) Consider the rule of parsimony: one diagnosis is probably responsible for the patient's complaint.
(c) Combine diagnoses which require the same treatment.

Rank the remaining active hypotheses: Rank the active hypotheses from the most likely to the least likely. List the evidence for each hypothesis. Committing your ideas to paper may remind you of some needed data, help to eliminate some hypotheses, and put the situation in perspective.

Example: Our patient with chest pain has substernal pain that is squeezing in character and occurs principally at night. These findings are consistent with either an atypical form of coronary artery disease or esophageal spasm. Pericarditis and musculoskeletal disease are much less likely, and other possibilities have no supporting evidence.

The rule of parsimony: According to the rule of parsimony, the patient's complaint is caused by only one disease, with rare exceptions. This rule is an application of a principle of logic, which states that simple explanations are generally to be preferred to complicated ones (Occam's razor). In a medical context, it implies that the clinician should eventually reduce the list of active hypotheses to a single disease.

The rule of parsimony is based on a basic theorem of probability theory: the probability that two unrelated events occur simultaneously is the probability of one event multiplied by the probability of the other event. The product of the two probabilities is a much lower number than the probability of either event occurring by itself. The rule of parsimony is probably reliable in previously healthy people but may be less reliable in persons with several chronic diseases. In this case, two diagnostic hypotheses are less likely to be independent of each other, which increases the probability that both are present.

The rule of parsimony should occasionally be ignored. First, the probability that two common diseases occur simultaneously may be greater than the probability of a single rare disease. Second, when delay in treating two hypothesized diseases might have serious consequences, it is better to treat both until it is possible to make a definitive diagnosis.

Example: If our patient with chest pain presented with fever, cough with blood-streaked sputum, a pleural friction rub, and a pulmonary infiltrate on a chest x-ray, he might have either pulmonary embolism or pneumonia. A suspected diagnosis of pneumonia requires 24 hours to confirm by culturing sputum or blood. Tests to diagnose suspected pulmonary embolism may not be available at all times. An experienced clinician will start therapy for both these life-threatening diseases while awaiting more information.

Combine diagnoses with the same consequences: "Clustering" is acting as if two diseases were really one disease because both have the same treatment. One should always consider whether to cluster several diseases on the list of active hypotheses in order to reduce the number that require independent evaluation.

Example: If our patient had nocturnal chest pain that is relieved by antacids, he might have either esophagitis or esophageal spasm. Distinguishing between these two hypotheses is unnecessary, because both diseases require treatment to reduce gastric acid secretion.

3. *A final step: testing how well the active hypothesis explains the patient's complaint*: At this point in differential diagnosis, one or two diagnostic hypotheses are still active. The next step is to decide between starting treatment, getting more information, or taking no immediate action (the subject of Chapter 9). One last step remains before deciding. After reviewing the patient's findings and the active hypotheses, the clinician should ask two questions:

(a) Do the hypothesized diagnoses explain all of the major clinical features of the case?
(b) Are any of the major clinical features inconsistent with the hypothesized diagnoses?

The purpose of these last questions is to assure a coherent and consistent explanation for the patient's findings. In effect, these questions remind the clinician to try to identify any "loose ends" that do not fit with the hypothesized diagnoses.

Example: Let us review the history of our patient with chest pain. The principal clinical features are:
- A chief complaint of "nocturnal chest pain for one month."
- The pain is a substernal tightness that begins an hour or so after lying down.
- It is unrelated to exertion and unaffected by antacids.
- There is no recent injury and no fever or cough.
- The physical examination is normal.

We have discarded several categories of illness because the patient's history is inconsistent with key features of these categories. Musculoskeletal causes are unlikely because the history does not include recent trauma and pressing on the chest does not reproduce the pain. Infection is unlikely since fever, chills, cough, and signs of pulmonary disease are all absent. Finally, the pain is not relieved by antacids. This finding reduces the likelihood of esophagitis or esophageal spasm but does not entirely eliminate this hypothesis, since the location and onset of the pain after lying down are consistent with this diagnosis. The remaining active hypothesis is an atypical form of coronary artery disease ("atypical angina pectoris").

Atypical coronary artery disease is a *coherent* explanation for the patient's complaint because it accounts for all of the findings. It is a *consistent* explanation because all findings are consistent with this hypothesis. Esophageal spasm is not a consistent explanation because antacids do not relieve the pain.

2.3.4 Selecting a course of action

When the active hypotheses have been ranked in order of plausibility, the clinician must decide what to do next. The three choices are:

- Treat.
- Gather more information now.
- Withhold treatment. Additional evidence may emerge as a hypothesized disease is allowed to follow its natural history.

The choice between these three alternatives is guided by probability (how likely is a disease?) and utility (how beneficial is prompt action and what are its harms?). The choice is obvious when a hypothesized illness is lethal, prompt treatment is safe and effective, and the patient is highly likely to have the disease. Despite a low probability of the disease, clinicians often treat if therapy is safe, and failure to treat has dire consequences. If a disease requires treatment that is expensive or dangerous, they should require stronger evidence.

Treating a disease has two elements of uncertainty. First, some patients with the disease do not respond to the treatment. Second, the patient may not have the disease. The patient is then exposed to the risk of harm from the treatment with no possibility of benefit. When the clinician is uncertain that the patient has the disease but starts treatment anyway, some patients will receive treatment for a disease that they do not have, a concept discussed at the beginning of Chapter 9.

Example: Our patient with chest pain has symptoms of two diseases – esophageal spasm and atypical coronary artery disease – that cannot easily be distinguished from one another by the history and physical examination. Further information must be obtained. The clinician has many options, ranging from performing a coronary arteriogram to initiating a therapeutic trial aimed at esophageal spasm.

The rest of this book is an exposition of the principles for making the best possible decision when the consequences of taking action are uncertain, so-called "decision making under uncertainty."

2.4 An extended example

The following scenario is a transcript of an imaginary interview between a clinician and a patient. We present the scenario to illustrate the concepts we have just presented. Kassirer *et al.* (2009) provide many examples of physicians "thinking out loud" as they work through a difficulty diagnostic problem.

Doctor: How may I help you today?
Patient: It's these headaches I've been having.

Doctor thinks: I'll have to think about tension headaches, vascular headaches, headache due to medications, brain tumor, and infection.

Comment: The clinician begins forming hypotheses as soon as the patient voices his chief complaint. At this point, the clinician will ask the patient to tell his story. After hearing the narrative, she cross-examines the patient to supply needed details and to test hypotheses.

Doctor: How long has this been going on?
Patient: For years, but it's worse now.
Doctor: How often are you getting these headaches?
Patient: I used to get them a few times a month, but now I it's almost
            every day.

Doctor thinks: This is a chronic problem that appears to have changed in severity. Either something has happened to exacerbate a pre-existing condition, or we are looking at a new process.

Comment: The clinician is beginning to ask screening questions that will help to exclude some diagnoses (e.g., many kinds of meningitis are unlikely with a chronic headache) and will serve to increase the likelihood of other diagnoses (e.g., both tension and vascular headaches are suggested by the present pattern).

Doctor: Have you noticed any other symptoms with the change in your
            headaches?
Patient: Well, yes. My vision has been rather blurry at times. Also, I don't
            think my appetite is as good, and I am not sleeping very well.

Doctor thinks: These are rather non-specific symptoms. I'd better ask a few questions that relate to causes of headache that are serious and treatable.

Doctor: Have you had any fever?
Patient: No.
Doctor: Have you had a lack of coordination or weakness or paralysis?
Patient: No.
Doctor: Have you noticed any numbness, weakness, or loss of sensation in
            a part of your body?
Patient: No.

Doctor thinks: Good. So far I see no evidence of any serious treatable disease, such as meningitis or brain tumor. Let's find out a little bit more about the headache itself.

Comment: With these initial screening questions, the clinician has efficiently tested and rejected a number of hypotheses. Tension headache and vascular headache remain likely explanations of the patient's complaint. Brain tumor and infection seem quite unlikely. As a result of responses to screening questions, the clinician has not pursued these hypotheses in depth. At this point, she will ask questions to test the hypotheses that the patient has tension headache or vascular headache.

For the sake of brevity, we will not repeat this entire conversation. Suffice it to say that, as the clinician tests hypotheses, she asks questions about aggravating or precipitating factors, ameliorating factors, and the relationship of the headaches to time of day and physical activity. Of course, the clinician also ascertains the location and nature of the headache, as well as its response to medications. Finally, she obtains a brief past medical history, including allergies and medication consumption, and use of alcohol, tobacco, or other stimulants.

At this point, the clinician moves to the physical examination. Because many hypotheses have already been rejected, she can focus her attention on seeking evidence for the remaining active hypotheses. She will take the blood pressure and will pay particular attention to the head, ears, eyes, nose, and throat. In addition, she will do a screening neurologic examination to look for evidence for brain tumor.

After completing the physical examination, the clinician reflects on what she has learned and lists the remaining active hypotheses. While she has been testing hypotheses throughout the examination, now she must weigh the evidence for the remaining active hypotheses and decide whether to do a diagnostic test, start specific treatment, or wait to see if the headache resolves spontaneously.

Doctor thinks: Let's see. So far, I know that the patient has had headaches for many years and that they have increased in frequency and intensity in the last few months. Nonetheless, they do not awaken the patient from sleep, and there are no other symptoms except for some blurred vision and some loss of appetite. The patient has not lost weight, and the physical examination is completely normal, including normal visual acuity. The patient also tells me that the headaches are diffuse, occurring over the entire top, front, sides, and back of the head. The headache seems to be least severe in the morning and most severe by the end of the day. Aspirin partially relieves the headache. Finally, he took a new job approximately six months ago and now spends most of his day at a computer terminal.

Of my active hypotheses, which are the most likely? What is the commonest cause of headache? Tension headache is not only the commonest cause of headache, but his findings fit the classic description of tension headache quite well. What about other possibilities?

What are the diseases that I cannot afford to miss? With a normal neurologic exam and a history of many years of headache, brain tumor is extremely unlikely. Could he have a chronic infection, such as tuberculous or fungal meningitis? The absence of nocturnal headache or other associated systemic signs or symptoms of a chronic illness makes infection very unlikely. There's not enough evidence to pursue these diagnoses.

What about other common causes of headache, such as vascular headache? He has none of the typical prodromal symptoms. Moreover, his headache is diffuse rather than unilateral and is frequently relieved by simple analgesic medication. He also has no family history for migraine. Thus, his symptoms do not fit my concept of vascular headache at all. Furthermore, there is evidence for tension headache: his new job is monotonous and associated with increased visual strain. At this point, I think that tension headache is the most likely diagnosis.

Comment: In following the clinician's analysis, you can see several features of clinical reasoning. First, she gave special weight to tension headache because it is a common diagnosis. Second, she gave consideration to the more serious and treatable but rare causes of headache. In each case, she considered the data for and against those diagnoses and ended up eliminating them as possibilities. Of course, as any good clinician, she will reconsider these possibilities at a later date if new information appears or if the patient does not respond to therapy. Finally, she did a pairwise comparison of the two leading diagnostic hypotheses, tension headache and vascular headache.

Now, the clinician must select a course of action. She must gather more information, observe the patient without treatment, or begin treatment.

Doctor thinks: At this point, I am fairly comfortable with the diagnosis of tension headache. I don't think any further tests are necessary. Instead, I will learn a little bit more about the patient's work environment and see if I can identify anything that could be changed.

Doctor: I think there are some things we can do to help improve your headache problem. Let's review your daytime activities and begin to develop a plan of action. In addition, I want you to return to my office in a month to re-evaluate the situation.

Patient: Fine.

Comment: The clinician will try to help relieve the tension headaches, and she will use the "test of time" to re-evaluate other diagnostic possibilities. If the headache has not disappeared or has changed in character when the patient pays an office visit in one month, the clinician may repeat part of the physical exam or may obtain diagnostic tests.

The clinician has chosen a relatively risk-free approach. She has not irrevocably excluded the possibility of a serious cause of headache. In deciding to forgo diagnostic tests, she has concluded that the likelihood of finding a treatable cause of headache is extremely low. Moreover, the expense and worry that diagnostic studies may engender appear to outweigh the remote possibility of a result that could benefit her.

Conclusion: Even the simplest of clinician–patient interactions contain the elements of rational decision making. Using these principles does not necessarily increase the amount of time required to evaluate the patient, especially if the screening and branching strategy is used to exclude hypotheses.

2.4.1 Clinical aphorisms

Clinical aphorisms are pithy, memorable distillates of clinical experience. Master diagnosticians rely on the following common-sense rules for clinical reasoning:

- If you hear hoofbeats, think of horses, not zebras.
- If a test result surprises you, repeat the test before taking action.
- Do not do a test if the result will not change your management.
- Rare manifestations of common diseases are often more likely than common manifestations of rare diseases.
- Your first priority is to think about the diseases you cannot afford to miss.

When you have read this book, you should be able to explain each of these aphorisms.

Summary

1. Experienced clinicians formulate and test diagnostic hypotheses from the moment they first see the patient. At any moment, they actively consider only a few hypotheses.
2. Research on how clinicians evaluate diagnostic hypotheses has shown that they compare their patient's findings to similar cases from their experience. Expert diagnosticians appear to have a larger, more easily recalled body of cases.
3. The process of clinical reasoning has four steps. The first three steps comprise the process of differential diagnosis, which is a cyclic process that goes on throughout the history and physical examination. The last step occurs when the clinical evaluation is complete.
   Step 1: Generate alternative hypotheses.
   Step 2: Gather data.
   Step 3: Use data to test hypotheses.
   Step 4: Select a course of action: treat, test, or observe.
4. Clinicians who wish to become master diagnosticians should remember that a systematic approach to differential diagnosis is much preferred to brilliant leaps of intuition. That said, mastery also involves learning the lessons of a wide exposure to patients. We learn best from our mistakes.

Bibliography

Elstein, A.S., Shulman, L.S., and Sprafka, S.A. (1978) *Medical Problem Solving: An analysis of clinical reasoning*, Harvard University Press, Cambridge, MA.

This book describes and analyzes experiments that were designed to uncover the basis for clinical reasoning. The authors propose a clinical problem-solving method based on their observations.

Gorry, G.A., Pauker, S.G., and Schwartz, W.B. (1978) The diagnostic importance of the normal finding. *New England Journal of Medicine*, **298**, 486–9.

A brief analytic paper showing how reducing the probability of one diagnosis increases the probability of all other active hypotheses.

Groopman, J. (2007) *How Doctors Think*, Houghton Mifflin, Boston, MA.

A physician wrote this engaging book for the general public. It uses extended examples to describe errors and triumphs of clinical cognition and judgment.

Kahneman, D. (2011) *Thinking, Fast and Slow*. Farrar, Straus & Giroux, New York.

Reflections on how the mind works with an emphasis on the perils of relying too much on a quick response.

Kassirer, J.P., Wong, J., and Kopelman, R. (2009) *Learning Clinical Reasoning*, 2nd ed., Lippincott, Williams and Wilkins, Baltimore, MD.

This book consists largely of analysis of case histories from the authors' experience. Excellent discussion of differential diagnosis.

Norman, G. (2005) Research in clinical reasoning: past history and current trends. *Medical Education*, **39**, 418–27.

A survey of the body of evidence about how clinicians reason.

Slovic, P., Fischoff, B., and Lichtenstein, S. (1977) Behavioral decision theory. *Annual Review of Psychology*, **28**, 1–39.

A thorough exploration of why decision makers act as they do.

CHAPTER 3

Probability: quantifying uncertainty

As we learned in Chapter 1, clinicians usually cannot directly observe the true state of the patient and must infer it from external, imperfect cues. These cues are the history, the physical examination, and diagnostic tests. In day-to-day clinical practice, the clinician relies on these imperfect indirect indicators of the patient's true state and accepts a degree of uncertainty when making decisions. Fortunately, many, perhaps most, decisions do not require certain knowledge of the true state of the patient.

Representing our uncertainty about the patient as a probability is an essential step in learning how to make decisions without certain knowledge. In this chapter, we will learn how to use the concept of probability to think clearly about the uncertainty inherent in most medical situations. This chapter has four parts.

3.1 Uncertainty and probability in medicine

This part of the chapter elaborates on concepts first introduced in Chapter 1. In the following four sections, we explore the meaning of probability and its importance in medicine.

3.1.1 The uncertain nature of clinical information

Imagine a clinical finding that occurred in a disease in the following way:

- **always** present in patients with the disease
  - therefore, if the finding is absent, the disease is absent;
- **never** present in patients who do not have the disease
  - therefore, if the finding is present, the disease is present.

Medical Decision Making, Second Edition. Harold C. Sox, Michael C. Higgins and Douglas K. Owens.
© 2013 John Wiley & Sons, Ltd. Published 2013 by John Wiley & Sons, Ltd.

We would not require clinical judgment to diagnose the disease; it would be sufficient to know if this finding were present.

This clinical finding is fictional, an illusion. No clinical finding has this perfect, one-to-one correspondence with a disease. Therefore, clinicians are seldom, if ever, certain what a finding implies about the patient's true state. They must recognize the following bleak truth:

> *The true state of the patient lies locked within the body, inaccessible to direct observation. The clinician must use external, imperfect cues to infer the patient's true state.*

The following three examples illustrate typical clinical situations in which the clinician cannot directly observer the patient's true state and must infer it by imperfect clinical cues:

Example 1: The patient complains of left leg pain four days after hip surgery. The left leg is not warm or tender and is the same circumference as the right leg. The clinician ignores these normal findings and obtains an ultrasound image of the leg veins, which shows a large blood clot.

Comment: Only one-third of patients with suspected deep venous thrombosis of the leg have physical signs of the disease.

Example 2: A 60-year-old man complains of retrosternal pain that radiates to the left arm. Exercise and emotional stress bring on the pain, which resolves promptly when the patient rests or calms down. The patient's clinician initially believes the pain is due to myocardial ischemia and obtains an exercise electrocardiogram. To the clinician's surprise, the exercise test is normal. A trial of medication for ischemic cardiac pain leads to resolution of the pain.

Comment: The patient's pain had the typical characteristics of ischemic pain, and his probability of coronary artery disease is at least 90%. A normal exercise test lowers this probability but not by much. The clinician could obtain a coronary arteriogram and observe the patient's true state directly, but chooses to start treatment while not completely sure of the diagnosis. The response to specific treatment confirms her judgment.

Example 3: Jimmy has a sore throat. A throat culture shows beta hemolytic streptococci. Does Jimmy have a streptococcal infection? Is he at risk for developing rheumatic fever?

Comment: Streptococci can reside on the pharyngeal mucosa without causing infection of the underlying tissue. Culturing a throat that is sore because of viral pharyngitis may disclose streptococci that are of no significance to the patient.

3.1.2   Probability: a language for expressing uncertainty

Clinicians' language reflects their understanding of uncertainty. In talking about a difficult decision, the clinician may say that she is treating the patient for a disease that is "possibly present" rather than a disease that is "probably not present." Most clinicians use such words to describe gradations of belief in a hypothesis. However, these words may interfere with clearly expressing uncertainty, for the following reasons:

- Clinicians choose different words to express the same judgment about the likelihood of a future event.
- Clinicians use the same word to express very different judgments about the likelihood of an event.
- Words cannot describe precisely how much to adjust one's belief in a diagnostic hypothesis as new information becomes available.

Clinicians who use words to communicate their uncertainty may feel secure that they have conveyed their meaning. In fact, *words are the enemy of clarity in expressing uncertainty*. When words are mapped onto a probability scale, the ranges of probabilities that correspond to different words overlap so much that the words do not have unique meanings. **Probability**, a quantitative means for expressing uncertainty, avoids this ambiguity.

Definition of probability: A number between 0 and 1 that expresses an opinion about the likelihood that a current state exists or a future event will occur.

Probability has the following properties:
- The probability of a present state or future event that is certain is 1.0.
- The probability that a state is certain to be absent or that an event is certain not to happen is 0.
- The probability of all possible mutually exclusive states or events is 1.0.

The meaning of probability: the present state vs. a future event

The definition of probability referred to a "present state" or a "future event" because uncertainty in medicine can be about the present state of the patient or about the occurrence of a future event. For example, the patient's history provides clues about whether the patient *has* coronary artery disease or whether the patient *will develop* coronary artery disease in the future.

The distinction between present state and future event carries over to the methods for using information about the present to quantify uncertainty. Discovering the predictors of the present state would involve a systematic history and physical examination, performing a definitive test (e.g., a coronary arteriogram) on the same day, and using statistical techniques to identify the predictors of the result of the arteriogram. This is a **cross-sectional study design**. To discover the predictors of a future event, one would obtain a systematic history and physical examination and then contact the patient periodically to see if he had experienced the outcome event of interest (e.g., a myocardial infarction). This is a **cohort study design**.

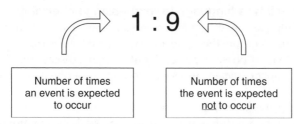

Figure 3.1 The meaning of the odds of an event.

In the next few chapters, we will focus on how to estimate the probability of the patient's present state before and after obtaining a diagnostic test. We will use the term "probability of the target condition" to represent uncertainty about the patient's present state. The term "target condition" refers to the hypothesized disease that the test is intended to detect.

Odds: an alternative way to express a probability

Some prefer to translate their uncertainty into a number by thinking in terms of **odds** rather than probability. They ask themselves, "for every time that this type of patient had cancer, how many times was cancer not present?" Figure 3.1 illustrates the concept of odds.

Definition of odds: The ratio of the probability of an event occurring over the probability of the event not occurring.

Odds and probability are equivalent. The relationship between the odds of an event and its probability is the following:

$$\text{odds} = \frac{p}{1 - p}$$

(where p is the probability that the event will occur).

Thus, if the probability of the event is 0.67, the odds of the event are 0.67 divided by 0.33, or 2 to 1. Another way to express the odds of an event is $p:(1 - p)$. Thus, writing 2:1 is equivalent to saying "2 to 1 odds."

Facility in doing arithmetic with odds is important because the simplest way to see the effect of new information on one's uncertainty is to multiply the odds of an event by a number called the *likelihood ratio* (see Chapter 5). Here are a few suggestions about using odds:

Convert odds written as 2:1 to a ratio or quotient (e.g., 2/1).

Multiply the quotient by another number (e.g., $6.0 \times 2/1 = 12/1$, or 12:1).

Convert odds to probability with the following relationship:

$$p = \frac{o}{1+o}$$

(where o is the odds of the event occurring).

Some find it especially useful to use odds to express their opinion about very infrequent events (1 to 99 odds, rather than a probability of 0.01) or very common events (99 to 1 odds, rather than a probability of 0.99).

3.1.3   Probability: a means for interpreting uncertain information

Why should a clinician adopt probability as a means of self-expression? Our answer to this question is that probability is the key to interpreting diagnostic information. The interpretation of new information is a conclusion about the certainty of an event in light of the new information. As clinicians, we are interested in questions such as the following:

- What is the probability that this patient with a warm, tender leg has a blood clot obstructing the deep veins of the leg *if* an indirect measure of venous blood flow (a Doppler ultrasound image) is abnormal?
- What is the probability that this patient with chest pain has significant coronary artery narrowing *if* an exercise electrocardiogram is abnormal?

These questions have a common theme: how much should one adjust the probability of disease to account for new information? Probability theory, which is a system of axiomatic relationships, provides the answer to this question. As shown in Chapter 4, these axioms lead directly to Bayes' theorem.

Bayes' theorem enables the clinician to answer this basic question:

"I have been concerned that my patient has cancer. How likely is cancer now, after this test is negative?"

One cannot answer this simple question without encountering a profound and subtle principle of clinical medicine:

The interpretation of new information depends on what you believed beforehand.

This fundamental assertion, perhaps the most important in this book, is a direct consequence of the axioms of probability theory (as shown in Chapter 4). Clinical observations lead to the same conclusion, as shown in the following table from a large study of patients with chest pain. Each patient had been referred for exercise testing and coronary arteriography. Prior to the tests, a cardiologist classified each patient's history into one of three categories (see Table 3.1).

This table shows that the probability of coronary artery disease when the exercise test is abnormal depends on the patient's history. In other words, *the interpretation of the test result depends on the probability of disease before the test.* Once you accept this principle, your life will never be the same again. Every time you start to ask, "what does this test result tell me about my patient?",

Table 3.1

Type of history	Probability of coronary artery disease	
	All men	Men with abnormal exercise test
Typical angina	0.89	0.96
Atypical angina	0.70	0.87
Non-anginal chest pain	0.22	0.39

Data from: Weiner, D.A. *et al.* (1979) Exercise stress testing: correlations among history of angina, ST-segment response, and prevalence of coronary-artery disease in the Coronary Artery Surgery Study (CASS). *New England Journal of Medicine*, **301**, 230–5.

you must first ask, "what did I think before I ordered the test?" Just as the physicist sees the world within a moving frame of reference in Einstein's theory of relativity, so a clinician should interpret new information in the context of her prior belief about the patient.

The next time someone asks you "what do you think this abnormal exercise test means?", your first response *must* be, "what kind of history did the patient give?" Then, and only then, can you answer the person's question.

Figure 3.2 depicts the relationship between the probability of disease before and after additional information. The two panels of Figure 3.2 illustrate how the characteristics of the patient influence the probability of colon cancer after a test result that increases the odds of colon cancer by a factor of nine.

Top panel (low pre-test odds): The odds of disease are low (1:9) ($P[D] = 0.10$) before doing the test. After the test, the odds of disease are 1:1 ($P[D] = 0.50$). In thinking about these probabilities the clinician may conclude, "before the test, I was pretty sure the patient did not have colon cancer. Now I'm not so sure."

Bottom panel (high pre-test odds): The odds of disease are intermediate (1:1) ($P[D] = 0.50$) before doing the test. Disease is as likely to be present as not, a toss-up. After the test, the odds of colon cancer are 9:1 ($P[D] = 0.90$).

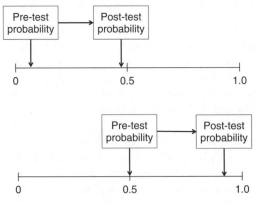

Figure 3.2 Relationship between probability before a test and after the test.

In thinking about these probabilities the clinician may reflect, "before the test, I was concerned about colon cancer. Now I'm pretty sure the patient has colon cancer."

These two examples show one very important reason for being concerned about estimating probability: the pre-test probability of disease affects the interpretation of the test result.

3.1.4   When to estimate probability

When in the diagnostic process should the clinician first think consciously about probability? During history taking and the physical examination, the clinician may categorize disease hypotheses according to their likelihood of being true (high, intermediate, and low) without assigning a probability to each. The time to estimate probability is when the clinician must choose one of the following actions:

1. **Do nothing** (do not test, do not treat).
2. **Get more information** (a test or a therapeutic trial).
3. **Treat** without obtaining any more information.

The choice between these options depends on the probability that a disease hypothesis is true. Chapter 9 describes a formal method for choosing between these options. If the probability of a disease is very low, doing nothing will be the best choice. Treating without further testing is the best choice if the probability of the target condition is relatively high. Testing is best when the probability of disease is intermediate.

The clinician should record the pre-test probability of disease at the time of ordering a test. The clinician can use then Bayes' theorem to calculate the post-test probability, as described in the following chapter. As computer-based medical information systems become an integral part of medical practice, clinicians will order tests and receive the results on a computer display. The computer can provide help in using the history and physical examination to estimate the pre-test probability. Prior to the test, it can calculate the probability of test results that might change the management of the patient. After the test, it can calculate and display the post-test probability of disease.

3.1.5   Objective and subjective probability

What is "the probability of an event?" This question can provoke a lively debate between two schools of thought. One holds that the probability of an event is a physical reality, such as the frequency of an event in a defined group of patients. Adherents to this interpretation of probability use the terms "objective probability" or "frequentist." An objective probability of a disease is the frequency of the disease in a defined group of patients, such as those with the same chief complaint (e.g., the frequency of coronary artery disease among those with chest pain).

Objective probability is important but only part of the story. A clinician should use all of the information in a complete history of the presenting complaint to estimate the patient's probability. To accomplish this task within the framework of objective probability would require knowing the frequency of a disease corresponding to each possible combination of symptoms, which would require studying a very large number of patients. More realistically, the clinician could use a clinical prediction rule, the most refined form of objective probability, as discussed later in this chapter. Even the probability estimate by a clinical prediction rule is just the starting point for estimating a patient's probability, as we shall see. A purist approach to using objective probability is neither realistic nor desirable.

In this book, we use a definition of probability that takes into account all of the information available to the clinician. For example, in a patient facing an open heart operation, this information would include the following:

1. Personal experience: When estimating probability, a clinician relies on personal experience with similar events. For example, a surgeon uses her experience with similar patients when she estimates the probability that Mr. Jones will survive an open heart operation.

2. Published experience: Published articles report the frequency of death after surgical procedures. These reports provide an average frequency for a large but not necessarily diverse population, raising questions about its applicability to a specific population.

3. Attributes of the patient: The experienced clinician uses published reports and personal experience to make an estimate that applies to the average patient. She then adjusts the estimate upward or downward starting from this average figure if the patient has unusual characteristics that might affect his risk (e.g., advanced age or many chronic conditions).

This chapter, and the two that follow, show how a clinician can integrate these three sources of information into a single number that expresses uncertainty about the likelihood of an event. This number is the **subjective probability**.

3.2 Using personal experience to estimate probability

Personal experience is the principal influence on a clinician's probability estimates. Experienced clinicians have seen so many patients that they have a good intuitive understanding of events that occur commonly and events that are unusual. Even in the hands of experts, however, these subjective estimates are prone to systematic error, as we will discuss in this chapter.

Probability assessment is the process by which a person elicits someone's probability that an event will occur. Probability assessment means asking a person to use a number to express how strongly they believe that an event will occur. At first thought, a process for translating a belief into a number may seem far-fetched. The following description will not put these thoughts to rest, but it should help the reader to assess someone's probability. There are two ways to assess probability: **direct** and **indirect**.

3.2.1 Direct probability assessment

Direct probability assessment: To assess a person's probability directly, one asks for the number between 0 and 1.0 that expresses the person's belief that an event will occur.

Experienced clinicians usually have little difficulty responding to this request, especially when they recall experience with similar patients. For example, after hearing a patient describe his chest pain, the clinician may use the following frame of reference: "How often was the coronary arteriogram abnormal in patients from whom I have obtained a similar history?"

Matching the patient's findings to prior patients is effective if the clinician can remember accurately and has a large experience. Figure 3.3 shows a clinician listening to the patient's history, recalling similar patients, and remembering how many of them had a positive arteriogram. The process would seem to require a prodigious memory, and the reader may wonder how a clinician could estimate a probability so that it truly reflected her actual experience.

3.2.2 Indirect probability assessment

Direct probability assessment is relatively easy but is subject to errors in recalling past experience. Next we describe an indirect probability assessment method that may help someone who has difficulty choosing a number to represent their opinion about the patient's present state.

To understand indirect probability assessment, consider the following example. Suppose you must assess a clinician's belief that a patient with weight loss has cancer. You ask her to choose between two wagers: betting that cancer is present or taking a wager at defined odds, such as a state lottery. If the two wagers are equally attractive to the clinician, her probability that the patient has cancer is the same as the probability of winning the lottery.

Indirect probability assessment is analogous to weighing an object. The event to be measured (the weight of the object) is compared to a standard of reference (a 1 kilogram weight). If the scale balances, the object weighs 1 kilogram. Indirect probability assessment allows the clinician to express a difficult concept (the probability that the patient has coronary artery disease) by comparing it to a more tangible event (the lottery).

Of course, the clinician wins the lottery only in her imagination, but she should take the game seriously. Therefore, the prize should be truly desirable, such as a tuition rebate, the internship of one's choice, or a three-month paid vacation!

The following scenario depicts the steps in the indirect assessment of probability. Imagine that a clinician has seen a patient with high blood pressure and asks your help in estimating the probability that the patient has a mineralocorticoid-secreting adrenal adenoma.

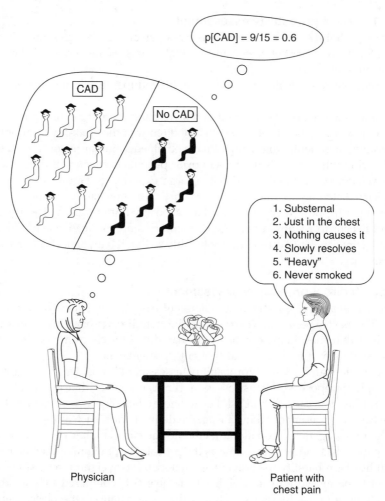

Figure 3.3 The clinician recalls her prior experience with similar patients as a patient describes his chest pain.

You　　Which would you prefer?
- Betting that the patient has an adrenal adenoma (if he does, you win a paid vacation).
- Drawing a ball from an urn containing 1 red ball and 99 white balls (if you draw a red ball, you win the paid vacation).

Clinician　I'd bet on the adenoma being present.

Interpretation: She believes that the probability of the patient having an adenoma is higher than 0.01 and prefers to bet on the event that is more likely to occur.

You   Which would you prefer?
- Betting that the patient has an adenoma (if he has one, you win a paid vacation).
- Drawing a ball from an urn containing 10 red balls and 90 white balls (if you draw a red ball, you win the paid vacation).

Clinician   I'd draw from the urn.

Interpretation: She believes that the probability of an adenoma is less than 0.10 and prefers the gamble with the higher chance of winning.

You   Which would you prefer?
- Betting that the patient has an adenoma (if he does, you win the paid vacation).
- Drawing a ball from an urn that has 5 red balls and 95 white balls (if you draw a red ball, you win the paid vacation).

Clinician   I really can't decide. The two wagers look equally good to me.

Interpretation: Since the prize for the two gambles is the same, her inability to choose between the two gambles means that she believes that the chance of winning is the same for both gambles. Since the chance of drawing a red ball from the urn is 0.05, the clinician's subjective probability that this patient has an adrenal adenoma is 0.05.

Probabilities obtained in this way must obey the laws of probability. Therefore, the probabilities of all possible causes of the patient's hypertension must add up to 1.0.

Subjective probability: a caution

Direct subjective probability estimation sounds easy to perform, but the results suggest otherwise. As part of a lecture, one of the authors asked several dozen audiences of clinicians to read a brief history and write down their individual estimates that the patient has a pulmonary embolism. He then asked members of the audience to indicate that included their probability estimate: 0 to 10, 11 to 20, 21 to 30, and so on. In every audience, roughly equal numbers raised their hand for every interval between 21–30 and 71–80. In other words, faced with the same history, experienced clinicians' subjective probability estimates varied widely.

This anecdote has an important lesson for clinicians: when conferring about a clinical problem that involves an element of uncertainty, begin by asking everyone to state their probability estimates. Disagreement about what to do may reflect differing levels of certainty about what is causing the patient's problem or the patient's prognosis.

3.2.3 Sources of error in using personal experience to estimate probability

Probability estimation seems dangerously prone to error for an activity that is so central to medical practice. Clinicians base their probability estimates on limited clinical data which they must recall from an all-too-fallible memory and then perform long division without recourse to pencil and paper. This section describes the methods for performing this mental task and the errors that can occur. The discussion has four parts:

- Heuristics defined
- The representativeness heuristic
- The availability heuristic
- The anchoring and adjustment heuristic.

Heuristics defined

Research shows that people use several types of cognitive processes (also called *heuristics*) for using past experience to estimate probability.

Definition of cognitive heuristic: A mental process used to learn, recall, or understand knowledge.

Research has also shown that we misuse our heuristics for estimating probability, which leads to systematic error (bias). If clinicians understand these heuristics and how to avoid using them incorrectly, their probability estimates might be more accurate.

We next define three heuristics and show how they can be misused. This material is easy to understand and is very important. The heuristics are:

1. Representativeness
2. Availability
3. Anchoring and adjustment.

Heuristic I: representativeness

In medicine, we often ask questions of the following kind: "What is the probability that patient A has disease B?" In order to answer such questions, we usually ask, *"how closely does patient A resemble the class of patients with disease B?"*

Definition of representativeness heuristic: A process for categorizing something by how closely its essential features resemble those of the parent population.

To evaluate the degree to which patient A is similar to a typical member of class B, we use a stereotypical picture of disease B as our standard of

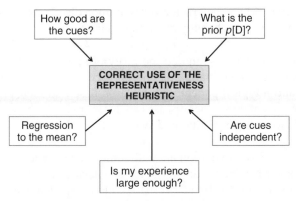

Figure 3.4 Factors that affect probability estimates derived from using the representativeness heuristic.

comparison. Consider a patient with symptoms of cholecystitis. Our estimate of the probability of cholecystitis will depend on how closely the patient's findings resemble the textbook description of cholecystitis (or patients from our own clinical experience with cholecystitis).

Clinicians often use the representativeness heuristic and must be aware of several ways that it can lead to mistakes. To avoid these errors, the clinician should ask the questions depicted in Figure 3.4.

Errors in using the representativeness heuristic: I. Ignoring the prior probability of the disease

The features of a case history that make it resemble the features of a disease are important, but they are not the only characteristics that affect the probability that the disease is present. An additional, frequently forgotten, feature is the prevalence of the disease in clinical practice. As seen in Figure 3.2, the probability of disease as new information becomes available is strongly influenced by the prior probability of disease. By analogy, *the prevalence of a disease in the population affects the probability of the disease when a patient's clinical features are taken into account*. Even if the patient's features match up well with the characteristic findings in a disease, the disease is unlikely if it seldom occurs in the population. One of the authors did a study of patients presenting with chest pain in different clinical settings. The results showed that the probability of coronary artery disease in patients with a similar history depends on the overall prevalence of coronary artery disease in the clinical setting.

The following examples illustrate the effects of ignoring the prior probability of disease:

Example 1: A long-time resident of Kansas presents to his community clinician with a history of intermittent shaking chills, sweats, and fever for one week. The physical examination is unrevealing. The examining clinician has just set up private practice after having spent two years as a staff clinician in a hospital in Southeast Asia, where malaria is a very common disease. She estimates that this patient has a 0.90 probability of having malaria.

Comment: The clinician has ignored the rarity of malaria in the usual North American patient and has made a diagnosis strictly on the similarity between her patient and a typical patient with malaria. Based on their prevalence in North American patients, other diseases are far more likely than malaria to be the cause of fever, shaking chills, and sweats.

Example 2: A 35-year-old woman with mild hypertension is obese and has prominent striae and moderately excessive facial hair. She does not take corticosteroids. The medical student clerk has just completed an endocrinology elective. He immediately suspects Cushing's disease and tells his preceptor that there is a 30% chance that the patient has this disease. He had written an order for a complete battery of tests of adrenal function. His preceptor asks him to cancel the order.

Comment: Cushing's disease is the cause of hypertension in fewer than 1 in 100 patients. The features of classic Cushing's disease occur in other conditions which are far more prevalent. Even when the patient's clinical features are quite representative of classic Cushing's disease, the diagnosis is still a long shot.

To avoid the mistake of ignoring prior probability, the clinician must ask, "how common is the hypothesized disease in my clinical setting?" The commonest error is to overestimate the prevalence of the disease. As clinicians increasingly care for a defined population and use electronic medical records to track its health, perhaps they will make more accurate estimates of disease prevalence in their practice.

Errors in using the representativeness heuristic: II. Using clinical cues that do not accurately predict disease

The cues that make up the textbook description of a disease are imperfect indicators of who has the disease. Cues are sometimes absent in diseased persons and sometimes present in persons who do not have the disease. One mark of an excellent diagnostician is to know how well clinical features do predict disease.

Example: A previously well patient comes to the emergency department with the sudden onset of shortness of breath. The clinician initially suspects a pulmonary embolism but discards the possibility because the patient's legs show no signs of blood clots. Furthermore, the patient does not complain of coughing blood. The clinician sends him home. Two days later, the patient's shortness of breath worsens and he goes to another hospital where the emergency department clinicians correctly diagnose pulmonary embolism.

Comment: The clinician who first saw the patient has underestimated the probability of pulmonary embolism because two of the classic features of pulmonary embolism were not present. She did not know that only one-quarter of patients with pulmonary embolism cough blood and only one-third have clinical evidence of blood clots in the leg. These findings, while part of the classic description of pulmonary embolism, are not accurate clues to the disease.

Knowing how well the classic features of commonly encountered diseases actually predict the disease is essential to a lean, safe style of medical practice. In the next two chapters, we will lay the foundation for understanding the **likelihood ratio**, which is the best measure of this characteristic. The best source for the likelihood ratios of common clinical findings is past issues of the *Journal of the American Medical Association*. Since 1998, the journal has published 60 articles that summarize how well the clinical findings of common diseases actually predict the disease. The feature is called The Rational Clinical Examination, which is also the name of the book that summarizes this series of articles (Simel and Rennie, 2008).

Errors in using the representativeness heuristic: III. Being too sure of a diagnosis when redundant predictors are present
When a patient has many of the classic predictors of a disease, the clinician is often very confident of the diagnosis because "the story holds together pretty well." This confidence is unjustified if the textbook predictors typically all occur together.

Internal consistency does not necessarily lead to accurate predictions. Consider this extreme case. If the classic predictors of disease *always* occur together, knowing that one predictor is present is the same as knowing that all are present. Therefore, more than one predictor does not add information, and the clinician should not be any more confident of the diagnosis than if only one predictor were present. Clinicians often assume that each additional finding increases the probability of disease proportionately. In fact, clinical cues may be less predictive in combination than the clinician expects.

Example 1: A 40-year-old woman has chest pain that is retrosternal, radiates to the left arm, and is crushing, squeezing, and pressure-like. The clinician hurriedly concludes that the pain is indicative of coronary artery disease and admits the patient to the intensive care unit. The patient is discharged the next day with an appointment for a test of her gall bladder.

Comment: The patient appeared representative of coronary artery disease, and the pain is indeed anginal in quality, but the probability that she had coronary artery disease would have been increased considerably by finding that the following independent predictors of coronary artery disease were present:

- A history of pain brought on by exertion and emotional stress.

- Pain relieved promptly by rest or nitroglycerin.
- Pain so severe that the patient had to stop all activities when the pain occurred.
- A history of smoking cigarettes for many years.
  These findings are independent predictors of coronary artery disease, whereas the location, radiation, and descriptors of anginal pain tend to occur as a group and are therefore highly correlated.

Information about which disease cues are uncorrelated (i.e., independent) predictors of disease is increasingly available. This information often is presented in the form of rules for interpreting clinical findings. We discuss these **clinical prediction rules** further on in this chapter.

Errors in using the representativeness heuristic: IV. Mistakenly using regression to the mean as diagnostic evidence

A change in the patient's condition is often used to test a diagnostic hypothesis. For example, a **therapeutic trial** consists of giving a treatment that is specific for a hypothesized disease. If the patient improves, the clinician's estimated probability of the disease increases accordingly. The drug's mechanism of action leads us to expect that it would affect the pathophysiology of the disease, and so the change in the patient's status becomes a diagnostic feature of the hypothesized disease. A response to specific treatment therefore increases the match between the patient's features and the classic features of the disease. **The test of time** is another form of therapeutic trial. Here, the clinician withholds treatment in order to test the hypothesis that the patient does not have a serious disease. If the patient improves without treatment, the probability of serious disease goes down. The response of the test of time also improves the match between the patient's features and the typical features of a self-limited illness. This type of hypothesis testing is widely used in clinical practice.

However, changes in disease status that coincide with giving a drug may mislead the clinician because the response to treatment is due to random variation rather than cause and effect. The name of this relationship is **regression to the mean**.

Example: A patient has mild hyperglycemia on a single measurement of serum glucose. The clinician puts the patient on a diabetic diet. The patient's blood sugar falls, and the clinician concludes that the patient had diabetes.

Comment: The patient may not have diabetes. Hyperglycemia on the first blood glucose test was a chance variation in this biological measure. The second measurement was simply another sample from the same frequency distribution of serum glucose for this patient rather than a sample from a new frequency distribution that reflects improved diabetes control.

What is the basis for this example? Most biological measurements vary randomly over time. These random values are often symmetrically distributed about a mean value as described by the normal distribution curve (Figure 3.5).

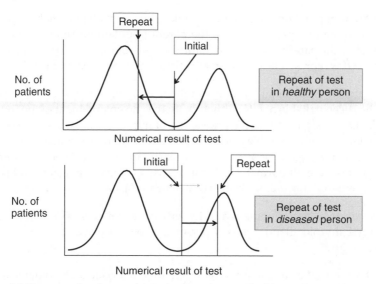

Figure 3.5 Two examples of regression to the mean: in normal individuals (top panel) and in diseased individuals (bottom panel).

The shape of the normal distribution curve shows that events whose value is close to the mean are much more common than events whose value is far from the mean. Thus, the value of a random event following an extreme value is likely to be closer to the mean because values close to the mean are more likely than extreme values. In a diseased patient, a low value is likely to be followed by a higher value, whereas in a well person a high value is likely to be followed by a low value. The event is consistent with either an effect of the drug or a random event. The clinician may therefore misinterpret random events as proving the success or failure of a therapeutic trial to test a diagnostic hypothesis. The "result" of treatment is actually a chance variation in a biological measurement, not an event that is representative of the hypothesized disease.

Errors in using the representativeness heuristic: V. Comparing a patient to a small, unrepresentative experience with a disease

When clinicians use the representativeness heuristic to judge the probability that a patient has a disease, they often compare the patient to their personal experience with the disease. In doing so, they usually do not take into account the size of their personal experience. When a person's experience with a disease is small, the principles of statistical sampling tell us that it is likely to be atypical. Thus, the clinician may mistakenly judge a patient with atypical clinical features of a disease as highly likely to have a disease with which she has a small, atypical experience.

Why is a small experience likely to be atypical? A clinician's personal experience with an event is a sample of the universe of all such events. From statistical theory, we learn that a small sample is more likely to deviate from the parent population than a large sample. Thus, a small personal experience may be quite unrepresentative of the parent population. An event which is unusual in the parent class, and therefore improbable, may be judged probable because it is representative of a small, atypical personal experience.

Example: Dr. V's patient has a heart rate of 100/min, has lost a little weight, and has been irritable of late. Although there is no enlargement of the thyroid gland, Dr. V estimates that the probability of hyperthyroidism is 0.50 because the patient closely resembles the only two cases of hyperthyroidism that Dr. V has ever diagnosed in his 10 years of primary care practice. When a battery of thyroid tests are all normal, Dr. V can scarcely believe the results and sends the patient to a consultant to help resolve this unusual case.

Comment: In a large population of hyperthyroid patients, 95% will have an enlarged thyroid gland. Dr. V's personal experience was too small to be representative.

Several mistakes in using the representative heuristic are avoidable. Clinicians should rely more on published accounts of the typical features of diseases and less on personal experience. Knowing more about the prevalence of diseases in one's practice would also help, as would a wider exposure to case histories and the resulting diagnoses.

This example concludes our discussion of the representativeness heuristic. The time spent in learning about the representativeness heuristic will be well repaid. Clinicians use his heuristic many times each day in clinical practice. Clinicians could avoid many errors in clinical reasoning by remembering the preceding examples.

The next heuristic is much easier to understand than the representativeness heuristic.

Heuristic II: availability
A second heuristic for using personal experience to determine probability is **availability**, the processes that enhance recall.

Definition of availability heuristic: Judging the probability of an event by how easily the event is remembered.

The availability heuristic leads to ascribing a higher probability to an easily remembered event than to an event that is difficult to recall. Availability is a valid clue for judging probability, due to experimental evidence that frequent events are easier to remember than infrequent events. However, factors other than frequency also affect availability in memory. They include vividness, consequences for clinician or patient, immediacy, recency, and rarity. These factors may distort the relationship of frequency and ease of recall, so that the clinician overestimates the probability that a patient has an unusual disease. The clinician vividly recalls a recent patient who had similar findings and had an unusual disease. The clinician assumes that the unusual disease is quite

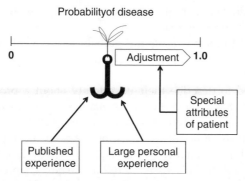

Figure 3.6 Schematic depiction of anchoring and adjustment.

common because its memory is so vivid. She remembers the similar patient with the disease but forgets the many similar patients who had other, more commonplace diseases.

Example 1: A clinician overestimates the probability that a patient with diarrhea has amoebiasis because she has recently seen a patient with amoebiasis (which is an unusual cause of diarrhea in the United States).

Example 2: A clinician recently made her first-ever diagnosis of subphrenic abscess by doing a white cell scan in a patient with fever and abdominal pain. For several months, whenever she had a patient with abdominal pain and low-grade fever, the clinician suspected subphrenic abscess and ordered a white cell scan. The patients all recovered uneventfully in a few days and wondered why they had to be hospitalized for a minor illness.

The third heuristic is the mental process by which special characteristics of the patient are used to estimate probability. This heuristic is called *anchoring and adjustment* (Figure 3.6).

Heuristic III: anchoring and adjustment

Clinicians often make a probability assessment by starting from an initial estimate and arriving at a final estimate by *adjusting* to take account of the patient's set of clinical features. This heuristic is very important and is often used incorrectly, typically by failing to adjust sufficiently for the patient-specific features. This bias toward the initial probability estimate is called *anchoring*. Different starting points for estimating probability lead to different estimates, which, because of the anchoring bias, are typically closer to the starting point than they should be.

There are several reasons why the anchoring bias leads to incorrect adjustment of probability estimates:

- People tend to *overestimate* the probability of events that are defined by the co-occurrence of several characteristics. This type of event is called **conjunctive**. The error in estimating probability may be due to overconfidence in redundant cues, as discussed in reference to the representativeness heuristic.

- People tend to *underestimate* the probability of events that are defined by the occurrence of any of several features. This type of event is called **disjunctive**.
- When asked to describe their uncertainty about a probability, people tend to overstate their certainty, as manifest by a narrower distribution of probabilities than is consistent with their actual level of certainty.
- People base the amount of adjustment on an incomplete assessment whose result is biased toward the starting point of the calculation.

Bayes' theorem, which is discussed in full in the next chapter, is an unbiased approach to adjusting probabilities from a starting point. Bayes' theorem indicates exactly how much to adjust an initial probability estimate when additional information becomes available.

Example: A patient with chest pain has atypical angina, and the clinician estimates the probability of coronary artery disease to be 0.70. The clinician orders an exercise electrocardiogram, which is very abnormal. Instead of diagnosing coronary artery disease, the clinician orders a costly radionuclide scan of the heart.

Comment: When the probability of disease prior to the test is estimated to be 0.70 and the exercise electrocardiogram is very abnormal, the probability of coronary artery disease is at least 0.95. At this point, most clinicians would tell the patient that he had coronary artery disease and begin treatment. Relying on intuition rather than Bayes' theorem, this clinician underestimated the effect of a very abnormal exercise ECG on the probability of coronary artery disease.

Correctly using heuristics for estimating probability

Using personal experience to estimate probability is among the most important topics in this book because it is a key part of the daily practice of medicine. To avoid the pitfalls of the methods that people use to estimate probability, the student of medicine must have a secure understanding of the heuristics for recalling experience.

Making precise, unbiased probability estimates from personal experience is beyond the cognitive ability of almost everyone. Clinicians do their best, and their best is often astonishing. The wisest seek guidance from published experience, which is our next topic.

3.3 Using published experience to estimate probability

Published experience is the second important influence on estimates of probability. The mortality rate from an operation, the probability of an adverse effect of therapy, and the prevalence of a severe form of coronary artery disease are examples of probability estimates obtained from published studies. Published studies are useful for several reasons:

- A published report about an uncommon disease usually reflects a much larger experience with the disease than most clinicians see in a lifetime in practice.
- Statistical analyses in published studies may organize the findings in a form that is useful for decision making.
- Published studies often report **prevalence**, which is the frequency of an event in a population of patients *at a specified instant in time*. The prevalence of disease is useful as a starting point to estimate its probability. Prevalence is often confused with **incidence**, which is the number of occurrences *during a specified period of time*.

The clinician is usually interested in the prevalence of disease in patients with a clinical finding or a pattern of findings. The prevalence of a disease appears in the published literature in the following ways:

1. Prevalence of a disease in a subgroup defined by a single clinical finding (e.g., chest pain).
2. Prevalence of a disease in a subgroup defined by several findings:
   - A patient is assigned to a subgroup by *intuitive interpretation* of the clinical findings (e.g., a syndrome such as heart failure).
   - A patient is assigned to a subgroup by a *formal process* for combining the clinical findings (e.g., a clinical prediction rule).

In the next several pages, we describe three ways to form a group of patients in which to measure the prevalence of disease. In each instance, the patients' common feature is a diagnostic problem.

3.3.1 Estimating probability from the prevalence of disease in patients with a symptom, physical finding, or test result

The prevalence of a disease in patients who have in common a symptom, physical finding, or diagnostic test result helps a clinician to diagnose the disease.

Example: A medical student evaluates a young man with abdominal pain. She is concerned about the possibility of appendicitis. The pain is present throughout the abdomen and is associated with loose bowel movements. The patient does not have localized abdominal tenderness, fever, or an increased blood leukocyte count. The medical student presents the patient to the chief surgical resident who, to the student's surprise, discharges the patient from the emergency room.

Comment: The chief surgical resident knows that the prevalence of appendicitis among self-referred adult males with abdominal pain is only 1%. The student should use this information as a starting point as she uses the patient's clinical findings to estimate the probability of appendicitis. If the history and physical examination do not suggest appendicitis, the probability of appendicitis is very low, since it was 1% in the average patient with abdominal pain. If the examination does suggest appendicitis, the student's estimate of probability must reflect the low prevalence of appendicitis in all men with abdominal pain.

3.3.2   Estimating the probability of a disease from its prevalence in patients with a clinical syndrome

After evaluating a patient, the clinician assigns the patient to a clinically defined syndrome (e.g., nephrotic syndrome) whose causes, and their prevalence, are known from published studies. To be sure that the prevalence of diseases in a study applies to a specific patient, the diagnostician needs to know if the study patients are similar to her patient. Because some published studies do not describe the process for choosing the patients to participate in the study, or list the findings that define the clinical syndrome, deciding that the study findings apply to a patient often requires clinical judgment.

Example: A resident is examining a 45-year-old man who came to the emergency room after experiencing retrosternal chest pain for the first time earlier in the day. The pain was pressure-like in quality and was confined to the chest. The pain came on after a hurried meal and lasted about 10 minutes. He has felt fine since then.

The resident is trying to decide whether to test for coronary artery disease. She knows that the decision about testing should depend on how well the patient's history fits the typical history for exertional angina pectoris, atypical angina, or non-anginal chest pain. The resident looks up an article which indicates the prevalence of coronary artery disease in each of these syndromes. Unfortunately, the article does not describe the criteria that the study used to classify a patient's pain as atypical angina or non-anginal. After consulting with a cardiologist, the resident decides that the patient's history is most consistent with non-anginal chest pain, counsels the patient against eating too fast, and schedules a follow-up visit in two weeks.

Comment: This method for estimating probability has one major drawback: it lacked a standardized process for assigning a patient to one of the three chest pain syndromes. Two clinicians may get the same history from this patient and yet differ on which anginal syndrome he has (if any). Therefore, they will make different estimates of the probability of coronary artery disease and perhaps disagree about whether to order a test. Clinicians might have fewer disagreements if the criteria for syndromes were standardized. Even so, this method for estimating probability is limited by the dearth of published information on the prevalence that cause a clinical syndrome.

3.3.3   Clinical prediction rules for estimating probability

Clinical prediction rules place a patient into a subgroup. The prevalence of disease in the subgroup is a starting point for estimating the probability of disease in the patient. Most clinical prediction rules are empirical. A typical study uses the following process:

1. Researchers obtain pre-specified clinical findings from many patients with the same clinical symptom, sign, or test result. The researchers then establish the final diagnosis by some means.
2. The researchers identify the predictors of disease by statistical methods that adjust the diagnostic weighting of each predictor to take into account the influence of the other predictors. The weighting of one factor does not depend on the presence of the other factors.
3. The prediction rule uses an explicit method for assigning patients to diagnostic subgroups based on their findings.
4. The prevalence of disease in a diagnostic subgroup is the number of patients in the subgroup with the target diagnosis divided by the total number of patients in the subgroup.
5. The prediction rule must be tested on additional patients to verify the prevalence of disease in the subgroups.

The following discussion focuses on how to create a clinical prediction rule. The details of the multivariate statistical techniques for identifying independent predictors of disease are interesting but beyond the scope of this book. A brief description will suffice. The principal statistical methods are **regression analysis** and **recursive partitioning**.

Regression analysis

Regression analysis describes the relationship between predictors (the independent variables or predictor variables) and the predicted event (the dependent variable). Regression analysis shows how the dependent variable changes when the value of a predictor changes while holding constant the values of the other variables. An important function of regression analysis is to test the hypothesis that a predictor variable is related to the dependent variable. It tries to answer the question, "independently of the value of the other potential predictors, is this predictor related to the dependent variable by anything more than a chance association?"

Regression analysis assigns a numerical weight to each predictor. The weight is a measure of its ability to discriminate between different values of the dependent variable (e.g., whether or not the patient has the target diagnosis). The larger the weight assigned to a variable, the better it discriminates.

The weights have practical value in diagnosis. To use a prediction rule derived by regression analysis, the clinician determines whether a predictor is present or not (e.g., she asks whether exertion causes a patient's chest pain). The clinician adds the numerical weights corresponding to the predictors that are present. The sum of the weights is a score. We will use the term

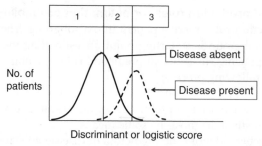

Figure 3.7 Hypothetical distribution of discriminant scores for diseased and non-diseased patients. The cut-off scores are represented by vertical lines.

discriminant score to represent this sum. The discriminant scores for diseased and non-diseased patients are distributed differently, as shown in Figure 3.7 for a hypothetical example.

As seen in Figure 3.7, the discriminant scores of diseased patients overlap with the scores of non-diseased patients. Typically, the researchers decide on a cut-off score below which most patients are not diseased and another cut-off score above which most patients are diseased. Between these two cut-off scores, the prevalence of disease is intermediate. The clinician uses a patient's discriminant score to put the patient into a group, as shown in Table 3.2.

The probability of disease in a patient assigned to a subgroup by his discriminant score is the prevalence of disease in that discriminant score subgroup. As a reminder of our terminology, this prevalence is an objective probability; its basis is a study of a population of patients.

Example 1: One of the authors performed a study of patients with chest pain. He found that seven findings in the history discriminate between patients with chronic chest pain who have significant narrowing of at least one coronary artery and chest pain patients with no significant narrowing (Table 3.3).

Interpretation: As in Table 3.4.

Example 2: A study of patients about to undergo non-cardiac surgery identified several predictors of cardiac complications of the surgery (Table 3.5). Depending on the discriminant score (the "cardiac risk score"), the prevalence of cardiac complications is very low, very high, or intermediate.

Table 3.2

Score group	Range of scores	Probability of disease
1	Low	Low
2	Intermediate	Intermediate
3	High	High

Table 3.3

Attribute	Diagnostic weight
Age >60 years	+3
Pain is brought on by exertion	+4
Patient must stop all activities when the pain occurs	+3
History of myocardial infarction	+4
Pain relieved within 3 minutes after taking nitroglycerin	+2
At least 20 pack-years of cigarette smoking	+4
Male gender	+5

Data from Sox *et al*. (1990).

Table 3.4

Chest pain score	Probability of coronary artery disease
0–4	0.10
5–9	0.39
10–14	0.67
15–19	0.91
20–25	1.00
All patients	0.76

Data from Sox *et al*. (1990).

Table 3.5

Clinical finding	Diagnostic weight
Patient's age is 70 years or greater	+5
Myocardial infarction in past 6 months	+10
Jugular venous distension or third heart sound	+11
Evidence of valvular aortic stenosis	+3
Arrhythmia on most recent electrocardiogram	+7
>5 ventricular premature beats/minute on any prior electrocardiogram	+7
Emergency surgery	+4
Intra-abdominal or thoracic surgery	+3
Laboratory evidence of organ dysfunction (Goldman *et al*., 1977) or patient is bed-ridden	+3

Interpretation: As in Table 3.6.

Recursive partitioning

Recursive partitioning is a statistical process that leads to an **algorithm** for classifying patients.

Definition of algorithm: Step-by-step instructions for solving a problem.

Table 3.6

Cardiac risk score	Fatal cardiac complication rate (%)
0–5	0.2
6–12	2.0
13–25	2.0
26 or greater	56.0

Data from Goldman *et al*. (1977).

The first use of clinical algorithms was to display the logic of diagnosis for medical corpsmen in the military, physician assistants, and nurse practitioners. Their use to describe a diagnostic or treatment strategy has spread to standard textbooks of medicine and journal articles. The term *algorithm* denotes a standard approach to a problem. A person can use an algorithm to describe their own logic in solving a problem. Our focus is on empirical algorithms which are based on a study in which researchers obtain pre-specified clinical findings from many patients and then establish the final diagnosis in each person. They then use statistical tests to decide which findings predict the final diagnosis.

In recursive partitioning, the diagnostic process is represented by a series of yes–no decision points. If a patient has a finding, he is placed in one group; if not, he is placed in a second group. Each of the two groups resulting from the first yes–no decision point is subjected to a second yes–no question about another finding. The process continues until it reaches a pre-defined stopping point. The goal of the process is to place each patient into a group in which the prevalence of disease is either very high or very low. Typically, the finding that is used at each yes–no decision point is the one that best discriminates between the diseased and non-diseased patients at that point in the partitioning process.

Example 1: A modified version of recursive partitioning was used to categorize adults with a sore throat as having a high, medium, or low probability of having a beta hemolytic streptococcal infection (Figure 3.8). According to some authors, patients with a high likelihood of infection should have treatment without obtaining a throat culture. In patients with a low likelihood of infection, neither throat culture nor treatment may be indicated.

Example 2: A tree of yes–no decision points is used to identify patients who are likely to have a myocardial infarction as the cause of their acute chest pain. Depending on which path the patient takes through the algorithm, the probability of acute myocardial infarction is high, intermediate, or low. The decision to admit the patient to the coronary care unit may depend on the probability of myocardial infarction (Figure 3.9).

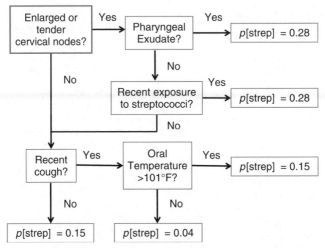

Figure 3.8 A recursive partitioning algorithm for classifying adults with sore throat (see Walsh *et al.*, 1975).

Strengths, shortcomings, and quality of clinical prediction rules

A clinical prediction rule is a powerful method because it imposes a formal, empirically derived method for grouping patients according to their clinical findings. Clinical prediction rules are statistical models of the diagnostic process. When a statistical model of experts' judgments is matched against the experts whose opinions were used in the model, the model usually outperforms the experts. Unlike the experts, the model is applied consistently from case to case without being diverted by information that seems useful but actually reduces diagnostic accuracy.

However, clinical prediction rules can lead to incorrect prevalence estimates if applied indiscriminately. The statistical techniques achieve optimum discrimination in the patient population that was used to create the rule (the **training set**). When the rule is used in other populations (the **test sets**), it typically discriminates less well. This outcome is known as over-fitting. Too many predictor variables and too few patients are a second cause of poor performance in a test set. A good general rule: Be cautious about using a prediction rule if the number of patients with the target condition in the training set is less than 10 for every candidate predictor in a regression analysis. The reason is that small numbers of patients are likely to be atypical samples of the universe of patients from which they are drawn.

A good general rule: Use an untested rule with caution!

The best way to test a prediction rule is to apply it to a large number of patients from a different setting than the training set patients, establish the final diagnosis, and calculate measures of **discrimination** and **calibration**. *Discrimination* is the ability of the rule to distinguish patients with the target diagnosis from everyone else. The *c*-statistic describes the probability that a

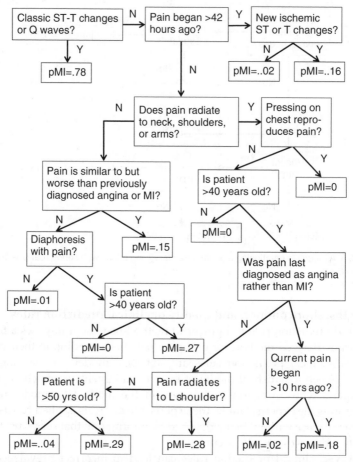

Figure 3.9 A recursive partitioning algorithm for estimating the probability of myocardial infarction (MI). The terms ST, T, and Q refer to different parts of the electrocardiographic tracing that reflects the electrical events in the heart during a single heart beat. Abnormalities in these electrical events occur during a myocardial infarction. (Data from Goldman *et al.*, 1982.)

patient with the target diagnosis will have a higher discriminant score than a patient with other diagnoses. A *c*-statistic of 0.50 denotes no discrimination. *Calibration* refers to the agreement between the probability of the target diagnosis in discriminant score subgroups of the training set and the test set.

Cross-validation uses a single data set to predict how well a prediction rule will perform in new test sets. Clinical studies are costly, so cross-validation is a good compromise between economy and the risks of using an untested rule. The principle is easy to understand. In its simplest form, the researcher randomly assigns patients from one study to two subsets, derives the rule from one set, and tests it on the other (noting the error rate). After reconstituting the original data set, the researcher repeats the cycle again and again. Hundreds of cycles are quickly performed on a computer. The computer can then calculate the mean error rate over the multiple test sets. If the entire process is repeated, each time increasing the number of predictor variables by 1, the error rate will decrease to a nadir point and then rise as the number of predictor variables increases further. The nadir point is the optimal number of predictor variables for the data set. The general name for this form of computer-intensive statistical analysis is the **bootstrap**.

The last topic in this section is quality standards for creating clinical prediction rules. Several articles have addressed this topic. Studies should clearly define the outcome to be predicted and the predictors. If possible, if the outcome is a diagnosis, it should be established by means other than the variables being assessed as predictors. A study should present the characteristics of the study population, so that a reader may judge its applicability to a specific clinical setting. A prediction rule should have *face validity*: it should make sense clinically. As noted in this section, the developers of a clinical prediction rule should, at a minimum, test the rule using cross-validation methods, preferably with a separate test set and ideally in another clinical setting with different patients and clinicians. The best test of a clinical prediction rule is its effect on patient care: it should be useful in practice. The findings should be reproducible, which means that when two clinicians examine the same patient independently, they should record the same findings.

3.3.4 Limitations of published studies

Published studies can mitigate the problem faced by the clinician with limited personal experience. However, a clinician faces several potential pitfalls when applying a published prevalence of disease to the clinician's own patients.

The most important source of error in published studies is **selection bias**. Selection bias is likely to be a problem when the criteria for selecting patients to participate in a published study are different than the conditions that brought the patient to whom the prediction rule will be applied to medical attention. Most published studies are performed on patients referred to academic medical centers. Patients are seen by specialists because a referring clinician suspects a disease in the specialist's sphere of expertise. Specialists are less likely to see patients with clinical findings that imply a low probability of disease. Therefore, the prevalence of serious disease in the specialist's practice will be higher than in the primary care clinician's practice.

One of the authors proved this point in a study of four different populations of patients with chest pain. He and his colleagues applied a clinical prediction rule developed in a training set consisting of patients referred for elective coronary arteriography (overall prevalence 76%) to three different test populations. One test population was having an elective coronary arteriogram, and two were primary care populations. When test set patients with similar chest pain scores – and therefore similar histories – were compared to the training set, the probability of coronary artery disease was the same in the coronary arteriography test set (overall prevalence 72%). However, the prevalence in patients with similar chest pain scores was lower in one primary care test set (overall prevalence 33%) and still lower in another primary care test set with an overall prevalence of 8%. The authors concluded that the probability of coronary artery disease in patients with a similar history varied according to the overall disease prevalence. In other words, the interpretation of the history depended on the overall prevalence of disease in the population.

Primary care clinicians should be cautious when applying the prevalence of disease from published reports to their practice. The following examples illustrate the consequences of uncritically applying published studies to primary care practice.

Example: A primary care internist feels a nodule in the prostate gland. How likely is prostate cancer? The only pertinent reference is a classic paper from the practice of a renowned urologist; in this study, half of the patients with a prostate nodule had prostate cancer.

Comment: Does the internist's patient have a 50% chance of having prostate cancer? Probably not. After all, the patients who were seen by the urologist who wrote the paper were seen first by primary care clinicians. These clinicians probably referred only when the patient's nodule was particularly suspicious for prostate cancer.

Example: A 40-year-old man has a blood pressure of 160/110 mm Hg. An internist who just completed training at a large referral center for hypertension orders a screening x-ray of the kidneys. A senior radiologist in the internist's practice calls to remind him to make the following research findings:

Comment: Studies in specialty practice showed that about 5% of hypertensive patients had surgically curable causes of hypertension, such as pheochromocytoma and aldosterone-secreting adrenal tumors. When a study of secondary hypertension in primary care patients was finally performed, the prevalence of curable causes was only about 1%. After this study was published, primary care clinicians became much more selective about launching an expensive work-up for secondary causes of hypertension.

Clinicians in referral practice have less reason for concern about the effects of selection bias on the accuracy of objective probability estimates in their practice. Their patients go through the same filtering process as the patients in most published studies.

Clinicians may disagree in their estimated prevalence of disease because they read different journals. The primary care clinician is more likely to read articles in primary care journals, which report the prevalence of disease in unselected patients. The surgeon reads surgical journals, which report studies of patients referred to surgeons. When consultant and referring clinicians discuss a patient, they must be aware of this reason for possible disagreement.

3.4 Taking the special characteristics of the patient into account when estimating probability

Patients often have special characteristics that must be taken into account when estimating probability. A patient may have a clinical finding that seems important in the circumstances but does not appear in a published clinical prediction rule. A patient's findings may differ from the clinician's prior experience with the suspected disease. The clinician must be prepared to adjust the estimated probability from the starting point provided by published studies and prior experience.

Example: A man in his mid-thirties has chest pain that has a few characteristics of anginal pain but is atypical. Clinical prediction rules and other published studies indicate that the probability of disease should be approximately 0.20. However, the patient's two siblings and his father all had a fatal myocardial infarction before the age of 40. Because of these unusual findings, the patient's internist sharply revises her estimate of the probability of coronary artery disease and initiates a search that ends with a diagnosis of severe coronary artery disease.

Comment: Having several young siblings die of coronary artery disease happens so seldom that multivariate statistical methods are unlikely to identify the finding as a significant independent predictor of coronary artery disease. This alarming family history should influence estimates of disease probability. Common sense ruled in this case.

Summary

1. Clinicians usually work in a state of uncertainty about the true state of the patient.
2. The clinical findings that clinicians use are imperfect. Almost invariably, negative results occur in patients with the target disease and positive results occur in patients who do not have the disease.
3. We define probability as an expression of opinion (on a scale of 0 to 1) about the likelihood of a future event or a present state. By expressing uncertainty as a probability it becomes possible to measure the effect of new information which opens the door to a hitherto unexplored realm of precise diagnostic reasoning.
4. Several factors influence a patient's probability of a disease: the clinicians' prior personal experience, published experience, the clinical setting of care, and special or unusual attributes of the patient.
5. Probability assessment can go astray when people misuse the mental methods for estimating probability (heuristics). The most important of these biased heuristics are:

- Neglecting the influence of disease prevalence just because the patient's findings match up nicely with the features of the disease.
- Matching the patient's characteristics against the least predictive features of the disease.
- Placing too much weight on information that is consistent with earlier information but redundant.
- Overestimating the probability of an event because it is easy to remember: it happened recently, it was especially vivid, or both.
- Initial estimates of probability are too high or too low and then they are not adjusted enough to take account of new information.
6. The usefulness of published disease prevalence and experts' probability estimates depends on how closely their patients resemble yours.
7. Clinical prediction rules provide a way to encode prior experience and thereby estimate probabilities reliably and reproducibly.

Problems

1. Suppose that an infectious disease expert gave you the following advice about various treatment alternatives for one of your patients:
   (a) The likelihood that the infection will respond to antibiotic A is greater than the likelihood that the infection will respond to antibiotic B.
   (b) The likelihood that the infection will not respond to antibiotic C is greater than the likelihood that the infection will not respond to antibiotic B.
   (c) The likelihood that the infection will respond to antibiotic C is greater than the likelihood that the infection will respond to antibiotic A.
   Does this advice make sense?
2. Are the following statements consistent? The probability that the patient will die sometime during the next seven days is 0.5, the probability that the patient will die after day 7 but on or before day 14 is 0.4, and the probability that the patient will survive beyond day 14 is 0.3.
3. Consider the following two treatments. The success of Treatment A depends on the successful completion of each of several intermediate steps. The successful application of the Treatment B can be achieved by any one of several alternative approaches. For which treatment are you more likely to overestimate the probability of success and for which treatment are you more likely to underestimate the likelihood of success?
4. Suppose that a colleague provides you with a large number of observations that you believe pertain to a particular patient. However, suppose that one of these observations, unknown to you, is incorrect. Which arrangement of these observations would be most misleading to you:
   (a) An arrangement in which the erroneous fact is presented first?
   (b) An arrangement in which the erroneous fact is presented last?

Bibliography

Bryant, G.D. and Norman, G.R. (1980) Expressions of probability: words and numbers (Letter). *New England Journal of Medicine*, **302**, 411.

An influential Letter to the Editor showing that the ranges of probabilities corresponding to the words used to express uncertainty overlap each other.

Goldman, L., Caldera, D.L., Nussbaum, S. *et al.* (1977) Multifactorial index of cardiac risk in non-cardiac surgical procedures. *New England Journal of Medicine*, **297**, 845–50.

A classic description of how a logistic rule was developed and used to estimate the risk of cardiac complications of surgery.

Goldman, L., Weinberg, M., Weisberg, M. *et al.* (1982) A computer-derived protocol to aid in the diagnosis of emergency room patients with acute chest pain. *New England Journal of Medicine*, **307**, 588–96.

The authors used recursive partitioning to develop an algorithm for diagnosing myocardial infarction (see Figure 3.9).

Kahneman, D. (2011) *Thinking*, Fast and Slow, Farrar, Straus & Giroux, New York.

A book written for the general public about two systems of thinking, fast and slow, and how faulty reasoning and biases can send the former off the track.

Kahneman, D., Slovic, P., and Tversky, A. (1982) *Judgment under Uncertainty: Heuristics and biases*, Cambridge University Press, Cambridge.

A collection of scientific papers on biased heuristics.

Laupacis, A., Sekar, N., and Stiell, I.G. (1997) Clinical prediction rules: a review and suggested modifications of methodological standards. *Journal of the American Medical Association*, **277**, 488–94.

The authors review prediction rules from a later era than Wasson *et al.* (see below) and propose modifications to the earlier standards and additional standards for producing them.

McGinn, T.G., Guyatt, G.H., Wyer, P.C., Naylor, C.D., Stiell, N.G., Richardson, W.S., and the Evidence-Based Medicine Working Group (2000) Users' guides to the medical literature: XXII: How to use articles about clinical prediction rules. *Journal of the American Medical Association*, **284**, 79–84.

One of the JAMA series of articles on the critical use of clinical information.

Simel, D.L. and Rennie, D. (2008) *The Rational Clinical Examination: Evidence-based Clinical Diagnosis*, McGraw-Hill Medical, New York.

A book with good information about test performance.

Sox, H.C., Hickam, D.H., Marton, K.I. *et al.* (1990) Using the patient's history to estimate the probability of coronary artery disease: a comparison of primary care and referral practices. *American Journal of Medicine*, **89**, 7–14.

This article describes the development and testing of a prediction rule for chest pain. The article supports the claim that the interpretation of the patient's history depends on the clinical setting (see Section 3.4).

Spetzler, C.S. and Stael von Holstein, C.A.S. (1975) Probability encoding in decision analysis. *Management Science*, **25**, 340–57.

A classic paper on probability assessment.

Tversky, A. and Kahneman, D. (1974) Judgment under uncertainty: heuristics and biases. *Science*, **185**, 1124–31.

A classic, readable article on biased heuristics in subjective probability estimation. Kahneman won the Alfred Nobel Memorial Prize in Economics in 2002. Tversky, his partner in research, died a few years earlier.

Walsh, B.T., Bookheim, W.W., Johnson, R.C. *et al.* (1975) Recognition of streptococcal pharyngitis in adults. *Archives of Internal Medicine*, **135**, 1493–7.

An empirical algorithm for classifying patients with sore throat using a modification of recursive partitioning (see Figure 3.8).

Wasson, J.H., Sox, H.C., Neff, R.K., and Goldman, L. (1985) Clinical prediction rules: applications and methodological standards. *New England Journal of Medicine*, **313**, 793–9.

The authors evaluate published clinical prediction rules and propose standards for developing and testing them.

Weiner, D.A., Ryan, T.J., McCabe, C.H. *et al.* (1979) Exercise stress testing: correlations among history of angina, ST-segment response, and prevalence of coronary-artery disease in the Coronary Artery Surgery Study (CASS). *New England Journal of Medicine*, **301**, 230–5.

CHAPTER 4

Understanding new information: Bayes' theorem

Clinicians must take decisive action despite uncertainty about the patient's diagnosis or the outcome of treatment. To help them navigate this wilderness, Chapter 3 introduced probability as a language for expressing uncertainty and showed how to "translate" one's uncertainty into this language. Using probability theory does not eliminate uncertainty about the patient. Rather, it *reduces uncertainty about uncertainty*. This chapter builds upon the preceding chapter to show how to interpret new information that imperfectly reflects the patient's true state. This chapter has eight parts:

4.1 Introduction

Why is it important to understand the effect of new information on uncertainty? Clinicians want to minimize their margin of error, in effect bringing probability estimates as close as possible to 1.0 or 0. Without knowing how new information has affected – or will affect – probability, the clinician may acquire too much information, too little, or the wrong information.

How does a clinician monitor progress toward understanding the patient's true state? Let us represent the process of diagnosis by a straight line (Figure 4.1). Probability provides a ruler for measuring progress along this line. Methods for estimating probability (Chapter 3) tell us where to put the first mark on the line. When we obtain more information, Bayes' theorem, which is the subject of this chapter, tells us where to put the next mark.

The following examples illustrate the importance of modifying one's estimate of probability as new information becomes available.

Medical Decision Making, Second Edition. Harold C. Sox, Michael C. Higgins and Douglas K. Owens.
© 2013 John Wiley & Sons, Ltd. Published 2013 by John Wiley & Sons, Ltd.

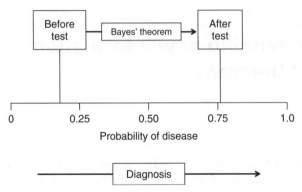

Figure 4.1 Role of Bayes' theorem.

Example 1: An intern on duty in the emergency department sees a man because of chest pain. The man has no health insurance.

The patient's history is as follows. He is 45 years old and has no cardiac risk factors. The pain began suddenly four days ago. The pain is in the left anterior chest, does not radiate to the arms, neck, or shoulders, has never occurred before, and is not accompanied by sweating. An electrocardiogram does not show ST segment changes indicative of myocardial ischemia or Q waves indicative of myocardial damage. The patient is admitted to cardiac intensive care. At the end of the first 24 hours, there have been no complications, the serum troponin (a measure of cardiac muscle death) is normal, and there is no change in the ECG. After two days in cardiac care, the patient's clinician tells him that he did not have a myocardial infarction and discharges him from the hospital. Later, he receives a $14 000 bill for this brief admission.

Comment: The intern was uncertain about whether the patient was having an infarction and admitted him in order to be on the safe side. If the intern had used the recursive partitioning algorithm shown in Figure 3.9 in Chapter 3, she would have known that the probability of acute myocardial infarction was only 0.01. Once admitted, the patient's clinicians were too cautious about interpreting what they had learned at the end of 24 hours. The complication-free course, the normal serum enzyme levels, and the unchanged ECG reduced still further the probability of infarction or hospital complication (Figure 4.2). They should have moved the patient to a less intense level of care, or even discharged him from the hospital, after the first 24 hours.

Example 2: The patient is a 60-year-old man with chest pain.

The pain began six months ago. It is a retrosternal sensation of pressure. When the pain is present, he cannot do anything. Exertion brings on the pain, and nitroglycerin relieves it within three minutes. The man has been a heavy cigarette smoker. The clinician interprets the history as "typical exertional angina pectoris" and obtains an exercise electrocardiogram to confirm her judgment. The patient is able to continue on the treadmill for 14 minutes, and there are no electrocardiographic indications of myocardial ischemia. The

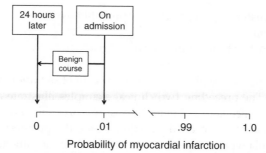

Figure 4.2 The effect of an uncomplicated hospital course on the probability of myocardial infarction.

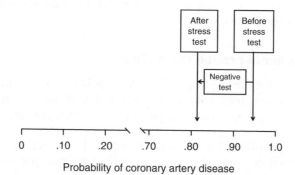

Figure 4.3 The effect of a normal exercise electrocardiogram on the probability of coronary artery disease.

clinician tells the patient that the treadmill test indicates he probably does not have coronary heart disease. After six months of continued pain, the patient obtains a second opinion. This physician tells him that the treadmill test result indicates that, although he has a relatively good prognosis, he probably does have coronary heart disease. To help the patient understand, he draws the diagram shown in Figure 4.3.

Comment: The second clinician correctly interpreted the history as indicating a high probability of coronary artery disease. The prevalence of coronary disease in 60-year-old men with typical angina is 0.95, which appears to apply to this patient. The exercise electrocardiogram is often normal in patients with coronary artery disease. If the test is negative, as in this patient, the probability of coronary artery disease is still 0.81.

Both of these examples involved estimating a probability before and after acquiring new information. The standard terminology for these two probabilities is:

Definition of prior probability: The probability of an event before acquiring new information.
   Synonyms: pre-test probability, pre-test risk.

Definition of posterior probability: The probability of an event after acquiring new information.

Synonyms: post-test probability, post-test risk.

In medicine, when we explain the meaning of an observation, we are said to "interpret" it. The preceding two clinical examples illustrate another usage of "interpret," which is to estimate the post-test probability of disease. While an interpretation of a test result should include the post-test probability, it should also explain other aspects of the test result in the patient.

In this context, the key to test interpretation is calculating the probability of disease corresponding to a clinical finding. Learning to make this important calculation requires a brief excursion into probability theory in order to learn a simple but helpful notation.

4.2 Conditional probability defined

Conditional probability is very helpful to clinicians who are interested in interpreting clinical information. The probability of disease given that a clinical finding is present is an example of a **conditional probability**.

Definition of conditional probability: The probability that an event is true given that another event is true (i.e., conditional upon the second event being true).

The notation of conditional probability is quite easy to understand. The conditional probability of **event A** given that **event B** is true is written:

P[A|B] which means "the probability of event A *conditional upon* event B."
The vertical line is read "conditional upon."

The formal definition of conditional probability is

$$P[A|B] = \frac{P[A \text{ and } B]}{P[B]}$$
(4.1)

which may be translated as "the conditional probability that A is true given that B is true is the ratio of the probability that both A and B are true divided by the probability that B is true."

A clinical example of a conditional probability is:

"What is the probability of coronary artery disease conditional upon an abnormal exercise electrocardiogram?"

This question is of great interest to the clinician who has just learned of a patient's exercise electrocardiogram findings. To obtain the answer to this question, she must translate Equation 4.1 into a form in which the probabilities can be measured. Each of the ways to calculate the posterior probability of disease is based on Bayes' theorem.

4.3   Bayes' theorem

Relatives of the Reverend Thomas Bayes (1702–61), an English clergyman, discovered his lasting contribution to knowledge when they were sorting his effects after his death. They discovered an unpublished manuscript that showed how, starting from Equation 4.1, to derive what came to be called Bayes' theorem. With Bayes' theorem, the clinician can calculate the posterior probability of a disease using the following quantities:

- the prior probability of the disease;
- the probability of a test result conditional upon the patient having the disease;
- the probability of the test result conditional upon the patient not having the disease.

4.3.1   Derivation of Bayes' theorem

Suppose we are trying to calculate the probability of disease D given that a particular test result (R) occurred. Using the notation of conditional probability, we must calculate

$$P[D|R]$$

where R represents a test result. This notation reads "probability of disease conditional upon the test result occurring."

We know from the definition of conditional probability (Equation 4.1) that

$$P[D|R] = \frac{P[R \text{ and } D]}{P[R]}$$

$P[R]$, the probability of a test result, is simply the sum of the probability of the test result in diseased patients and its probability in non-diseased patients:

$$P[R] = P[R \text{ and } D] + P[R \text{ and no } D]$$

Thus, we get

$$P[D|R] = \frac{P[D \text{ and } R]}{P[R \text{ and } D] + P[R \text{ and no } D]} \qquad (4.2)$$

By the definition of conditional probability (Equation 4.1)

$$P[R|D] = \frac{P[R \text{ and } D]}{P[D]}$$

and

$$P[R|\text{no } D] = \frac{P[R \text{ and no } D]}{P[\text{no } D]}$$

Rearranging these expressions, we get

$$P[R \text{ and } D] = P[D] \times P[R|D] \tag{4.3}$$

$$P[R \text{ and no } D] = P[\text{no } D] \times P[R|\text{no } D] \tag{4.4}$$

Substituting Equations 4.3 and 4.4 into 4,2, we obtain Bayes' theorem:

$$P[D|R] = \frac{P[D] \times P[R|D]}{(P[D] \times P[R|D] + P[\text{no } D] \times P[R|\text{no } D])} \tag{4.5}$$

4.3.2 Clinically useful forms of Bayes' theorem

Bayes' theorem when a test result is *positive*

To translate Equation 4.5 into a clinically useful form, we will make several changes.

First, we express the test result (R), which could potentially have any biologically reasonable value, as a dichotomous variable (positive or negative). Why? Most test results are expressed as a continuous variable (e.g., the concentration of an enzyme in the blood or the size of a lung mass on a chest radiograph). To act on a test result, we must choose a threshold value for taking action (e.g., the smallest lung mass that experts feel should be biopsied rather than monitored to see if it grows). All values of the test result above the threshold we call "positive." All values below the threshold, we call "negative." Choosing the cut-point that defines positive and negative is an important topic that we take up in Chapter 5.

Second, since the probability of all causes of a diagnostic problem must add to 1, $P[\text{no } D]$ is equivalent to $1 - P[D]$.

Third, we will express $P[+|D]$, the probability of a positive test result given that the patient is diseased, as the **sensitivity** of the test. Articles about the performance characteristics of tests use the term "sensitivity" rather than its equivalent in conditional probability notation:

$$\text{sensitivity} = \frac{\text{number of diseased patients with positive test}}{\text{number of diseased patients}}$$

Fourth, we will rewrite $P[+|\text{no } D]$, the probability of a positive test result given that the hypothesized disease is absent, in terms of the **specificity** of the test, which is the probability of a negative test if the hypothesized disease is absent. The reason for rewriting $P[+|\text{no } D]$ in terms of specificity is that studies of diagnostic test performance customarily report their findings as specificity. The probability of all test results in patients who do not have the hypothesized disease must add up to 1. Therefore, $P[+|\text{no } D]$ (see Equation 4.5) is equivalent to $(1 - P[-|\text{no } D])$ or $(1 - \text{specificity})$:

$$\text{specificity} = \frac{\text{number of non-diseased patients with negative test}}{\text{number of non-diseased patients}}$$

Combining these four changes, we have Bayes' theorem in a useful form:

$$P[D|+] = \frac{(P[D] \times \text{sensitivity})}{P[D] \times \text{sensitivity} + (1 - P[D]) \times (1 - \text{specificity})} \qquad (4.6)$$

A note on navigating this book: Diagnostic tests and Bayes' theorem are closely related, so that it is difficult to describe one without describing the other. This book has separate chapters for these two topics. In this chapter, we provide just enough information about sensitivity and specificity to support the in-depth presentation of Bayes' theorem. We present methods for measuring the sensitivity and specificity of a diagnostic test in Chapter 5. Some readers may prefer to read Chapter 5 before reading Chapter 4.

A simplification: We explain why we use "disease" and "no disease," which are the terms that we will use to simplify the presentation here and in other chapters. In applying Bayes' theorem to medicine, people often combine the potential causes of a diagnostic problem into two mutually exclusive states,

1. The disease that is hypothesized to be present (often labeled simply "disease" or "target condition").
2. All other states that are known to cause the diagnostic problem (including states in which no disease is demonstrable). This abstract state means "the hypothesized disease is absent" and is often labeled "no disease." Since the probability of all possible causes must add up to 1, the probability of the "no-disease" state is

{1 − the probability of the hypothesized disease}

Later in the chapter, we will consider what to do when several diseases are under consideration and a test can detect each of them.

Bayes' theorem when a test result is *negative*
To calculate the probability of disease if a test result is negative (i.e., below the threshold result for taking action), we use Equation 4.5 after substituting minus signs (to denote a negative test result) for R in Equation 4.5. Thus, $P[D|+]$ becomes $P[D|-]$:

$$P[D|-] = \frac{P[D] \times P[-|D]}{(P[D] \times P[-|D] + P[\text{no } D] \times P[-|\text{no } D])} \qquad (4.7)$$

To translate Equation 4.7 into clinically useful form, note that:

$P[-|D]$ is the probability of a negative test result given that the patient has the target condition, which is 1 − the probability that the test is positive when the patient has the target condition.

$P[-|no\ D]$ is the probability of a negative test result given that the patient does not have the hypothesized disease, which is the *specificity* of the test.

$$P[D|-] = \frac{P[D] \times p(1 - \text{sensitivity})}{(P[D] \times P(1 - \text{sensitivity}) + P[no\ D] \times \text{specificity})} \qquad (4.8)$$

Probability of a test result

As noted earlier, the probability of a positive test result ($P[+]$) is the sum of its probability in diseased patients and its probability in non-diseased patients:

$$P[+] = P[+\ and\ D] + P[+\ and\ no\ D]$$

In the previous section, we rearranged the definition of conditional probability to show that

$$P[+\ and\ D] = P[D] \times P[+|D]$$

$$P[+\ and\ no\ D] = P[no\ D] \times P[+|no\ D]$$

Since $P[+|D] = \text{sensitivity}$ and $P[+|no\ D] = 1 - \text{specificity}$,

> probability of a positive result
>
> $= P[D] \times \text{sensitivity} + (1 - P[D]) \times (1 - \text{specificity})$ $\qquad$ (4.9)

> probability of a negative test result
>
> $= [1 - \text{probability of a positive test result}]$ $\qquad$ (4.10)

Example: For illustration, imagine a 55-year-old man with hemoptysis and a long history of smoking cigarettes. Based on the clinical findings and her personal experience, the clinician suspects lung cancer and estimates the pre-test probability of lung cancer to be 0.4. The interpretation of the chest x-ray is "mass lesion in the right upper lobe."

The performance of the chest x-ray in patients with suspected lung cancer is
   sensitivity: 0.60
   specificity: 0.96
How should the clinician interpret the finding of a "mass lesion in the right upper lobe?"

$$P[D|+] = \frac{P[D] \times \text{sensitivity}}{(P[D] \times \text{sensitivity} + (1 - P[D]) \times (1 - \text{specificity}))}$$

$$= \frac{0.4 \times 0.60}{(0.4 \times 0.6 + (1 - 0.4) \times 0.04)} = 0.94$$

What if the chest x-ray had *not* shown a mass lesion?

$$P[D|-] = \frac{P[D] \times (1 - \text{sensitivity})}{(P[D] \times (1 - \text{sensitivity}) + (1 - P[D]) \times (\text{specificity}))}$$

$$= \frac{0.4 \times 0.4}{0.4 \times 0.4 + (1 - 0.4) \times 0.96} = 0.22$$

Explanation: Since the chest x-ray showed a mass lesion, the patient probably has lung cancer, although further confirmation will be required before starting treatment. If the chest x-ray had shown no evidence of lung cancer, the clinician should have still been suspicious, since the pre-test and post-test probabilities of lung cancer were so high. Some patients with lung cancer do not have chest radiographic evidence at the time the disease is first detected. Recent studies have compared screening to a chest radiograph to screening with a low-dose CT scan; the latter is more sensitive but less specific.

4.4 The odds ratio form of Bayes' theorem

One disadvantage of Bayes' theorem is that most people need a calculator. A second disadvantage is that sensitivity and specificity do not convey information about the effect of a test result on probability. The solution to both of these problems is to rewrite Bayes' theorem to calculate the post-test odds, which is equivalent to the post-test probability. The odds ratio form of Bayes' theorem is easy to remember and involves multiplying just two numbers, of which only one must be memorized.

Expressing the pre-test probability of disease in terms of the *pre-test odds* of disease achieves a powerful simplification of Bayes' theorem. Using the odds ratio format of Bayes' theorem, anyone can easily update probabilities after learning of new information. Moreover, expressing Bayes' theorem in its odds ratio format leads directly to a simple, intuitive way to describe the effect of new diagnostic information. This is the **likelihood ratio**, and it is one of the most important ideas in this book.

4.4.1 Derivation

To derive the odds ratio form of Bayes' theorem, start with Bayes' theorem in its familiar form (here we use R to denote any test result)

$$P[D|R] = \frac{P[D] \times P[R|D]}{(P[D] \times P[R|D] + P[\text{no } D] \times P[R|\text{no } D])} \tag{4.5}$$

Now, convert $P[D]$, a probability, to odds using the relationship learned in Chapter 3:

$$P[D] = \frac{\text{odds}[D]}{1 + \text{odds}[D]}$$

Instead of odds[D], we write O[D]. Substituting $O[D]/(1 + O[D])$ where we see $P[D]$ in Bayes' theorem (Equation 4.2), we get the expression

$$P[D|R] = \frac{\left(\dfrac{O[D] \times P[R|D]}{1 + O[D]}\right)}{\dfrac{O[D] \times P[R|D]}{1 + O[D]} + \left(1 - \dfrac{O[D]}{1 + O[D]} \times P[R|\text{no } D]\right)}$$

Remembering that

$$P[D|R] = \frac{O[D|R]}{1 + O[D|R]}$$

this long expression for $P[D|R]$ simplifies to:

$$\frac{O[D|R]}{1 + O[D|R]} = \frac{O[D] \times P[R|D]}{O[D] \times (P[R|D] + P[R|\text{no } D])}$$

Multiplying the numerator and denominator of the right side by $1/(O[D] \times P[R|D])$,

$$\frac{O[D|R]}{1 + O[D|R]} = \frac{1}{1 + \left(\dfrac{P[R|\text{no } D]}{O[D] \times P[R|D]}\right)}$$

Cross-multiplying,

$$O[D|R] + O[D|R] \times \frac{P[R|\text{no } D]}{O[D] \times P[R|D]} = 1 + O[D|R]$$

$$O[D|R] \times \frac{P[R|\text{no } D]}{O[D] \times P[R|D]} = 1$$

Rearranging terms, we obtain the odds ratio form of Bayes' theorem:

$$\boxed{O[D|R] = O[D] \times \frac{P[R|D]}{P[R|\text{no } D]}} \tag{4.11}$$

Look carefully at Equation 4.11. It is telling you that the post-test odds of disease conditional upon test result R ($O[D|R]$) are equal to the pre-test odds ($O[D]$) times a number. That number is the amount that the odds change after the test result, R. An expression that tells you how much the odds of disease change after new information is so useful that it (i.e., $P[R|D]/P[R|\text{no } D]$) has a name: *the likelihood ratio*.

Definition of likelihood ratio: A number that shows how much the odds of disease change after getting new information.

Another way to state the odds ratio expression of Bayes' theorem is

$$\boxed{\text{post-test odds} = \text{pre-test odds} \times \text{likelihood ratio}}$$

The likelihood ratio is convenient and powerful: a single number that shows how much one's uncertainty should change after new information, such as a test result.

Table 4.1

Test result (mm ST segment depression)	Likelihood ratio for coronary artery disease
<1.0	0.40
1.0–1.49	2.09
1.5–1.99	4.50
2.0–2.49	10.80
≥2.5	38.00

Data from Diamond and Forrester (1979).

4.4.2 The likelihood ratio: a measure of test discrimination

We saw in the previous section that

$$\text{likelihood ratio} = \frac{P[\text{result in diseased persons}]}{P[\text{result in non-diseased persons}]}$$

The likelihood ratio is a very useful way to characterize clinical information. Any clinical finding may be characterized by its likelihood ratio. Different amounts of ST segment depression during an exercise stress test indicate different likelihoods of coronary artery disease on an arteriogram, as shown in this example (Table 4.1).

In contrast to this example of a continuous variable having likelihood ratios for each of several results, a binary result (result above a threshold for taking action) or result absent (result below the action threshold), which translate into "positive" and "negative," can also have likelihood ratios. For example, physicians often treat the amount of ST segment depression on a stress electrocardiogram as a dichotomous variable. Less than 1 mm ST segment depression is a negative test; ST segment depression of ≥1 mm is a positive test, one that may require additional testing. Table 4.2 shows the likelihood ratio for all amounts of ST segment depression that are at least 1 mm.

Each of these two findings has a likelihood ratio, one corresponding to ≥1 mm ST segment depression (abbreviated LR+), and one corresponding to

Table 4.2

Test result (mm ST segment depression)	Likelihood ratio for coronary artery disease
<1.0	0.41
≥1	7.45

Data from Rifkin and Hood (1977).

<1 mm ST segment depression (abbreviated LR−):

$$LR+ = \frac{P[\text{finding present in \textbf{diseased} persons}]}{P[\text{finding present in \textbf{non-diseased} persons}]}$$

From the definitions of sensitivity and specificity, this definition takes the following form:

$$LR+ = \frac{\text{sensitivity}}{1 - \text{specificity}} \tag{4.12}$$

$$LR- = \frac{P[\text{finding absent in \textbf{diseased} persons}]}{P[\text{finding absent in \textbf{non-diseased} persons}]}$$

From the definitions of sensitivity and specificity, this definition takes the following form:

$$LR- = \frac{1 - \text{sensitivity}}{\text{specificity}} \tag{4.13}$$

The likelihood ratio is especially useful for expressing the discriminatory power of a test result because the clinician needs to remember only one number (the likelihood ratio) instead of two numbers (sensitivity and specificity).

4.4.3 Using the odds ratio form of Bayes' theorem

The likelihood ratio is used in the odds ratio form of Bayes' theorem. To understand the odds ratio format, recall the following definitions from Chapter 3:

$$\text{odds of event} = \frac{P[\text{the event will occur}]}{P[\text{the event will not occur}]}$$

$$\text{odds of event} = \frac{p}{1 - p}$$

Thus, if the probability of an event is 0.33, the odds that the event will occur are

$$\text{odds of event} = \frac{p}{1 - p} = \frac{0.33}{1 - 0.33} = \frac{1}{2} \text{ or } 1 : 2$$

If a finding is present, the amount that the pre-test odds increase may be calculated with the odds ratio form of Bayes' theorem:

$$\boxed{\text{post-test odds} = \text{pre-test odds} \times \text{likelihood ratio}}$$

The first example of the odds ratio form of Bayes' theorem shows how to calculate the post-test probability with a test result that is one point on a continuum of results. The test is a stress electrocardiogram, a test whose results can be expressed as a continuous variable, the amount of ST segment depression.

Example 1: What is the post-test probability of coronary artery disease in a middle-aged man with a history of atypical angina pectoris? His exercise stress electrocardiogram showed 2.0 mm ST segment depression.

Step 1: Determine the likelihood ratio for the patient's stress test result. From Table 4.1, we know that 2.0 mm ST segment depression has a likelihood ratio of 10.8.

Step 2: Calculate the pre-test odds of coronary artery disease. From Table 3.1 in Chapter 3, we know that a male with a history of atypical angina pectoris has a pre-test probability of 0.70. To convert this probability to odds, we do the following:

$$\text{odds of event} = \frac{p}{1-p} = \frac{0.7}{1-0.7} = \frac{0.7}{0.3} = 2.3 : 1$$

Step 3: Use the odds ratio form of Bayes' theorem to calculate the post-test odds:

$$\boxed{\text{post-test odds} = \text{pre-test odds} \times \text{likelihood ratio}}$$

$$\text{post-test odds} = \frac{0.7}{0.3} \times 10.8 = 25.2 : 1$$

In this case, the very positive stress test result has increased the probability of coronary artery disease to a virtual certainty.

In the second example of using the odds ratio form of Bayes theorem, the test result is a dichotomous variable: a lung mass is either present (a positive test) or it is not (a negative test). In this example, the mass is present.

Example 2: How should a radiologist interpret a lung mass on a chest radiograph taken in a man whose pre-test probability of lung cancer is 0.4?

Step 1: The first step in answering this question is to calculate the likelihood ratio for the radiographic finding of a lung mass:

$$\text{LR+} = \frac{P[\text{finding present in \textbf{diseased} persons}]}{P[\text{finding present in \textbf{non-diseased} persons}]}$$

The probability that a lung mass is present in persons with lung cancer is 0.6, which is the **sensitivity** of the chest radiograph for lung cancer. The probability that a lung mass is present in persons who do not have lung cancer is 0.04, which is **1 − the specificity** of the chest x-ray.

According to Equation 4.12, *when a finding is present*, the likelihood ratio is

$$\text{LR+} = \frac{\text{sensitivity}}{1 - \text{specificity}}$$

The likelihood ratio for cancer when a lung mass is present on chest x-ray is

$$LR+ = \frac{0.60}{0.04} = 15.0$$

Step 2: For the post-test odds convert the pre-test probability to the pre-test odds:

$$\text{odds of event} = \frac{p}{1-p} = \frac{0.4}{1-0.4} = \frac{0.4}{0.6} = 0.67 : 1$$

Step 3: Use the odds ratio form of Bayes' theorem to calculate the post-test odds:

> post-test odds = pre-test odds × likelihood ratio

$$\text{post-test odds} = \frac{0.4}{0.6} \times 15.0 = 10 : 1$$

Thus, the post-test odds are higher than the pre-test odds when the chest x-ray shows a mass. The expression "post-test odds = 10:1" is read, "with this chest radiographic finding, for every 10 persons who have cancer, 1 person will not have cancer."

Thinking in terms of odds of events and likelihood ratios for tests simplifies computation. The odds of an event may be converted back to the probability of the event, if desired:

$$\text{probability} = \frac{\text{odds}}{1+\text{odds}} = \frac{10:1}{1+10:1}$$

$$\text{probability} = \frac{10}{11} = 0.91$$

In the third example of using the odds ratio form of Bayes' theorem, the test result is a dichotomous variable: either a lung mass is present (a positive test) or it is absent (a negative test). In this example, the mass is absent despite a high pre-test probability.

Example 3: How should a radiologist interpret a normal chest radiograph taken because of concern about lung cancer? The patient had a pre-test probability of lung cancer equal to 0.4.

Step 1: The first step in answering this question is to calculate the likelihood ratio for the lung cancer when the chest radiograph does not show a lung mass:

$$LR- = \frac{P[\text{finding absent in \textbf{diseased} persons}]}{P[\text{finding absent in \textbf{non-diseased} persons}]}$$

The probability that the chest radiograph shows a lung mass in persons with lung cancer is 0.6 (the sensitivity of the chest radiograph), which means that the probability that a lung mass is absent is 0.40 (1 − **sensitivity**), (Explanation: since a lung mass is either present or absent, the sum of the two probabilities must add to 1.0.)

The probability that a lung mass is absent in persons who do not have lung cancer (0.96) is by definition the **specificity** of the chest x-ray.

From Equation 4.13, *when a finding is absent*, the likelihood ratio is

$$LR- = \frac{1 - \text{sensitivity}}{\text{specificity}}$$

The likelihood ratio when a lung mass is absent on a chest x-ray is

$$LR- = \frac{0.40}{0.96} = 0.42$$

Step 2: For the post-test odds convert the pre-test probability to the pre-test odds, as in the second example:

$$\text{odds of event} = \frac{p}{1-p} = \frac{0.4}{1-0.4} = \frac{0.4}{0.6} = 0.67 : 1$$

Step 3: Use the odds ratio form of Bayes' theorem to calculate the post-test odds:

$$\boxed{\text{post-test odds} = \text{pre-test odds} \times \text{likelihood ratio}}$$

$$\text{post-test odds} = \left(\frac{0.4}{0.6}\right) \times 0.42 = 0.28 : 1 = 1 : 3.5$$

Thus, the post-test odds are lower than the pre-test odds when the chest x-ray does not show a mass. The expression "1:3.5" is read, "in this patient with this normal chest radiograph, for every 1 person who has cancer, 3.5 people with the same pre-test level of concern about lung cancer will not have the disease."

Note that the post-test probability of lung cancer is quite high – surprisingly high perhaps – despite the normal chest radiograph. We will return to this point later in the chapter.

While using odds of events and using likelihood ratios for tests simplifies computation, many people find probability an easier language to express uncertainty. We can convert the odds of an event back to the probability of the event:

$$\text{probability} = \frac{\text{odds}}{1 + \text{odds}} = \frac{0.28 : 1}{1 + 0.28 : 1} = 0.22$$

4.5   Lessons to be learned from Bayes' theorem

4.5.1   Insights about interpreting diagnostic tests

Clinicians can learn about interpreting diagnostic tests by applying Bayes' theorem to various clinical situations. Some of these lessons emerge from studying a graph of the post-test probability for all possible pre-test probabilities (Figure 4.4).

The relationship depicted in Figure 4.4 highlights one of the two most important ideas in this book: the post-test probability depends on the pre-test probability. Evidently, test interpretation depends on the pre-test probability of disease.

More generally, we may say:

The interpretation of new information depends on what we already knew about the patient.

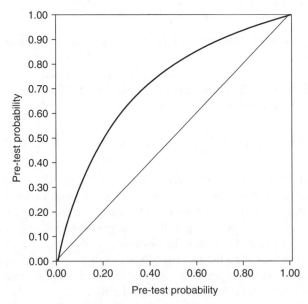

Figure 4.4 Post-test probability corresponding to a positive test result, calculated for all possible pre-test probabilities. Test sensitivity set at 0.8. Specificity set at 0.8.

If you understand the implications of this statement, you will respond as follows to a typical clinical situation:

Colleague: The radiologist says that Mr. Smith's liver scan shows metastatic disease.

You: What was the probability of metastases before we got the scan?

Colleague: I don't know exactly. I guess we didn't think he had metastases.

You: Well, I wouldn't take the positive scan too seriously if the pre-test probability was low. The post-test probability is still quite low. Let's review the findings with the radiologist and decide how to confirm the findings on the scan. Also, let's talk some more with the patient. Maybe we underestimated the pre-test probability of cancer.

Figure 4.4 shows that the effect of a test on disease probability depends on the pre-test probability. When the pre-test probability equals the post-test probability, the point falls on the 45 degree diagonal line. Thus, the 45 degree line represents a hypothetical test result that does not change the probability of disease at all. The farther the curved line lies above the 45 degree line, the greater is the effect of the test result on the probability of disease. At low pre-test probabilities, the post-test probability is much higher than the pre-test probability. As the pre-test probability approaches 1.0, the post-test probability is only slightly higher than the pre-test probability.

Why would we want to do a test on a patient with a very high pre-test probability? The gain in diagnostic certainty after a positive test would be small when the pre-test probability is so high. Surely, a *positive* test result would not change the next steps in managing the patient. On the other hand, a *negative* test result might reduce the probability of disease enough to change our management. *The possibility of a negative test result* is the reason for considering testing even when the pre-test probability is very high.

In fact, the probability can decline steeply after a negative test, as shown in Figure 4.5. The figure shows that the post-test probability for a test result that reduces the probability of disease (a "negative" result) is also affected by the pre-test probability. As the pre-test probability decreases, the probability of disease is affected less and less by a negative result, so that when the pre-test probability is quite low, the post-test probability changes very little after a negative result.

These observations lead to a generalization:

When the clinician is nearly certain prior to a test (i.e., the pre-test probability is close to 0 or to 1.0), a test result that confirms prior suspicions has little effect on the probability of disease.

We may therefore question whether much can be gained by doing a test in order to confirm one's expectations. **Confirmation** of one's expectations has

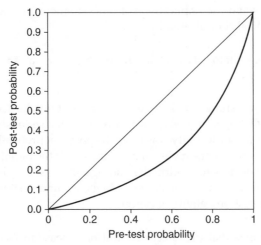

Figure 4.5 Post-test probability for a negative test result. Test sensitivity set at 0.8. Specificity set at 0.8.

little effect on the probability of disease. **Disconfirmation** of strong clinical suspicions can be quite useful, however. An unexpected negative test result (one occurring in a person with a high pre-test probability of disease) may reduce the probability of disease considerably, perhaps enough to reverse a decision about starting treatment. An unexpected positive result can have a similar effect if the clinician was on the verge of deciding against a diagnostic hypothesis. Does this observation mean that we should be ordering tests routinely when the pre-test probability is very low or very high? The answer is no, in part because the probability of a surprising test result is very low when the pre-test probability is at the extreme ends of the probability scale. This topic is the subject of Chapter 9.

4.5.2 The clinical significance of test specificity

The test with the highest sensitivity and specificity is always preferred if other factors, such as the harms of testing and cost, are equivalent. However, a highly sensitive and specific test is often more expensive. The clinician should ask, "Is the added benefit of a highly specific or sensitive test worth the extra cost?" One way to answer this question is to ask if the "better" test leads to a clinically significant difference in the post-test probability of disease. Chapter 9 presents an alternative approach to answering the same question.

The significance of the specificity of a test may be appreciated by calculating the post-test probability corresponding to a highly specific test and comparing it to the post-test probability after a relatively non-specific test (Figure 4.6).

Figure 4.6 has several lessons to impart:
* *The specificity of a test strongly affects the interpretation of a **positive** result.* As the specificity increases, so does the post-test probability of disease. When the pre-test probability is very low, only a test result with a very low specificity will raise the probability of disease to 0.90 or greater.

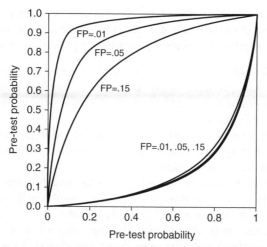

Figure 4.6 Effect of the specificity of a test on post-test probability of disease. The sensitivity of the test was set at 0.90. The post-test probability was calculated when the specificity was 0.99, 0.95, and 0.85 (in the figure, labeled FP = .01, FP = .05, and FP = .15 respectively). Curves that are concave upward denote a negative test result. Curves that are concave downward denote a positive test result.

> **Example**: Non-invasive tests for coronary artery disease are ineffective in patients with a low pre-test probability because their specificities range from 0.80 to 0.95. In these patients, the highly specific coronary arteriogram is required to make a secure diagnosis.

- *When the pre-test probability of disease is low, a positive test result is usually not diagnostic.*
- *When the pre-test probability is very high, the specificity of a test is not important.* When the pre-test probability of disease is high (0.70 or greater), the post-test probability of disease is high across the range of specificities shown in the figure. Thus, a test with a very high specificity has little advantage when the clinician strongly suspects a disease.

> **Example**: In patients with typical angina, the pre-test probability of coronary artery disease is 0.90 or more. The post-test probability after a more expensive myocardial scan is 0.99, only slightly higher than after the less expensive exercise electrocardiogram (0.98).

- *Most screening tests have a low yield of disease.* Screening tests are performed on patients who have no symptoms or findings of disease. Typically, the pre-test probability of disease is very low (often 1 or 2 patients per 1000 tested). Figure 4.7 shows that the post-test probability of disease is usually quite low. When the cost of screening includes evaluating patients who prove to have false-positive results, routine use of screening tests may be very costly. Also, the probability of a positive screening test is typically low because of the low pre-test probability.

Example: Routine use of the erythrocyte sedimentation rate in patients with a normal history and physical examination will lead to an unsuspected diagnosis in fewer than 6 patients in 10 000.

- *The specificity of a test has little or no effect on the interpretation of a negative test result.* Interpreting a negative test result may be possible even if the specificity of the test is not known precisely, as seen in the lower family of curves in Figure 4.6.

The importance of specificity can be understood intuitively by realizing that all non-diseased patients are candidates for false-positive results. This fact has two implications:
- When the pre-test probability is *low*, non-diseased patients far outnumber diseased patients. Therefore, false-positive results will outnumber true-positive results unless the test is highly specific.
- If the pre-test probability is *high*, diseased patients who are candidates for true-positive results far outnumber non-diseased patients who are candidates for false-positive results. Consequently, true-positive results will outnumber false-positive results, and the specificity of a test is not very important.

4.5.3 The clinical significance of test sensitivity

The significance of test sensitivity may be appreciated by comparing the post-test probability after a positive result with a test with very high sensitivity to the post-test probability after tests with a lower sensitivity (Figure 4.7).

Figure 4.7 illustrates several concepts:
- *The sensitivity of a test strongly affects the probability after a **negative** test result.* The higher the sensitivity of a test, the lower is the post-test

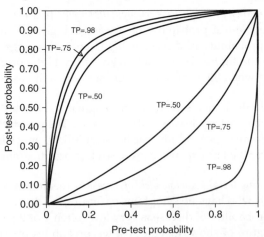

Figure 4.7 Effect of the sensitivity of a test on post-test probability of disease. The specificity of the test was set at 0.95. The post-test probability was calculated when the sensitivity of a test was set at 0.98, 0.75, and 0.50. Here, TP denotes sensitivity. Curves that are concave upward denote a negative test result. Curves that are concave downward denote a positive test result.

probability of disease. This relationship is strongest when the pre-test probability of disease is high.

> **Example**: Non-invasive imaging tests for coronary artery disease typically have a sensitivity of 0.70 to 0.80. For patients with exertional angina pectoris, the probability of coronary artery disease after a negative imaging test is far too high to exclude coronary artery disease.

- *When the pre-test probability of a diagnosis is high, the post-test probability after a negative test result is usually too high to discard the diagnosis.* When the pre-test probability is high (greater than 0.80), a clinician may order a test in the hope that a negative result will show that the disease is not present. This rationale is usually wrong, since a negative result on a highly sensitive test does not reduce the probability of disease below 0.10. This generalization does not apply to a perfectly sensitive test (no false-negative results), but few such tests exist, and they are generally expensive and often risky.

> **Example**: In patients with proven lung cancer, the sensitivity of computerized tomography of the chest is 0.88 for detecting metastases to the mediastinum. If suspicion of metastases is high (pre-test probability = 0.90), the post-test probability of metastases if the scan is negative is 0.70, and an invasive test would be required to rule out metastases prior to performing potentially curative surgery. Since a positive test would not affect a very high pre-test probability, doing a scan would not avoid an invasive test. However, the test could still be helpful in identifying enlarged nodes to biopsy.

- *When the pre-test probability of disease is low, the sensitivity of a test is relatively unimportant.* When the prior probability of disease is low (0.20 to 0.10), using a test to rule out disease is often possible, depending on what probability you think is low enough to "rule out" a disease (Chapter 9 addresses this topic). The need for a highly sensitive test depends on the clinician's requirements. The clinician who needs the strong reassurance of a very low post-test probability usually has to spend more to get it.

> **Example**: In searching for mediastinal metastases from primary lung cancer, the sensitivity of computed tomography (CT) of the chest is lower (0.61) than PET scan (0.85). However, in patients whose pre-test probability of metastases is low (0.10), the post-test probability after a negative test is 0.055 for the CT scan and 0.02 for the PET scan. The clinician would have to weigh the importance of a slightly lower probability of mediastinal metastases (0.02 vs. 0.05) against the much greater cost of a PET scan. Would the next step in management differ because of that small difference in post-test probability?

- *The probability after a positive test is not affected by the sensitivity of the test.* As seen by comparing the upper family of curves in Figure 4.7, the sensitivity of a test has relatively little effect on the post-test probability corresponding to a positive test result. If the clinician's goal is to raise the probability of disease, a less expensive, less sensitive test will do as well as a more expensive, more sensitive one.

4.6 The assumptions of Bayes' theorem

Bayes' theorem requires us to make several assumptions. To understand them, we shall express Bayes' theorem in conditional probability notation:

$$P[D|R] = \frac{P[D] \times P[R|D]}{(P[D] \times P[R|D] + P[\text{no } D] \times P[R|\text{no } D])} \tag{4.5}$$

where R = test result, D = disease present, no D = disease absent.

Assumption no. 1: *The conditional probability of a test result is independent of the prior probability of disease*
We assume that this relationship is true whenever we substitute the same sensitivity and specificity into Bayes' theorem regardless of the prior probability of disease. The following example shows that this assumption may sometimes be incorrect. Imagine a radionuclide scan of the liver that detects metastases from colon cancer. This scan detects all metastases that are larger than 2 cm. Now consider two patients with recently discovered colon cancer. Unbeknownst to their clinicians, both patients have metastases to the liver.
- One has lost weight. His liver is considerably enlarged and has a stony hard consistency. This patient's prior probability of metastases is high. If a pathologist could examine this patient's liver, most of the metastases would be larger than 2 cm, easily detectable by the liver scan. If the liver scan were evaluated in patients like this one, its sensitivity would be close to 1.0.
- The other patient feels and looks well, and his liver is not enlarged. The patient's prior probability of liver metastases is low. If a pathologist could examine this patient's liver, the metastases would probably be smaller than 2 cm, and would not be detected by the liver scan. If the liver scan were evaluated in patients like this one, its sensitivity would be quite low.

In this hypothetical example, the sensitivity of the test depends on the prior probability of disease, in violation of the assumption that the sensitivity and specificity are both constant. Few examples of this phenomenon exist, principally because few researchers stratify their measurement of diagnostic test performance in a way that would detect it (principally because investigators seldom measure the pre-test probability of the target disease when they measure sensitivity and specificity). A study of the exercise electrocardiogram

Table 4.3

	Type of chest pain	No. of patients	P[CAD]	Sensitivity	Specificity
Men	Typical angina	487	0.88	0.84	0.71
	Atypical angina	443	0.67	0.72	0.80
	Non-anginal pain	203	0.22	0.46	0.79
Women					
	Typical angina	67	0.58	0.57	0.57
	Atypical angina	153	0.35	0.69	0.69
	Non-anginal pain	175	0.05	0.81	0.81

Data from Weiner *et al*. (1979).

showed that the sensitivity of this test in men increased as the prior probability of coronary artery disease increased (Table 4.3). The authors did classify each patient by the type of chest pain syndrome. As shown in Table 4.3, the pre-test probability of coronary artery disease varied according to the type of chest pain syndrome. This study enrolled hundreds of men, which meant that the authors could reliably measure the sensitivity in subgroups of patients with a different pre-test probability. The number of women was smaller, and the differences in test performance are less likely to be statistically significant (Table 4.3).

Assumption no. 2: *The conditional probability of a test result is independent of prior test results*
To understand this assumption, imagine that two tests have been done in sequence (first $R1$ and then $R2$) and calculate the probability of disease after the second test:

$$P[D|R1, R2] = \frac{P[D] \times P[R2|D, R1]}{(P[D] \times P[R2|D, R1] + P[\text{no } D] \times P[R2|\text{no } D, R1])}$$

where $R1$ = result of test 1, $R2$ = result of test 2, D = disease present, no D = disease absent, and

$P[D|R1, R2]$ = probability of disease given the results of test 1 *and* test 2

$P[R2|D, R1]$ = probability of result on test 2 conditional upon the patient

being diseased *and* the result on test 1.

As discussed in the next section, few investigators have studied several diagnostic tests done always in the same sequence. Diseased patients would be divided into those with a normal result on the first test and those with an abnormal result. Then see if the sensitivity of the second test depends on the results of the first test, the frequency of a result on the second test should be measured in both of these groups of patients with the target disease. Since this information is seldom available, *clinicians must assume that the frequency of a result on the second test in diseased patients is the same regardless of the results of the first test.* This assumption is the same as saying that

$$P[R2|D, R1] = P[R2|D]$$

which is often called *the assumption of conditional independence.*

When measuring the post-test probability after a sequence of tests, one must also assume conditional independence for test specificity. We illustrate the principle of conditional independence in an extended example in the next section.

4.7 Using Bayes' theorem to interpret a sequence of tests

Diagnostic tests are often used in sequence. An abnormal finding on one test may raise concerns that can only be resolved by a second test. For example, when a test is performed in an asymptomatic person, an abnormal finding may raise concerns, and a second test seems necessary. What method should be used to interpret the results of the second test? The reader who has absorbed the lessons of this chapter will answer as follows:

> Use the *post-test* probability following the **first** test as the *pre-test* probability for the **second** test. Then, use the sensitivity and specificity of the second test and Bayes' theorem to calculate the post-test probability for the second test.

We illustrate this concept for an exercise electrocardiogram (hereafter exercise ECG) that has been done in an asymptomatic 45-year-old man who is about to begin an exercise training program (Figure 4.8). The pre-test probability of coronary artery disease is 0.06 in asymptomatic men in the fifth decade of life. The sensitivity of the exercise ECG is 0.58 and its specificity is 0.88. The probability of coronary artery disease if the exercise test provokes ≥1 mm ST segment depression is 0.24, as calculated with Bayes' theorem. Thus, following an unexpected abnormal stress test, the odds are 1 in 3 that the patient

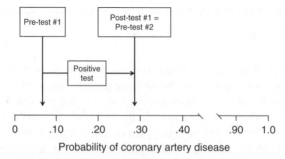

Figure 4.8 Interpreting a sequence of tests for coronary artery disease.

has significant coronary artery disease. The clinician has three alternatives: ignore the finding, do a non-invasive diagnostic test, or perform coronary arteriography. Many clinicians would take the middle course and perform an exercise radionuclide scan of the myocardium or a stress echocardiogram.

Before using Bayes' theorem to calculate the post-test probability of coronary artery disease, the clinician must answer two questions:

1. What should I use for the pre-test probability of coronary artery disease?

   This question is easily answered. The probability of coronary artery disease after the positive exercise ECG *is* the probability of disease prior to a second test.

2. What is the sensitivity and specificity of the exercise radionuclide scan of the myocardium?

   This question seems even more straightforward than the first. The apparently correct answer is the sensitivity and specificity of the exercise radionuclide scan in a large study of patients who had the scan and a definitive test, such as a coronary arteriogram. In reality, the answer is more complicated because the ideal study population should be similar to the patient who had the abnormal exercise ECG. Therefore, all study patients should have an exercise ECG followed by an exercise radionuclide myocardial scan and then a definitive test for coronary artery disease. With this study design, it is possible to calculate the sensitivity and specificity of the exercise radionuclide myocardial scan in two groups of patients, those with a positive exercise ECG and those with a negative exercise ECG.

A large series of patients in whom the sensitivity and specificity of the radionuclide scan following an exercise ECG are measured will have two subgroups:
- those in whom the exercise ECG is *abnormal*;
- those in whom the exercise ECG is normal.

If the sensitivity and specificity of the scan are exactly the same in these two subgroups, the scan is said to be *conditionally independent* of the exercise ECG.

Definition of conditional independence: Two tests are conditionally independent if the sensitivity and specificity of one test do not depend upon the result of the other test.

When the sensitivity and specificity of the scan in the entire population are applied to those with a positive exercise ECG, the clinician is *assuming* that the scan and the exercise ECG are conditionally independent.

When Bayes' theorem is used to interpret a sequence of tests, most people assume that the sensitivity and specificity of each test are conditionally independent of the results of the other tests. Opportunities to test the conditional independence assumption occur infrequently because most studies

Table 4.4

	Number of patients					
	$E+T+$	$E-T+$	$E+T-$	$E-T-$	$E?T+$	$E?T-$
CAD present	110	19	21	8	54	14
CAD absent	3	3	16	77	6	58

CAD = coronary artery disease; E+ = positive exercise ECG; E− = negative exercise ECG; T+ = positive radionuclide scan; T− = negative radionuclide scan; E? = equivocal exercise ECG.
Reprinted from Sox HC, Exercise testing in suspected coronary artery disease. Disease-a-Month, 1985; 31 (12): 1−70 (December 1985) with permission from Elsevier.

of test performance have studied one test rather than several. Luckily, several studies have performed an exercise ECG and a radionuclide scan prior to coronary arteriography. The findings of three studies are summarized in Table 4.4.

If the two tests are conditionally independent, the sensitivity and specificity of the scan should be the same in patients with an abnormal exercise ECG as in patients with a normal exercise ECG. We will test this assumption using the data from these three studies (Table 4.5). A pair of asterisks (*) denotes two values that are statistically significantly different from one another ($p < 0.05$).

The specificity of the scan is significantly higher when the exercise ECG is normal than when it is abnormal. Therefore, the assumption of conditional independence does not hold for these two tests.

Likewise, the sensitivity and specificity of the exercise ECG in patients with a normal scan may be compared to the sensitivity and specificity of the exercise ECG in patients with an abnormal scan (Table 4.6). The

Table 4.5

Results of exercise ECG	Sensitivity of radionuclide scan	Specificity of radionuclide scan
Abnormal	0.84	0.84*
Normal	0.70	0.96*
Equivocal	0.79	0.91

Table 4.6

Results of radionuclide scan	Sensitivity of exercise ECG	Specificity of exercise ECG
Abnormal	0.85	0.50*
Normal	0.72	0.83*

Table 4.7

Pre-test probability of CAD after positive exercise ECG	Probability of CAD if scan and exercise ECG are both positive	
	Conditional independence assumed*	Conditional independence not assumed**
0.25	0.76	0.64
0.50	0.90	0.84
0.75	0.97	0.94

*To calculate the post-test probability after the second test in the sequence, $P[T_2+|D]$ and $P[T_2+|$no $D]$ were substituted in Bayes' theorem.
**To calculate the post-test probability after the second test in the sequence, $P[T_2+|T_1+,D]$ and $P[T_2+|T_1+,$no $D]$ were substituted in Bayes' theorem (Table 4.4).

specificity differs according to the results of the scan, while the sensitivity does not differ.

Thus, although the sensitivity of each test is independent of the results of the other test, the specificity of each test is dependent on the results of the other test. The effect of incorrectly assuming conditional independence of the two tests is shown by calculating the post-test probability of coronary artery disease (CAD) (Table 4.7).

The consequences of assuming that the scan and the exercise ECG are conditionally independent depend on the prior probability of CAD, as would be expected from inspecting Figure 4.7. The probability of CAD if both scan and exercise ECG are positive is consistently lower with conditional independence not assumed (i.e., when the test performance of the second test was measured separately in patients with positive results and patients with negative results on the first test, rather than assuming that the performance of the second test does not depend on the results of the first test).

Tests are often used in sequence, and it is important to be able to interpret the results. Using the post-test probability of disease from the first test as the prior probability of disease for the second test is reasonable. However, failing to take account of the results of the first test in measuring the performance of the second test may lead to error because the appropriate population for measuring the performance of the second test depends on the results of the first test. As the number of tests in a sequence increases, errors due to assuming conditional independence of test performance increase simply because more tests in a sequence mean more opportunities for error.

Before succumbing to despair over the potential for errors of this kind, the reader should remember two facts. First, for a wide range of pre-test probabilities, Bayes' theorem tells us that the post-test probability is largely independent of errors in measuring test performance (see Figures 4.6 and 4.7). Second, the post-test decisions depend on the post-test probability of disease relative to a treatment-threshold probability. If the post-test probability is close to the treatment-threshold probability, accuracy is important, because a small error could move the post-test probability to the other side of the treatment threshold. It is less important if the post-test probability is far above or below the threshold, since a much larger error would be required to change the post-test probability enough to move it past the treatment threshold and alter the decision about how to manage the patient.

4.8 Using Bayes' theorem when many diseases are under consideration

This section contains advanced material and can be skipped without loss of continuity.
Heretofore, we have learned how to calculate the conditional probability of a disease vs. all other possible diseases (expressed as "no disease"). In doing so, we express the probability of other diseases only as $(1 - P[A])$, where A is the target condition. In effect, we are saying that the contribution of other diseases to the denominator of Bayes' theorem is a constant that reflects the frequency distribution of other diseases in the differential diagnosis in the entire population of patients with the suspected condition A.

Assuming that disease rates in a study population apply to a specific patient can lead to error. If, in addition to the suspected target condition, a specific patient has another condition that causes the test to be positive, the frequency of positive results on the test might be much higher than in the study population. Accordingly, we might overestimate the post-test probability of the target condition after a positive test.

If we have information about the probability of other individual diseases, we should use it. In this section, we derive Bayes' theorem in its most general form, one which can show the contribution of every "other disease" to the denominator of Bayes' theorem individually (rather than lumping all of them under the term "no disease").

Suppose a clinician is considering three diseases (A, B, and C) as the possible cause of a patient's symptoms. The clinician's goal is to calculate the probability of disease A given the presence of a clinical finding.

In this instance, we know the prevalence of diseases A, B, and C, and we also know the frequency of findings x, y, and z in these diseases (e.g., $P[x|A]$). Instead of representing two of the diseases (e.g., B and C) as "no disease," we can list them separately and gain additional precision in estimating the conditional probability that disease A is present.

The prior probabilities of these diseases are $P[A]$, $P[B]$, and $P[C]$, where $P[A] + P[B] + P[C] = 1$. The clinician makes three observations (x, y, and z). The relationships between these observations and the three diseases are given in Table 4.8 by the conditional probabilities.

Table 4.8

Disease	Probability of observation given disease A, B, or C		
	x	y	z
A	$P[x|A]$	$P[y|A]$	$P[z|A]$
B	$P[x|B]$	$P[y|B]$	$P[z|B]$
C	$P[x|C]$	$P[y|C]$	$P[z|C]$

The probability that one of these findings occurs in a patient with one of these diseases (e.g., $P[x$ and $A]$) arises from the definition of conditional probability:

$$P[x|A] = \frac{P[x \text{ and } A]}{P[A]}$$

$$P[x \text{ and } A] = P[A] \times P[x|A]$$

The probability of observation x occurring in all patients suspected of having diseases A, B, or C is the sum of the probability of its occurrence in each disease:

$$P[x] = P[A] \times P[x|A] + P[B] \times P[x|B] + P[C] \times P[x|C]$$

The probability of disease A given that observation x has occurred, $P[A|x]$, follows from the definition of conditional probability:

$$P[A|x] = \frac{P[x \text{ and } A]}{P[x]}$$

Substituting the expressions for $P[x$ and $A]$ and $P[x]$ into the expression for $P[A|x]$, we obtain Equation 4.14, which is what the clinician is interested in:

$$P[A|x] = \frac{P[A] \times P[x|A]}{P[A] \times P[x|A] + P[B] \times P[x|B] + P[C] \times P[x|C]} \qquad (4.14)$$

From this three-disease case, it is a small step to express Bayes' theorem in its most general form, with n diseases. In Equation 4.13, j refers to a clinical finding, and the subscript i refers to a disease:

$$P[D_1|j] = \frac{P[D_1] \times P[j|D_1]}{\sum_{i=1}^{n} (P[D_i] \times P[j|D_i])} \qquad (4.15)$$

Summary

1. The most compelling reason to use probability to express uncertainty is to gain access to Bayes' theorem, thereby to calculate post-test probability.
2. Bayes' theorem takes two equivalent but not identical forms:
   - The algebraic form of Bayes' theorem is especially useful when several diseases are being considered, but it does require a calculator.
   - With the odds ratio form of Bayes' theorem, calculating the post-test odds requires multiplying two numbers. Moreover, a test's likelihood ratio is easy to remember.
3. Perhaps the most important idea in this book is the following: *the interpretation of a test result depends on the pre-test probability of disease.*
4. Bayes' theorem provides other insights about interpreting test results and deciding when a test is likely to be useful:
   - Rare is the test that will *rule out* disease when the pre-test probability is quite high.
   - Still rarer is the test that will *rule in* disease when the pre-test probability is quite low.
   - If you screen for occult disease, take particular care to avoid tests that have a low specificity.

Problems

1. If the pre-test probability of disease is 0.1, the true-positive rate for the test is 0.8, and the specificity for the test is 0.15, what is the probability that the patient does not have disease, once you learn that the test is positive?
2. If the following statements are true, is the probability of symptom A independent of the probability of symptom B?

    The probability of symptom A alone is 0.2, the probability of symptom B alone is 0.5, and the probability that both symptoms occur together is 0.1.

3. Can the probability that symptoms A and B are both present be greater than the probability that symptom A is present in a patient in whom it is known that symptom B is present?
4. Suppose that the probability that neither disease A nor disease B is present is 0.1, the probability that only disease A is present is 0.3, and the probability

that only disease B is present is 0.2. Do you have enough information to determine the probability that both diseases will be present?

5. Suppose that, based on your findings during the initial evaluation of a patient, you believe the probability of disease is 0.25. You would be willing to start a specific treatment if the probability of disease is greater than 0.5. What is the minimum likelihood ratio for a test result that will change your treatment of this patient?

6. Suppose that you have installed a pacemaker in a patient. It will be necessary to replace the battery in 10 years; however, experience has taught you that the probability of failure in some other component in the device during a one-year period is 0.05. That is, if the pacemaker is functioning at a point in time, the probability that it will still be functioning one year later is 0.95. Assume that this annual failure probability stays constant throughout the life of the device. What is the probability that this pacemaker will fail before the battery needs to be replaced?

Bibliography

Diamond, G.A. and Forrester, J.S. (1979) Analysis of probability as an aid in the clinical diagnosis of coronary-artery disease. *New England Journal of Medicine*, **300**, 1350–8.

Fagan, T.J. (1975) Nomogram for Bayes' formula. *New England Journal of Medicine*, **293**, 257.

Gorry, G.A. and Barnett, G.O. (1968) Sequential diagnosis by computer. *Journal of the American Medical Association*, **205**, 849–54.

A description of the sequential use of Bayes' theorem to interpret several clinical findings.

Gorry, G.A., Pauker, S.G., and Schwartz, W.B. (1978) The diagnostic importance of the normal finding. *New England Journal of Medicine*, 1978; **298**: 486–9.

A clear discussion of how a negative test result can be evidence against one disease and evidence for another.

Raiffa, H. (1968) *Decision Analysis: Introductory Lectures on Choices Under Uncertainty*, Addison-Wesley, Reading, MA.

Chapter 2 of this classic book contains a derivation of Bayes' theorem.

Rifkin, R.O. and Hood, W.B. (1977) Bayesian analysis of electrocardiographic stress testing. *New England Journal of Medicine*, **297**, 681–6.

Probabilistic reasoning in test selection has become particularly well accepted in cardiologic practice. This article was very influential.

Simel, D.L. and Rennie, D. (2008) *The Rational Clinical Examination: Evidence-based Clinical Diagnosis*, McGraw-Hill Medical, New York.

A book with good information about test performance.

Sox, H.C. (1985) Exercise testing in suspected coronary artery disease. *Disease-a-Month*, **31**(12), 1–70.

Weiner, D.A., Ryan, T.J., McCabe, C.H. *et al.* (1979) Exercise stress testing: correlation among history of angina, ST-segment response and prevalence of coronary artery disease in the Coronary Artery Surgery Study (CASS). *New England Journal of Medicine*, **301**, 230–5.

This study illustrates how measuring the true-positive rate and false-positive rate in subgroups of patients can yield new insights. This study showed that the test performance of the exercise ECG depends on the patient's history.

CHAPTER 5

Measuring the accuracy of diagnostic information

Introduction

Clinicians rely upon information to make decisions. When taking a history, they interpret the answer to a question as evidence for or against a diagnostic hypothesis. As we learned in the preceding chapters, diagnostic information is usually imperfect. Interpretive errors occur when:

- *the clinician assumes that a negative response means that the disease is absent.* A **false-negative** finding occurs when a patient has a disease but does not have the finding.
- *the clinician assumes that a positive response means that the disease is present.* A finding that is associated with a disease sometimes occurs in patients who do not have the disease: it is a **false-positive** result.

In Chapter 4, we learned that the interpretation of a clinical finding depends in part on its false-negative rate and false-positive rate. This chapter is about measuring the frequency of these misleading findings and evaluating published reports of diagnostic tests. There are eight parts in the chapter:

5.1 How to describe test results: abnormal and normal, positive and negative

This part of the chapter is about a language for describing test results. We first describe the distribution of test results in patients with the target condition and in those who do not have the target condition. Building on this knowledge, we then consider several ways to describe test results.

Most test results are expressed as continuous variables. For example, the serum concentration of troponin I and T (protein constituents of heart muscle

Medical Decision Making, Second Edition. Harold C. Sox, Michael C. Higgins and Douglas K. Owens.
© 2013 John Wiley & Sons, Ltd. Published 2013 by John Wiley & Sons, Ltd.

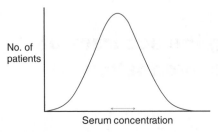

No. of patients

Serum concentration

Figure 5.1 Results of a hypothetical test in a healthy population.

cells) is a measure of cardiac muscle damage. The serum cardiac troponin can be any value from less than 0.01 ng/ml to greater than 100 ng/ml, depending on the amount of damaged muscle. In a patient with a suspected myocardial infarction, each point on this scale indicates something about the probability that the patient has had a myocardial infarction. To understand this claim, first consider the results of a test in a population of healthy individuals. Figure 5.1 shows the distribution of values around the central value.

Figure 5.1 shows a symmetric distribution of values. It closely resembles the **normal distribution curve**, which has many important statistical properties. The most important of these are the **mean** of the distribution, which is the unweighted average of all individuals' results, and the **standard deviation**, which is a measure of the degree of spread around the mean of the distribution. The normal curve has another important feature: the test results for 65% of the population fall within one standard deviation of the mean value. The test results for 95% of the population fall within two standard deviations of the mean (Figure 5.2).

Test results in a healthy population are often distributed normally (i.e., have a symmetric distribution that has the properties of the normal distribution curve). Figure 5.2 shows the mean of the distribution in normal people and the values for two standard deviations above and below the mean.

Definition of target condition: The disease that the clinician wants to diagnose.

We use "target condition" instead of "disease" because it is more specific to the clinician's purpose. A clinician uses a test to test a specific hypothesis: "does this patient have the target condition?"

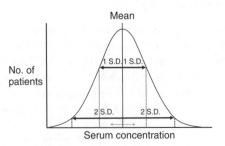

Mean

1 S.D. 1 S.D.

No. of patients

2 S.D.   2 S.D.

Serum concentration

Figure 5.2 The standard deviation of a normal distribution.

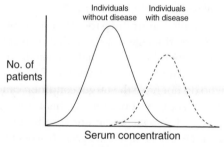

Figure 5.3 Distribution of test results in individuals with the target condition and individuals who do not have the target condition.

Principle: When describing the performance of a test (sensitivity, specificity, likelihood ratio), always specify the target condition.

The distribution of values in patients with the target condition often overlaps the values in individuals without the target condition (Figure 5.3). The interpretation of a test result depends on knowing the shape of the distribution curves in persons with and without the target condition and where the curves overlap. Very low values indicate no disease, and very high values indicate disease. Uncertainty is not a problem with extreme values. Uncertainty is a problem for values in the range where the two distribution curves overlap, because the patient could either have the target condition or not have it. Interpreting these intermediate values requires Bayes' theorem.

5.1.1   Defining a test result

- A test result as a dichotomous variable:
  - Below and above the upper limit of normal.
  - Normal vs. abnormal.
  - Positive vs. negative.
- A test result as a continuous variable.

A test result as a dichotomous variable
The language commonly used to describe test performance uses terms that place test results into two categories: above and below a threshold value for taking action. The most used terms are sensitivity, the frequency of a "positive" test in patients with the target condition, and specificity, the frequency of a "negative" test in someone who does not have the target condition. If the test result is expressed as a continuous variable (like serum troponin, a test for heart muscle damage), we will need a thoughtful way to decide on the cut-point test result that divides test results into "positive" and "negative."

Definition of cut-point: The test result that divides the spectrum of test results into a positive region and a negative region.

Using the upper limit of normal as the cut-point

Clinical laboratories usually report the patient's test result (e.g., 35 units/ml) and, as a guide to interpretation, the test result that corresponds to the "upper limit of normal." The "upper limit of normal" is usually all values up to two standard deviations above the mean. As shown in Figure 5.3, the distribution curve for persons who do not have the target condition can overlap the curve for patients with the target condition. Often, this means that patients with the target condition have test results that are within the "range of normal." Therefore, using the range of normal to interpret a test result can be misleading.

We should avoid using the "upper limit of normal" as a point of reference for defining a test result for several reasons:

- The label "upper limit of normal" encourages simplistic reasoning. Clinicians may assume that a value above the upper limit of normal means the disease is present and a value below it means that the disease is absent.
- The best cut-point value for dividing "positive" from "negative" results will depend on the clinical situation, not simply on the distribution of results in healthy people, as we shall see at the end of this chapter.

Using normal and abnormal as the cut-point

Clinicians often hear the following: "That chest radiograph is abnormal." Or, "this MRI scan is perfectly normal." Or, "that tuberculin skin test is abnormal." Here, the clinician has not categorized a test result in reference to a cut-point along a continuous scale of test result values. Instead, the point of reference seems to be the normal condition. Some specialists may define the abnormal condition according to strict criteria, but in practice most clinicians probably define it as "not normal." When the boundary that defines a test result that requires action is fluid, or at least vague and personalized, applying the methods described in this book is far more difficult. So, we will not use the terminology of normal and abnormal.

Using positive and negative as the cut-point

In practice, most of the ideas that define the discipline of medical decision making depend on expressing numerical results as a dichotomous variable. Perhaps this usage reflects the nature of decision making: it is the act of choosing one action and not another. The cut-point that defines action should reflect the characteristics of the decision problem. Toward the end of this chapter, we will show how aspects of the decision problem – the patient, the disease, and the treatment – play a role in defining the cut-point that is the threshold for taking action. We follow the conventions of the scientists who conceived the ideas in this book and define the two categories on either side of the cut-point as "positive" and "negative." The cut-point therefore divides the range of possible values into "positive" and "negative" regions.

As a practical matter, we define a "positive" test result as one that is at or above the cut-point. It increases the probability that the patient has the target condition. A "negative" result is below the cut-point, and it decreases the probability of the target condition.

A test result as a continuous variable

Dividing the range of values into a positive and negative region is important, but it has an important shortcoming. It disregards the information contained in the magnitude of the numerical result. In general, a larger value of the serum troponin means a greater probability that the patient has a myocardial infarction, and a very low value means a lower probability. A result that moves the probability of the target condition closer to 1.0 or 0 – one that reduces uncertainty to a minimum – is useful for many reasons. However, as we will see in later chapters, passing a threshold probability for taking action is a sufficient rationale for taking that action. Reducing uncertainty any further will not change management, so the resources required are not well spent.

Referring to Figure 5.4, within the range of test results that occur in both patients with the target condition and patients who do not have the target condition (the overlap region), a test result is consistent with either having the target condition or not having it. If the overlap region contains the cut-off value that defines a positive and negative test result, patients with the target condition can have a negative result (false-negative), and patients who do not have the target condition can have a positive result (false-positive) (Figure 5.4).

Thinking about the overlap region leads us to a fundamental, powerful principle:

For a particular test result, the frequency of false-positive results and false-negative results is both necessary and sufficient to describe how much the test result changes the probability of the target condition.

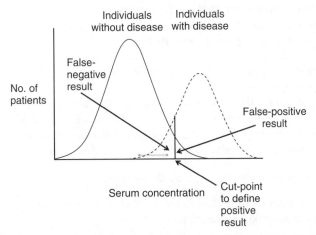

Figure 5.4 The distribution of results in patients with and without the target condition. The cut-point defines a positive (or negative) result and divides the overlap region in which results occur in patients with and without the target condition into false-negative results and false-positive results.

To convince yourself that this principle is true, imagine moving the vertical line that represents the cut-point to the right along the horizontal axis. The relative proportion of false-positive and false-negative results changes. So does the relative proportion of the patients who have a test result above the cut-point and also have the target condition, which determines the probability of the target condition in patients with a result above the cut-point. Section 5.2 of this chapter will describe exactly what this important principle means in practice.

In this part of the chapter, we have acquired a language for describing test results. It applies to any information that might affect our certainty about the patient's true state: history, physical examination, or diagnostic test result. We have adopted a language that categorizes test results into "positive" and "negative." This decision deprives us of some information but is in keeping with our focus on getting just the information we need to make a decision – no less and no more.

5.2   Measuring a test's capability to reveal the patient's true state

The key measure of any diagnostic information is its ability to discriminate between the target condition and all other conditions. What do we mean by "discriminate?" A test that perfectly discriminates between the target condition and all other conditions is positive in all patients with the target condition and negative in all patients who do not have it. Most tests fall far short of this ideal.

Definition of test performance: A test's ability to discriminate between patients with a disease and all other patients.

5.2.1   How to measure test performance
Bayes' theorem defines the measures of test performance. The odds ratio form of Bayes' theorem (Chapter 4) states that

$$\boxed{\text{post-test odds} = \text{pre-test odds} \times \text{likelihood ratio}}$$

This form of Bayes' theorem reminds us that *the function of diagnostic information is to change the probability of disease*. The likelihood ratio is the most meaningful measure of diagnostic information because it shows the effect of the information on the probability of disease. In other words:

To know the performance of a test, know its likelihood ratios.

Recall the definition of the likelihood ratio, as it emerges from the derivation of the odds ratio of Bayes' theorem:

$$\boxed{\text{likelihood ratio} = \frac{P[R|D]}{P[R|\text{no } D]}}$$

where $P[R|D]$ is the probability of a test result in patients with the target condition and $P[R|no\ D]$ is the probability of the result in people who do not have the target condition.

This line of argument leads us to the following method for measuring test performance:

1. To measure the performance of a test for a disease, first perform the test in patients who are known to have the target condition and in patients who are known to be free of the target condition (but might have other diseases).
2. Then, calculate the frequency of a result in patients with the target condition and in patients who do not have the target condition.

This simple prescription is hard to achieve in practice. Many studies of test performance have serious flaws. These flaws can lead to inaccurate test performance measurements that can lead in turn to incorrect interpretation of test results and mistakes in patient care.

We will first learn how to measure test performance. Then, we will learn how to evaluate articles about test performance and identify studies that we can rely upon.

Recall that the first step in measuring the performance of a test is to determine the frequency of a test result in patients with a target condition and in patients known to be free of the disease. Deciding if the patient has the disease requires doing another test, which is usually called the "gold standard" test (also "diagnostic reference standard"). We will return to the desired characteristics of a good gold standard test.

Definition of "gold standard" test: The procedure that defines the true state of the patient in a study of test performance (also known as "diagnostic reference standard").

Definition of index test: The test whose performance is being measured.

Definition of source population: The patients whose findings lead the doctor to order the index test. (also known as the "clinically relevant population.")

Definition of verified sample: Patients who receive the gold standard test to *verify* their disease status (ideally, identical to the source population but, too often, either a *sample*, or subset, of the source population or entirely unrelated to the source population).

In the ideal study of a test, each patient in a source population containing N patients undergoes both the index test and the gold standard procedure. If the test results are a dichotomous variable (positive or negative), a 2 by 2 table is a convenient way to display the results of the study. In Table 5.1 the name "2×2" refers to the array of the four lightly shaded cells that contain the primary test results, labeled TP, FP, FN, and TN.

Table 5.1

Results of the index test	Results of the gold standard test		Totals
	Positive	Negative	
Positive	True positive (TP)	False positive (FP)	TP + FP
Negative	False negative (FN)	True negative (TN)	FN + TN
Totals	TP + FN	FP + TN	$N = $ TP + FN + FP + TN

We may use the 2×2 table to define several important terms:

TP = number of **true-positive** results
  (index test positive and disease present)

FP = number of **false − positive** results
  (index test positive and disease absent)

FN = number of **false − negative** results
  (index test negative and disease present)

TN = number of **true − negative** results
  (index test negative and disease absent)

If the index test and the patient's true state were perfectly concordant, we would have that elusive animal, the perfect test, one with no false-positive results and no false-negative results. Most tests have misleading test results. Measures of concordance and discordance, such as the **true-positive rate** and **false-positive rate** of a test, are part of the basic vocabulary of medicine.

5.2.2   Measures of concordance between index test and disease state

Two types of test results reflect the true state of the patient: **true-positive** results and **true-negative results**. The relative frequency of these two types of results completely characterizes the performance of a test.

True-positive rate of a test

Definition of true-positive rate (TPR; also called "sensitivity"): The likelihood that a diseased patient has a positive test.

In conditional probability notation, the true-positive rate of a test result is

P[positive test result|disease] or $P[+|D]$

which means the "probability that an abnormal test result will occur if the patient has the target condition":

$$\text{true-positive rate} = \frac{\text{no. diseased patients with positive test}}{\text{no. diseased patients}}$$

To measure the true-positive rate of a test, perform the index test and the gold standard test in a source population. In terms of the 2×2 table, the true-positive rate (TPR) of a test is as given in Table 5.1 (In Tables 5.1 through 5.4, the numerator and denominator of the definitions of test performance are highlighted).

$$TPR = \frac{TP}{TP + FN}$$

True-negative rate of a test

Definition of true-negative rate (TNR): The likelihood that a patient that does not have the target condition has a negative test. Also called "specificity".

In conditional probability notation, the true-negative rate of a test result is

P[negative test result|no disease] or $P[-|$ no $D]$

which means the "probability that a negative test result will occur if the patient does not have the target condition":

$$\text{true-negative rate} = \frac{\text{no. non-diseased patients with negative test}}{\text{no. non-diseased patients}}$$

To measure the true-negative rate of a test, perform the index test and the gold standard test in a source population. In terms of the 2×2 table, the true-negative rate (TNR) of a test is given in Table 5.2.

Table 5.2

Results of the index test	Results of the gold standard test		Totals
	Positive	Negative	
Positive	True positive (TP)	False positive (FP)	TP + FP
Negative	False negative (FN)	True negative (TN)	FN + TN
Totals	TP + FN	FP + TN	N = TP + FN + FP + TN

$$TNR = \frac{TN}{FP + TN}$$

5.2.3 Measures of discordance between index test and disease state

The two types of test results that do not reflect the true state of the patient are **false-negative** results and **false-positive** results.

False-negative rate of a test

Definition of false-negative rate (FNR): The likelihood that a patient who does not have the target condition has a negative test.

In conditional probability notation, the true-positive rate of a test result is

P[negative test result|no disease] or $P[-|\text{ no } D]$

which means the "probability that a negative test result will occur if the patient has the target condition":

$$\text{false-negative rate} = \frac{\text{no. diseased patients with negative test}}{\text{no. diseased patients}}$$

To measure the false-negative rate of a test, perform the index test and the gold standard test in a source population. In terms of the 2×2 table, the false-negative rate (FNR) of a test is as given in Table 5.3.

Table 5.3

Results of the index test	Results of the gold standard test		Totals
	Positive	Negative	
Positive	True positive (TP)	False positive (FP)	TP + FP
Negative	False negative (FN)	True negative (TN)	FN + TN
Totals	TP + FN	FP + TN	N = TP + FN + FP + TN

$$\text{FNR} = \frac{\text{FN}}{\text{TP} + \text{FN}}$$

In diseased patients, a test result is either positive (a true-positive result) or negative (a false-negative result). Therefore, the false-negative rate is the complement of the true-positive rate:

$$\text{FNR} = 1 - \text{TPR}$$

False-positive rate of a test

Definition of false-positive rate (FPR): The likelihood that a patient that does not have the target condition has a positive test.

In conditional probability notation, the true-negative rate of a test result is

P[positive test result|no disease] or $P[+|\text{no } D]$

which means the "probability that a positive test result will occur if the patient does not have the target condition":

$$\text{false-positive rate} = \frac{\text{no. non-diseased patients with positive test}}{\text{no. non-diseased patients}}$$

To measure the false-positive rate of a test, perform the index test and the gold standard test in a source population. In terms of the 2×2 table, the false-positive rate (FPR) of a test is as given in Table 5.4.

Table 5.4

Results of the index test	Results of the gold standard test		Totals
	Positive	Negative	
Positive	True positive (TP)	False positive (FP)	TP + FP
Negative	False negative (FN)	True negative (TN)	FN + TN
Totals	TP + FN	FP + TN	$N =$ TP + FN + FP + TN

$$\text{FPR} = \frac{\text{FP}}{\text{FP} + \text{TN}}$$

In patients without the target condition, a test result is either positive (a false-positive result) or negative (a true-negative result). Therefore, the false-positive rate is the complement of the true-negative rate:

$$\text{FPR} = 1 - \text{TNR}$$

Predictive value

Predictive value is another way to describe the results of performing the index test and the gold standard test in terms of the 2×2 table. Unlike the measures of test performance, for which the columns of the 2×2 table contain the key measures, the calculation of predictive value uses the rows. Predictive value is, effectively, a *post-test probability*. The two types of predictive value are **positive predictive value** and **negative predictive value.**

Definition of positive predictive value (PV+): The fraction of patients with a positive test who also have the target condition. See Table 5.5.

Table 5.5

Results of the index test	Results of the gold standard test		Totals
	Positive	Negative	
Positive	True positive (TP)	False positive (FP)	TP + FP
Negative	False negative (FN)	True negative (TN)	FN + TN
Totals	TP + FN	FP + TN	$N =$ TP + FN + FP + TN

$$PV+ = \frac{\text{no. diseased patients with positive test}}{\text{no. patients with positive test}}$$

In terms of the 2 × 2 table in Table 5.6,

Table 5.6

Results of the index test	Results of the gold standard test		Totals
	Positive	Negative	
Positive	True positive (TP)	False positive (FP)	TP + FP
Negative	False negative (FN)	True negative (TN)	FN + TN
Totals	TP + FN	FP + TN	$N =$ TP + FN + FP + TN

$$PV+ = \frac{TP}{TP + FP}$$

Definition of negative predictive value (PV−): The fraction of patients with a negative test result who do not have disease.

$$PV- = \frac{\text{no. non-diseased patients with negative test}}{\text{no. patients with negative test}}$$

In terms of the cells in the 2×2 table (Table 5.6),

$$PV- = \frac{TN}{TN + FN}$$

Difference between predictive value, post-test probability, and posterior probability

Posterior probability is a general term for the probability after an event. *Post-test probability* is the special case of posterior probability in which the event is a diagnostic test result.

Predictive value and posterior probability appear to be very similar. Both answer the all-important question, *"as a result of this test result, what is the likelihood that my patient has this disease?"* However, posterior probability and predictive value are different in important ways. Posterior probability is far more useful than predictive value. Moreover, it is self-defining, in the sense that its definition says exactly what it is. Unfortunately, predictive value has become established as the preferred term for the probability of disease after a test result. Table 5.7 summarizes the differences between posterior probability and predictive value.

The authors urge readers of this textbook to use the term "post-test probability" when in a medical context.

Thus, *the predictive value is an observable number obtained from a defined population. It does not necessarily apply to another population.*

An important caution: A reader might mistakenly believe that predictive value is a measure of test performance. It is not. It reflects test performance because the sensitivity and specificity of a test affect the number of true-positive and false-positive test results, which in turn affect the predictive

Table 5.7

Posterior probability	*Predictive value*
Defined as the probability of disease after taking into account new information	Defined as the proportion of patients with a test result who have disease (or no disease)
A mathematical relationship (Bayes' theorem) makes it possible to calculate the posterior (or post-test) probability in *any* population	Calculated from a 2×2 table of results in a specific population of patients
According to Bayes' theorem, the posterior probability depends on the prior probability of disease, which is defined as an **opinion** about the likelihood of an event in a specific situation prior to obtaining new information	Depends on the prevalence of disease in the specified population It is not possible to calculate the predictive value in another population
Caveat: Requires the assumption that the sensitivity, specificity, and likelihood ratios obtained from published research apply to the patient in the specific situation	*Caveat*: Because it refers to a test as used in a particular population, using a published predictive value for a disease in a population with a different prevalence of the disease will cause potentially serious errors

value. However, the prevalence of the target condition also affects predictive value through its effect on the number of patients that can have a true-positive result (those with the target condition) or a false-positive result (those who do not have the target condition). The prevalence of the target condition therefore *confounds* the relationship between predictive value and test performance, making the one a poor reflection of the other.

The next several sections will illustrate the pitfalls of using predictive value as a surrogate for posterior probability.

5.3 How to measure the characteristics of a diagnostic test: a hypothetical case

5.3.1 Description of study

You must evaluate a new radionuclide scanning test for splenomegaly. The purpose of the test is to detect spleen enlargement that is too slight to be detected by palpating the abdomen. The scan uses radioactively labeled macroaggregated iron particles. When injected in the bloodstream, these particles attach preferentially to splenic macrophages, which ingest and then digest them. You decide to measure the accuracy of this test by comparing the size of the radionuclide scan image of the spleen to the weight of the spleen, which is a good gold standard test for splenomegaly. In order to weigh the spleen, someone must remove it. Therefore, you perform the spleen scan on all patients who are to undergo elective splenectomy.

A description of your study of the radionuclide spleen scan should contain the following information:

- **Index test**: Macroaggregated iron scan of the spleen.
- **Gold standard test**: Weighing the spleen after surgical removal.
- **Definition of abnormal index test**: Spleen silhouette as seen on the scan is more than 1.5 times normal size.
- **Definition of disease (splenomegaly)**: Splenic weight >250 grams.
- **Source populations**:
  - Patients whose clinicians cannot agree on the size of the spleen; some clinicians can feel it, but others cannot.
  - Patients whose spleen is not palpable, but they have a disease that is often accompanied by splenomegaly.
- **Verified sample**: patients who are about to undergo splenectomy usually because their spleen is so large that it interferes with survival of the formed elements of the blood.

A description of the flow of patients through the study appears in Figure 5.5.

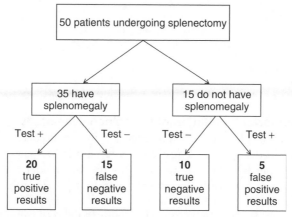

Figure 5.5 Flow of patients through an illustrative study of a hypothetical test for splenomegaly.

5.3.2 Description of results

The results of using the scan in 50 study patients appear in Table 5.8.

Table 5.8

Results of the spleen scan	Number of patients		Totals
	Spleen weighs >250 grams	*Spleen weighs <250 grams*	
Positive	True positive $N=20$	False positive $N=5$	$N=25$
Negative	False negative $N=15$	True negative $N=10$	$N=25$
Totals	$N=35$	$N=15$	$N=50$

As shown in the table, 35 of the patients (70%) have splenomegaly. Of these 35 patients, 20 have a positive radioactive iron scan. Of the 15 patients with normal-size spleens, 10 have a normal scan. Therefore,

$$\text{true-positive rate (TPR; } P[+|D], \text{sensitivity)} = \frac{20}{35} = 0.57$$

$$\text{true-negative rate (TNR; } P[-|\text{no } D], \text{specificity)} = \frac{10}{15} = 0.67$$

Similarly,

$$\text{false-negative rate} = \frac{15}{35} = 0.43$$

$$\text{false-positive rate} = \frac{5}{15} = 0.33$$

Predictive value:

$$PV+ = \frac{20}{25} = 0.80$$

$$PV- = \frac{10}{25} = 0.40$$

5.3.3 An important limitation of the spleen scan study

Your study of the spleen scan will be of little value to anyone. The study has a major error in design, one that occurs often and is the major reason why studies of test performance can mislead the unwary reader. Everyone who reads a study of test performance must be alert to its occurrence:

The commonest study design error is the choice of the verified sample.

Recall these definitions:

Definition of source population: The patients whose findings lead the doctor to order the index test. (Also known as the "clinically relevant population.")

Definition of verified sample: Patients who receive the index test and the gold standard test (usually a subset of the source population and sometimes entirely unrelated to the source population).

When the verified sample is identical to the source population, the reader can be sure that the data obtained in the study apply to patients whose description matches that of the source population. When, as in the spleen scan study, the verified sample differs from the source population, the reader cannot confidently use the findings in patient care.

In the spleen scan study, the verified sample is not the same as the source population:

Source population: Patients whose doctors cannot agree on the size of the spleen; some can feel it, but others cannot; also, patients whose spleen is not palpable, but they have a disease that is often accompanied by splenomegaly.

Verified sample: Patients who are about to undergo splenectomy, usually because their spleen is so large that it is causing medical problems.

In fact, patients in the verified sample have such large spleens that they do not need a spleen scan at all! In this example, the verified sample is not a subset of the source population.

So far, in this section, we have learned an important paradox of technology assessment:

The patients in a study of test performance often differ from the patients who typically get the test.

The difference between the source population and the verified sample leads to two errors, which are easily mistaken for one another:

- *The predictive value in the verified sample is not necessarily the same as the post-test probability in the source population,* for two reasons. First, the patients in the verified sample have different clinical characteristics than the source population (in this case, very large spleens). Second, the prevalence of the target condition is different in the verified sample (in this case, higher). Therefore, the predictive value calculated from the verified sample is not necessarily the same as the post-test probability in the source population.
- *The measurements of test performance in the verification sample may not apply to the source population.* The patients in the verified sample have different clinical characteristics than the source population. These clinical characteristics can affect the sensitivity and specificity of the index test, which are therefore different than in the verified sample.

Both of these errors are important. We address the first in the next section of this chapter, which is entitled "Pitfalls of predictive value." We focus in depth on avoiding the second error in the following section, which is entitled "Sources of biased estimates of test performance and how to avoid them."

5.4   Pitfalls of predictive value

Applying the predictive value in one population to another risks error because different prevalences of disease in the two populations can dramatically affect the predictive value of a test. Here, we use the true-positive rate (0.57) and false-positive rate (0.33) of the spleen scan in the verified population to calculate the predictive value of the test in a primary care population of patients with suspected splenomegaly, in which the prevalence of splenomegaly is only 20%. Using the scan in 1000 patients from this population, the distribution of positive and negative test results among diseased and non-diseased patients would be as shown in Figure 5.6.

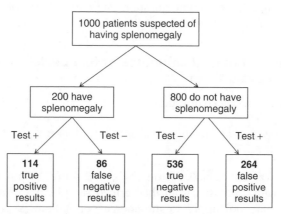

Figure 5.6 Results of applying test for splenomegaly to a hypothetical population of primary care patients with a pre-test probability of 20% of having splenomegaly.

Using the numbers from Figure 5.6, the predictive value of the test is

$$\text{PV}+ = \frac{114}{114 + 264} = 0.30$$

$$\text{PV}- = \frac{536}{536 + 86} = 0.86$$

The predictive value in the two populations is quite different, as seen in Table 5.9.

Table 5.9 Predictive value in a verification sample population and the source population.

	Prevalence of splenomegaly in population	Positive predictive value	Negative predictive value
Verified sample	0.70	0.80	0.40
Source population	0.20	0.30	0.86

The positive predictive value of the spleen scan is much lower (and the negative predictive value much higher) in the source population than in the verified sample. Therefore, *if the prevalence of the target condition differs in two populations, their predictive value of a test will differ.*

As discussed in Chapters 4 and in this chapter, predictive value is a number derived from a 2×2 table of results from a study of a test. The predictive value obtained in one population usually does not apply to another population unless the two populations are very similar.

A final point about using the term "predictive value": the words "predictive value" do not precisely describe the meaning of the term. A person who is unsure of the meaning of "predictive value" would have to look it up. In contrast, consider the precision of the language of probability: "probability of disease if the test is positive." More words to be sure, but no ambiguity. In this book, we will not use predictive value when we mean post-test probability.

Now we turn to the following question: *do biased estimates of sensitivity and specificity lead to serious errors in interpreting tests?*

5.5 Sources of biased estimates of test performance and how to avoid them

We now return to a crucial question:

Do measurements of the sensitivity and specificity of a test apply to the source population?

The brief answer is "not necessarily." If some source population patients are systematically excluded from the verified sample, the measures of test performance may not apply to the source population. A propensity for systematic error is called *bias.*

The odds ratio form of Bayes' theorem states that the post-test probability of disease depends on the likelihood ratio of the test (or, equivalently, its sensitivity and specificity):

$$\text{post-test odds} = \text{pre-test odds} \times \text{likelihood ratio}$$

The clinician might well ask, "if I use Bayes' theorem to interpret a test result, can I use the likelihood ratio from a published study to calculate the post-test odds in my patients?" The purpose of this section is to answer this question.

First, consider features of the ideal study of a diagnostic test:

Characteristics of the ideal study of a test:
- The selection of study patients reflects test ordering decisions in usual practice.
- Assembly of the study cohort is prospective which means that each study patient joins the study before undergoing the index test and gold standard test.
- A standard set of pertinent clinical features is obtained from each patient.
- Test results are defined in advance of the study.
- The gold standard test is an accurate measure of the patient's true state.
- Interpretation of the index test and gold standard test occurs independently of each other and without knowledge of the clinical features of the patient.
- If the test is a visual image, several different people interpret the image independently.
- The number of enrolled patients, both with the target condition and free of the target condition, is sufficient to ensure precise measurements of the sensitivity and specificity of the test.
- The index test and gold standard test are both performed within a short time period.
- Every patient who has the index test also has the gold standard test.

We will discuss each of these features in the next few pages.

5.5.1   Study characteristics that help to insure that the results apply to usual practice

- **The assembly of the study cohort reflects test ordering decisions in usual practice.**

Insofar as possible, study patients should be similar to patients in typical patient care settings.

Of course, there are often several typical settings for testing. For example, many primary care physicians order a stress electrocardiogram when they suspect coronary artery disease in a patient with chest pain. Cardiologists also see patients with chest pain but usually after a primary care physician has evaluated the patient. Taken as a group, specialists' patients are often very different than primary care physicians' patients. The results of a study of exercise test performance may apply to a cardiologist's practice but not necessarily to primary care.

What to look for in a study: Read the description of the practice settings from which the source population came. Is it typical of your practice? Who actually ordered the index test?

- **Assembly of the study cohort is prospective.**

The ideal study enrolls patients in the clinical setting, not at the point of testing. The journal article states the inclusion and exclusion criteria for participating in the study. In the ideal study, patients enroll as their care reaches a pre-identified point so that data collection occurs according to a protocol that enforces the discipline needed for good clinical research. Retrospective assembly of a study cohort is a much weaker design. In a typical retrospective study, someone identifies all patients who had a test during a defined prior time interval. A good retrospective study is planned in advance and has a study protocol. The study protocol should include a pre-defined standard set of pertinent clinical features. However, some of the items are typically missing from a patient's medical record.

What to look for in a study: A description of the enrollment process. Were patients enrolled prospectively in the clinical setting where the test ordering decisions occurred? Were inclusion and exclusion criteria stated clearly?

- **Each patient provides a standard set of pertinent clinical features.**

A list of the frequency of clinical features in the source population helps clinicians to decide if test performance measures apply to their practice. A full description of the source population should include gender, average age, reasons for testing, duration and severity of illness, and other illnesses. By comparing the list from the source population to the list from the verified sample, the reader can ascertain possible selection biases.

What to look for in a study: A table listing key clinical features and their frequency in the source population and the verified sample. Each item in this table should list the number of patients with missing data.

5.5.2 Study characteristics that insure unbiased, reproducible interpretation of the index test and the gold standard test

- **Test results are defined in advance of the study.**

The raw data of a study of test performance are four numbers in a 2×2 table: the number of true-positive, false-positive, true-negative, and false-negative results. Getting these numbers right is the objective of a good clinical study of test performance. The sources of these numbers are the results of the gold standard test and the index test. One essential step is being sure that the people who interpret the gold standard test and index test use the same criteria *each time they classify a test result*. The study protocol should state the rules of interpreting the tests.

Suppose the index test is an imaging test, such as a chest radiograph. A radiologist looks at this image and sees a pattern. This pattern has certain characteristics that experience has shown to predict the underlying disease. The radiologist must decide how to classify the image and then label it correctly (e.g., "patchy honeycomb appearance"). The leaders of a study want to be sure that the radiologist classifies similar patterns in the same way each time. To accomplish this goal, they must decide which characteristics of the chest radiograph pattern should cause the specialist to classify the pattern in a particular way and assign the appropriate label to it.

The leaders of a study should specify a system for classifying patterns on an image, reflecting the clinical reality that several patterns may reflect the underlying disease, often to a differing extent with some features more accurate than others. Alternatively, they may decide to classify the pattern as "positive" or "negative" for a target condition, in which case they must define "positive."

What to look for in a study: Do the authors define the criteria for deciding how to label a result, either with a name or by calling it "positive" or "negative?" Did they double-check to be sure that the specialists were using their criteria consistently? Do their criteria correspond to the system used in your hospital?

- **The index test and gold standard test are both performed within a short time interval.**

  A study to measure the performance of a test is cross-sectional. Its intent is to see how well the index test reflects the actual state of the patient, so both tests must be performed before the patient's target condition has changed.

What to look for in a study: Look for the average time elapsed between doing the index test and doing the gold standard test. Is the interval reasonable, given the likelihood that the target condition may have improved or worsened since the index test?

- **The index test is interpreted independently of the gold standard test and both are interpreted without knowing the clinical features of the patient.** Following this principle will help to avoid biased interpretation of the index test and the gold standard test. These biases have names: test-review bias and diagnosis-review bias

An example of test-review bias: The physician interprets an exercise electrocardiogram result that is on the borderline between normal and abnormal. The call depends on the clinician's judgment. Knowing the very abnormal results of the patient's coronary arteriogram (the gold standard test) may influence the clinician toward calling the exercise electrocardiogram abnormal.

An example of diagnosis-review bias: The physician is interpreting a coronary arteriogram. She must classify the result as abnormal or normal, but is uncertain which interpretation to make. Knowing that the patient had very abnormal results on an exercise electrocardiogram may influence the clinician toward calling the coronary arteriogram abnormal.

Test-review bias and diagnosis-review bias have similar effects on measured test performance. When an observer allows the interpretation of one test to be influenced by the results of the other test, the two tests are more likely to agree. Why?

The definition of a true-positive result is a positive index test result in someone with a positive gold standard test. If you are in doubt about the interpretation of the index test and know that the gold standard test was positive, you may be more likely to interpret the index test as a positive result. Repeated many times, this form of biased interpretation will increase the true-positive rate of the index test.

Similarly, the definition of a true-negative result is a negative index test result in someone with a negative gold standard test. If you are not sure how to interpret the index test and know that the gold standard test was negative, you may lean toward interpreting the index test as a negative result. This tendency to interpret the two tests concordantly will increase the true-negative rate of the index test.

Should the person who interprets the gold standard or the index test know the clinical history? What do you think and why?

What to look for in a study: Look for a statement that the study protocol required blinding the people who interpreted the index test to the results of the gold standard test and vice versa. Those who interpreted one of the tests should not have had any information about the result of the other test.

- **If the test is a visual image, several different people should interpret the image independently.**

Many index tests and gold standard tests require someone to look at an image of a disease process, place the pattern into a category, and assign the correct label to the category. This process is prone to error, and many studies have shown that physicians often disagree about the interpretation of a visual image. These interpretive errors will lead to incorrect numbers in the cells of the 2×2 table that describes the performance of a test.

The best way to avoid errors in interpretation is to have several people interpret the same image without knowing each other's interpretation. If they disagree, the usual procedure is to discuss the disagreement and come to a consensus interpretation or to ask a third person to participate in forming a consensus opinion.

This error will not occur with numerical test results, such as the serum thyroxine level or a measure of airway resistance, such as the forced vital capacity at 1 second.

What to look for in a study: Evidence that several people interpreted the gold standard test independently of each other and settled any disagreement by consulting with one another and reaching a consensus. A separate group should follow the same procedure for the index test. The study should report a measure of the disagreement rate. The best measure is the kappa statistic, which takes into account agreement by chance alone (any kappa statistic above +0.5 is good agreement; kappa equal to 0 is agreement due to solely to chance).

- **The number of enrolled patients, both with the target condition and free of the target condition, is sufficient for precise measurements of the sensitivity and specificity of the test.**
  The 95% confidence interval for a proportion such as the true-positive rate is given by the following relationship:

$$95\% \text{ confidence interval} = \pm 1.96\sqrt{\frac{p(1-p)}{N}}$$

where p is the proportion in question. p might be $P[+|D]$, the sensitivity of a test. N is the number of patients with the target condition. A larger N means a narrower confidence interval and a more precise estimate of sensitivity and specificity.

Figure 5.7 shows the relationship between the number of diseased patients used to calculate the true-positive rate and the half-width of the 95% confidence

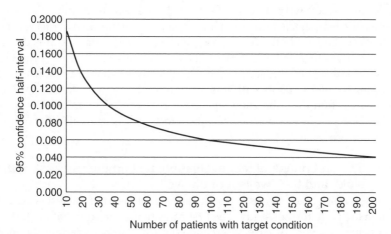

Figure 5.7 Relationship between 95% confidence interval for the sensitivity of a test and the number of patients used in a study to measure the sensitivity of a test. In this calculation, the sensitivity of the test is 0.90.

interval. With more than 100 diseased patients, the width of the confidence interval remains essentially the same as the number of patients increases.

What to look for: The study should enroll at least 100 patients who have the target condition and 100 patients who do not have the target condition.

- **Every patient who has the index test also has the gold standard test.**

The most important source of error in measuring test performance is due to differences between the verified sample and the source population, which contains the patients that undergo the test in usual practice. In the example of the splenic scan, we have seen the contrast between the source population and the verified sample. This extreme example of spectrum bias helps to understand the concept, which we discuss in detail in the next part of the chapter.

A well-reported study of the sensitivity and specificity of a test will address all of the key characteristics of a well-designed and carefully executed study. The STARD (Standards for Reporting of Diagnostic Accuracy) statement describes a 25-item checklist of the important features (see References).

5.6 Spectrum bias

Definition of spectrum bias: Differences in test performance caused by differences in the spectrum of disease presentation and severity in different study populations.

When applied to the study of diagnostic test performance, spectrum bias usually refers to differences between the type of patients in the source population and the verified sample in a study. As a result, the measurements of test performance may not apply to the source population. Spectrum bias may also refer to between-study differences in the spectrum of patients. As a result, the studies will not get the same results for sensitivity and specificity.

Spectrum bias affects measurement of test performance in two phases of the evaluation of a test. In the first phase, the test is unproven, and it is difficult to find patients to enroll in a study of the test. In the second phase, physicians are overconfident of the accuracy of the negative index test result and are unwilling to refer patients with this result to undergo the gold standard test. The next section describes how spectrum bias can occur in studies of test performance. Later sections describe the effects of spectrum bias on measures of test performance.

5.6.1 The first phase of test evaluation: testing the "sickest of the sick" and the "wellest of the well"

The first studies of a diagnostic test are attempts to learn if the test is accurate enough to justify further study. The first concern is to be sure that the test will be positive in severe disease. A second concern is to be sure that the test is not positive in everyone. The easiest way to accomplish this limited goal is to study the test in two entirely different populations of patients:

"**The sickest of the sick**": One population is the very sickest patients who, because they have advanced disease, are ideal for learning if the test can detect disease. The sensitivity of the test is apt to be very high in these patients because their advanced disease is easy to detect. When patients representing a broader spectrum of illness undergo the test, the sensitivity usually falls.

"**The wellest of the well**": The other convenient study population consists of healthy volunteers. In many situations, it is reasonable to assume the absence of the target condition because the volunteers are in excellent health. Therefore, performing a gold standard test to prove the absence of the target condition is unnecessary. The volunteers are often much younger than patients who would usually undergo the test in practice. Volunteers are also usually free of diseases that might cause a false-positive index test. As the test is evaluated with a broader spectrum of patients, the false-positive rate of the test usually increases (and the specificity falls).

Both of these verified samples can lead to spectrum bias – systematic error due to differences in the spectrum of disease – because the members of both populations do not resemble the source population, in which the test is used to resolve diagnostic uncertainty.

5.6.2   The second phase of test evaluation: testing patients who have been referred for the gold standard test

The diffusion of a new diagnostic test into clinical practice usually precedes careful research to establish its place in practice. Manufacturers use the results of the first phase of test evaluation to convince an eager, often uncritical, audience of physicians to adopt the new test. With few government pre-marketing regulations, new tests quickly appear on the market after completing the first phase of evaluation.

Adoption of new diagnostic technology occurs remarkably quickly. Testing in patients who are typical of clinical practice usually occurs after physicians have begun to rely upon the test. Typically, patients in the verified sample have had the index test and have been referred for the gold standard procedure. Because physicians have begun to believe in the new test, they are more likely to refer patients who have an abnormal result on the test and are less likely to refer patients with a normal result. Because of selective referral of patients to undergo the gold standard test, many studies of test performance are not credible.

Using the index test to decide who should receive the gold standard procedure is a special form of spectrum bias, called *test-referral bias*. Test-referral bias is the most common form of bias in studies of test performance, and it is therefore very important to understand.

Definition of test-referral bias: Systematic error in measuring test performance because an abnormal index test influences the decision to refer a patient for the gold standard test.

Significant differences between the verified sample and the source population often occur. How might these differences affect the applicability of the sensitivity and specificity of a test (as measured in the verified sample) to the source population? These effects are the subject of the next two sections.

5.6.3   Effects of spectrum bias

Effect of spectrum bias on the sensitivity of a test

Spectrum bias causes the verified sample to have a different spectrum of disease than the source population. Two forms of spectrum bias affect test **sensitivity.**

To illustrate the problem of spectrum bias due to selective referral of patients, consider how a patient would become a member of the verified sample for our hypothetical spleen scan to detect splenomegaly. Remember that the index test is the spleen scan and the gold standard test is the weight of the spleen after surgical removal.

- **Disease severity bias:** One reason for referral is a spleen that has grown so large that it is causing symptoms and is at risk for complications. Many people who undergo splenectomy have very large spleens that a scan can detect more easily than the normal or nearly normal-sized spleens of most patients in a source population. This form of spectrum bias leads one to overestimate the sensitivity of the scan because the scan detects a greater proportion of enlarged spleens than it could detect in the source population.
- **Test referral bias:** An enlarged spleen on the index test is another reason for referral and enrollment in the verified sample. Clinicians are more likely to refer a patient for splenectomy when the spleen scan is abnormal. A negative index test reassures clinicians, so that they are less willing to refer patients to obtain the gold standard test. Patients with negative index test results are often under-represented in studies of test performance.

To see how test-referral bias works, we revisit the study of the spleen scan, in which the verified sample comprised patients who had been referred for splenectomy because their spleens were very large and needed surgical removal. The results of the study appear in Table 5.10.

Table 5.10 Hypothetical results of doing the spleen scan in the verified sample.

Results of the spleen scan	Number of patients		Totals
	Spleen weighs >250 grams	Spleen weighs <250 grams	
Positive	True positive $N = 20$	False positive $N = 5$	$N = 25$
Negative	False negative $N = 15$	True negative $N = 10$	$N = 25$

Thus

$$\text{true-positive rate (TPR; } P[+|D], \text{sensitivity)} = \frac{20}{35} = 0.57$$

$$\text{true-negative rate (TNR; } P[-|no\ D], \text{specificity)} = \frac{10}{15} = 0.67$$

Imagine doing the study in the source population. The source population of patients with suspected splenomegaly contained 230 patients, of whom only the 50 shown in Table 5.10 made it into the verified sample. Now suppose that we could also learn the true state of the spleen in the 180 primary care patients whose physicians did not refer for splenectomy because the spleen scan (the index test) was negative. Table 5.11 shows the hypothetical results. The number of source population patients not referred for the gold standard procedure appears in bold-face type: 45 of them had an enlarged spleen and 135 had a normal-sized spleen.

Table 5.11 Hypothetical results of studying the spleen scan in the source population.

Results of the spleen scan	Number of patients		Totals
	Spleen weighs >250 grams	Spleen weighs <250 grams	
Positive	20	5	25
Negative	15 + **45**	10 + **135**	205
Totals	80	150	230

Thus

$$\text{true-positive rate (TPR; } P[+|D], \text{sensitivity)} = \frac{20}{35+45} = 0.25$$

$$\text{true-negative rate (TNR; } P[-|\text{no } D], \text{specificity)} = \frac{10+135}{15+135} = 0.97$$

The verified sample contained all the patients with positive index test results but only a few patients with negative index test results. The patients who did not get referred to the verified sample (bold-face type) would have had true-negative or false-negative results. The denominators of the true-positive rate and true-negative rate in the verified sample (see Table 5.10) are smaller than in the source population (Table 5.11). Since all patients with positive tests were referred and therefore were in the verified sample, the numerator of the true-positive rate is the same as in the index population. Therefore, the true-positive rate (sensitivity) in the verified sample is higher than in the index population. Figure 5.8 illustrates this point graphically.

Thus, as a general rule:

When test-referral bias is present, the true-positive rate is higher in the verified sample than in the source population.

5.6.4 Effect of spectrum bias on the false-positive rate of a test

Spectrum bias due to selective referral also affects the false-positive rate of a test, causing it to be higher in the verified sample than it would be in the source population.

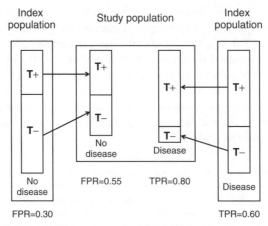

Figure 5.8 The effect of preferential referral of patients with positive tests on measurements of true-positive rate (TPR) and false-positive rate (FPR). T− denotes a negative index test; T+ denotes a positive index test.

Disease severity bias: When a patient is very sick, a physician is likely to refer the patient for the gold standard procedure, even though the index test is negative. This natural tendency enriches the verified sample with sick patients, relative to their number in the source population. Regardless of whether they have the target condition or other diseases, sick patients are more likely to have positive index test results. When measuring the performance of a test for the target condition, a positive index test in a patient with another disease is a false-positive result. Therefore, disease severity bias increases the false-positive rate (and decrease specificity).

Test-referral bias: Physicians are less likely to refer a patient with a negative index test for a gold standard test. Therefore, the verified sample has relatively few patients with a negative index test, which means relatively few true-negative test results. A reduction in the true-negative rate (specificity) means an increase in the false-positive rate, since the two must sum to 1.0. Therefore,

Test referral bias causes the false-positive rate to be higher (and therefore the specificity to be lower) in the verified sample than it would be in the source population.

Table 5.12 uses the spleen scan study to illustrate the effect of test-referral bias on the measures of test performance.

Table 5.12 Summary of the effects of test-referral bias.

	Verified sample	Source population
True-positive rate	0.57	0.25
False-positive rate	0.33	0.033

Also, refer to Figure 5.8 for a graphical representation of the effect of test-referral bias on the false-positive rate.

Because of these referral biases and stringent inclusion and exclusion criteria, the verified sample may contain as little as 3% of the source population (Philbrick *et al.*, 1982). Readers must scrutinize reports of test performance characteristics for evidence of these biases. One important clue to spectrum bias is a retrospective study, in which the decision to order a test is up to the clinician rather than built into a study protocol. A positive index test provides a rationale for ordering a dangerous or costly gold standard test. In contrast, it is difficult to convince the patient who has had a negative index test to undergo a potentially dangerous gold standard test or the patient's insurance company to pay for a costly gold standard test after the negative index test. The best clues to a trustworthy study are prospective design, an accounting of how many source population patients dropped out and why, and a comparison of the clinical characteristics of the source population and the verified sample.

Spectrum bias is a serious problem, but remediation is possible. The next section contains advice about how to adjust the true-positive rate and false-positive rate for spectrum bias.

5.6.5 How to adjust for biased estimates of sensitivity and specificity

How should the clinician adjust published estimates of the true-positive rate and false-positive rate so that they apply to the source population? The following discussion outlines some general principles.

Review of general principles

Sensitivity and specificity are **conditional probabilities:**

Sensitivity is the probability of a positive test given that the patient has the target condition: $P[+|D]$.

Specificity is the probability of a negative test given that the patient does not have the target condition: $P[-|no\ D]$.

In Chapter 3, we defined probability as a statement of opinion about the likelihood that a current state exists or a future event will occur. To estimate the probability of disease in a patient, we **anchor** on the prevalence of disease in the subgroup to which our patient belongs and **adjust** to take account of the special characteristics of our patient. Likewise, we can use the anchoring and adjustment heuristic to adjust a published sensitivity or specificity to take account of differences between the verified sample and the population to which the patient belongs.

Heuristics for adjusting published reports for disease severity bias

These heuristics assume that the target population for the test is the average patient in a primary care practice. Test performance measured in a prospective study in which everyone in the source population received the gold standard test would apply directly to the source population without any adjustment. Applying this study to a very sick inpatient population might require adjustments in the opposite direction to the following two suggestions:

Sensitivity: When patients in the verified sample are especially sick in comparison to the target population, the sensitivity as measured in the verified sample should be adjusted farther downward.

Specificity: If the verified sample consists of healthy volunteers, adjust the specificity downward. If the verified sample is mostly very sick patients, adjust the specificity upward.

These rules of thumb beg the question of *how much* to adjust the true-positive rate and false-positive rate estimates. Techniques for exact adjustment are the next topic.

Exact adjustment for spectrum bias

This material is advanced. The reader may want to skip to Section 5.6.5.3.

Exact correction for spectrum bias is possible, subject to two related assumptions (Gray *et al.*, 1984):
- Selection for the gold standard test depends *only* on the index test result.
- Selection for the gold standard test depends on disease severity only through the correlation between test result and disease severity.

These assumptions are probably valid for screening tests, since healthy people do not have clinical findings that might influence selection for the gold standard test. The assumptions are less likely to be valid when the patient has symptoms and signs that might influence the clinician to refer the patient for the gold standard test even after a negative index test.

Begg *et al.* (1984) showed that the unbiased estimate of $P[R|D]$ is

$$P[R|D] = \frac{P[R] \times P[D|R, S+]}{P[D]}$$

where $P[R|D]$ is the probability of result R if the target condition is present, $P[D]$ is the prevalence of the target condition in the verified sample, $P[R]$ is the probability of the result in the source population, and $P[D|R, S+]$ is the post-test probability of the target condition in the verified sample.

Another approach is to focus on estimating the likelihood ratio in the entire population that underwent the index test (the source population) (Gray *et al.*, 1984).

If $L[R]$ is the likelihood ratio for result R in the source population, and $L^*[R]$ is the likelihood ratio in the verified sample, then

$$L[R] = c \times L^*[R]$$

The correction factor, c, depends only on the odds of disease in the verified sample and in the source population (Gray *et al.*, 1984), and it is the same for all test results:

$$c^* = \frac{\text{odds of disease (verified sample)}}{\text{odds of disease (source population)}}$$

So, an author of a study of test performance should do more than give the odds of the target condition in the verified population, which would appear in a 2×2 table. The author should try to make a final diagnosis in all patients in the source population (those undergoing the index test) by either long-term follow-up through the medical record or calling each patient to ascertain the final diagnosis. From this information, the author could calculate the odds of the target condition in the source population and in the verified sample, calculate c, and then calculate the likelihood ratio in the source population.

When to be concerned about inaccurate measures of test performance
At this point in the chapter, the reader should be concerned about whether it is possible to measure test performance so that the results apply to the source population. Our focus on test performance should not obscure the real goal, which is making accurate estimates of post-test probability. For this purpose, accurate measurements of test performance are sometimes important but not always necessary because, across a range of sensitivity or specificity, the post-test probability may to make a difference clinically. Figures 5.9 and 5.10 illustrate this point.

When is accurate measurement of the true-positive rate important?
Figure 5.9 shows the post-test probability for any value of the true-positive rate, three values of the pre-test probability, and a false-positive rate of 0.20. Remember that most tests have a true-positive rate that is larger than 0.75, which is the region of greatest interest in Figure 5.9 (see shaded area).

Figure 5.9 shows that accurate measurement of the true-positive rate is not very important most of the time because the post-test probability does not change very much as the true-positive rate changes in the range above 0.75, where many test sensitivities lie. Accurate measurement is important in the following circumstance:
- If your patient has an intermediate to high pre-test probability and a negative test result.

Figure 5.9 shows that a change in the true-positive rate has little or no effect on the post-test probability for positive tests in any patient and for negative tests when the pre-test probability is low.

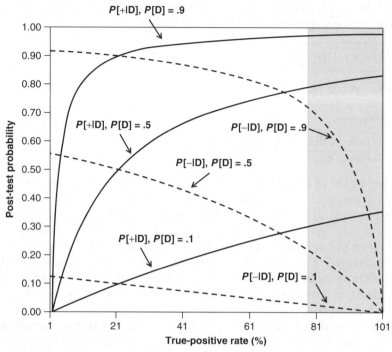

Figure 5.9 Change in post-test probability because of changes in the true-positive rate. The false-positive rate was 0.2 for all calculations. The pre-test probability (denoted by $P[D]$) was 0.1, 0.5, and 0.9 in successive calculations using Bayes' theorem and varying the true-positive rate of the test from 0 to 1.0. The post-test probabilities after a positive test ($P[+|D]$) are denoted by the solid lines. After a negative test ($P[-|D]$), they are denoted by the dashed lines. The shaded section denotes the range of true-positive rates typically present in clinical practice.

When is accurate measurement of the false-positive rate important?

Figure 5.10 shows the post-test probability for various values of the false-positive rate, three values of the pre-test probability, and a true-positive rate of 0.80. Remember that most tests have a false-positive rate that is smaller than 0.2, the region to pay attention to in Figure 5.10.

Figure 5.10 shows that accurately measuring the false-positive rate within the range commonly seen in practice is not very important for decision making in many situations, but it is important in the following circumstance:

- If your patient has a low to intermediate pre-test probability and a positive test result.

The false-positive rate has little or no effect on the post-test probability for negative test results in any patient. It has little effect when the test is positive and the pre-test probability is high.

Bottom line

- *Worry about accurate measurements of test performance when your patient has an unexpected result:*

- When the pre-test probability is high and the test is negative.
    - When the pre-test probability is low and the test is positive.
- Worry about test performance when your patient has an intermediate probability (i.e., when you are the most uncertain about the diagnosis).
- Otherwise, do not worry.

A moment's reflection should tell you that accurate measurements of test performance are important in all the situations in which a test result can change the probability a lot.

5.7   Expressing test results as continuous variables

In most of this chapter, we have described test results as "positive" and "negative." Often, we use these terms because the clinical laboratory provides only the "upper limit of normal" as information to guide test interpretation (by now, you should be feeling impatient with clinical laboratories that do not provide the information that you need to interpret test results!). Now that

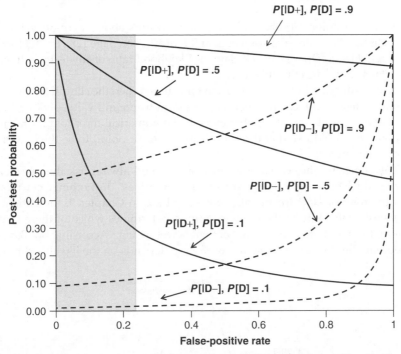

Figure 5.10 Change in post-test probability because of changes in the false-positive rate. The true-positive rate was 0.9 for all calculations. The pre-test probability (denoted by $P[D]$) was 0.1, 0.5, and 0.9 in successive calculations using Bayes' theorem and varying the false-positive rate of the test from 0 to 1.0. The post-test probabilities after a positive test ($P[-|D]$) are denoted by the solid lines. After a negative test, ($P[-|D]$), they are denoted by the dashed lines. The shaded section denotes the range of true-positive rates typically present in practice.

you have adopted a probabilistic approach to test interpretation, a test result has become simply an engine to move the probability of disease. We want to know the likelihood ratio corresponding to a test result, and we recognize that *the more extreme the result, the greater the effect on the probability of disease*. This part of the chapter describes some of the advantages of expressing test results as a continuous variable (a number within a range) rather than a dichotomous variable (positive or negative).

5.7.1 The distribution of test results in diseased and well individuals

As discussed earlier in this chapter, the distribution of test results in diseased patients often overlaps the distribution in non-diseased patients (Figure 5.11).

When published reports provide information about the distribution of test results in diseased and non-diseased patients, we can express the conditional probabilities of test result R ($P[R|D]$ and $P[R|\text{no } D]$) in several ways:

- The conditional probabilities of a range of values of test results in diseased and non-diseased patients (x_1 to x_2 in Figure 5.12). From $P[R|D]$ and $P[R|\text{no } D]$, we can calculate the likelihood ratio of a test result that falls in this range.
- The conditional probabilities of all test results above a cut-off value in diseased and non-diseased patient (Figure 5.13 on page 128). From $P[R|D]$ and $P[R|\text{no } D]$, we can calculate the likelihood ratio of any test result that falls above the cut-off value.

Test results should link to a decision for action. When the clinical laboratory reports a test result as a number (e.g., a serum troponin I value of 50 ng/dl), we have to decide if that number exceeds the numerical threshold for taking action. We would like that threshold value (the cut-point) to be the best one for the patient.

The clinician who learns of a test result should always ask the question, "what do I do now?" There are three alternatives: do nothing, get more information, or start treatment. As we shall see in Chapter 9, the patient's post-test probability of the target condition determines which of these three alternatives will maximize the patient's well-being. According to Bayes' theorem, the post-test probability of disease depends on the likelihood ratio,

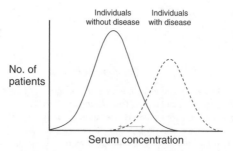

Figure 5.11 Distribution of test results in healthy and diseased individuals.

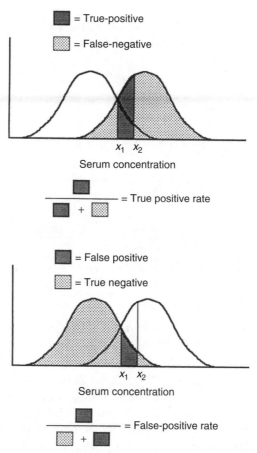

Figure 5.12 Calculation of $P[R|D]$ (top panel) and $P[R|$no $D]$ (bottom panel) for a range of test results.

which in turn depends on the cut-off value for the test. Our goal in this section is to lay the groundwork for determining the test result cut-off value that maximizes the patient's well-being.

Establishing a criterion for taking action will require making a tradeoff (Figure 5.14 on page 129):

- To obtain a test that detects all patients with the disease, reduce the cut-off value until all test results in patients with disease lie above it. As the cut-off value falls, more and more patients who do not have the disease will have results that lie above it and are therefore false-positive results. Thus, to be sure of detecting all diseased patients, one must accept the tradeoff of an increased false-positive rate.
- To obtain a test that is abnormal only in persons with a target condition, increase the cut-off value until all test results in patients who do not have the target condition lie below it. As the cut-off value increases, however,

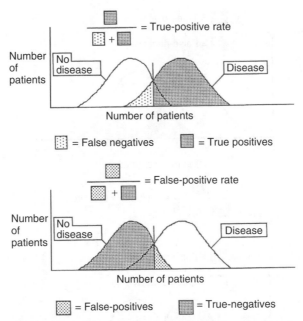

Figure 5.13 Calculation of $P[R|D]$ (top panel) and $P[R|no\ D]$ (bottom panel) for all test results above a cut-off value (denoted by the vertical line).

more and more patients who have the disease will have results that lie below the cut-off and are therefore false-negative results. Avoiding false-positive results means accepting more false-negative results.
In the terminology of game theory, adjusting the definition of an abnormal test result is a "zero-sum game": one goal is achieved at the expense of another.

5.7.2 The receiver operating characteristic curve

The ROC (Receiver Operating Characteristic) curve is a graphical method for depicting the tradeoff between the true-positive rate and the false-positive rate of a test. To obtain a ROC curve, one first calculates the conditional probability of a test result in diseased and non-diseased patients ($P[R|D]$ and $P[R|no\ D]$) for each definition of the test result. As shown in Figure 5.15 on page 130, the ROC curve is a plot of $P[R|D]$ (on the vertical axis) and $P[R|no\ D]$ (on the horizontal axis). In Figure 5.15, each point represents one of the three definitions of a test result, as defined by three different cut-off values (as shown on the inserts).

The area of the graph has three parts:

- **The 45 degree line:** This line is the locus of points for test results in which $P[R|D]$ equals $P[R|no\ D]$. Therefore, the likelihood ratio for such points is 1.0. According to Bayes' theorem, the post-test odds equal the pre-test odds times the likelihood ratio. Therefore, these results have no effect on the probability of disease.

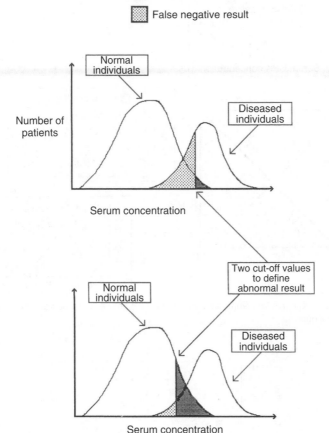

Figure 5.14 Effect of altering the cut-off value that defines an abnormal test result.

- **The area above the 45 degree line:** The likelihood ratio for test results that fall above the 45 degree line is greater than 1.0, indicating that the test result increases the probability of disease.
- **The area below the 45 degree line:** The likelihood ratio for points below the 45 degree line (shaded area in Figure 5.15) is less than 1.0, indicating that the test result decreases the probability of disease.

Figure 5.16 displays the ROC curve for ST segment depression on an exercise electrocardiogram. One measure of an abnormal exercise electrocardiogram is how far the ST segment falls during exercise as compared to the baseline value prior to exercise. A cut-point corresponding to deeper ST segment depression means a lower false-positive rate but also a lower true-positive rate.

This ROC curve illustrates the tradeoffs involved in defining the threshold test result that leads to different actions. To illustrate this point, suppose that the exercise electrocardiogram result determines whether a patient receives a

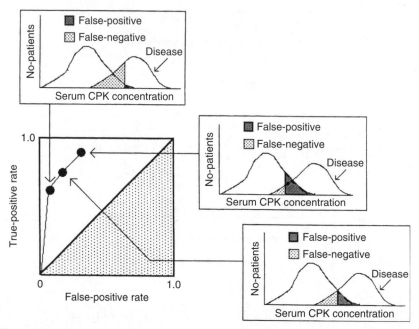

Figure 5.15 ROC curve for serum troponin levels as used to detect myocardial infarction (hypothetical data).

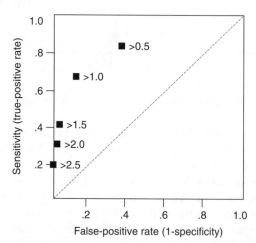

Figure 5.16 ROC curve for ST segment depression on an exercise electrocardiogram. Each point represents a different amount of ST segment depression, as indicated on the graph by the number of millimeters of ST depression. ROC curve created by the authors using data from Diamond and Forrester (1979).

coronary arteriogram. Setting the cut-point at ≥ 2 mm of ST segment depression would result in fewer false-positive results (thus fewer negative coronary arteriograms), more false-negative results (thus many more coronary artery disease patients who were not selected for a coronary arteriogram), and fewer coronary arteriograms (thus lower costs). Setting the cut-point at 1.0 mm of ST segment depression would result in more costs but fewer coronary artery disease patients who experience delay in treatment.

5.7.3 Using the ROC curve to compare tests

The ROC curve is useful for comparing tests. The area under the ROC curve is a measure of test performance. Of several tests for the same target condition, the best test is the one with the greatest area under its ROC curve. This method has become the preferred method for comparing tests. A shortcoming is the requirement for knowing $P[R|D]$ and $P[R|\text{no } D]$ for each definition of a test result. Two ROC curves could have different shapes and yet enclose the same area. As seen in the next section, the *shape* of the ROC curve is often the decisive factor in deciding to use a test for an indication of a specific clinical situation.

5.7.4 Setting the cut-off value for a test

The preceding parts of this section have prepared us to learn about a method for setting the cut-off value for a test. This method takes into account two characteristics of the patient: the pre-test probability of disease and the importance to the patient of avoiding false-negative and false-positive results. The principle is as follows:

The cut-off value of a test is the test result corresponding to the point on the ROC curve at which the slope of the tangent to the ROC curve satisfies the following relationship:

$$\text{slope of ROC curve} = \frac{H}{B} \times \frac{1 - P[D]}{P[D]}$$

where $P[D] =$ the pre-test probability of disease, $H =$ the net harms of treating patients who do not have the target condition (the harms of a false-positive result), and $B =$ the net benefit of treating patients with the target condition.

The appendix to this chapter contains a derivation of this relationship. The principle underlying the derivation is maximizing the patient's expected utility. Thus, *to maximize the patient's well-being, make the cut-point the test result that corresponds to the point on the ROC curve where the tangent to the curve has a slope that satisfies this relationship*. The principle of maximizing the patient's well-being is very powerful and is a compelling reason to use this method to determine the cut-point of a test.

Chapter 9 contains a description of the method for determining the harms (*H*) and benefits (*B*) of treatment. In the examples in this chapter, we will use subjective judgment to estimate the ratio of *H* to *B*.

Example: Imagine a test for serum antibodies against an infectious disease of serious consequence. The concentration of antibodies can have any value. A reliable research group has measured the likelihood ratio of each serum concentration.

There are two potential target populations for this test: those who have clinical findings of active disease (*disease confirmation*) and those who have no evidence for the disease but wish to donate blood that could transmit the infection (*screening*). The net harms and benefits of treatment depend on the target population.

Cut-off value for disease confirmation: Patients requiring disease confirmation may or may not have disease. Suppose the probability of disease is 0.50. Patients with a positive test undergo a treatment that is very toxic to the bone marrow, putting the patient at risk of other infections for a period of several months. Patients with the disease derive considerable benefit from disease detection because, although the disease is incurable, treatment can prolong survival by up to a year. Patients who do not have the disease but have a positive test receive the very toxic treatment but cannot benefit from it. Thus, the ratio of harms to benefit for disease detection is 2 to 1. In this population, the test result that divides "negative" from "positive" corresponds to the point on the ROC curve where the tangent has the following slope:

$$\text{slope of ROC curve} = \frac{H}{B} \times \frac{1 - P[D]}{P[D]} = \frac{2}{1} \times \frac{1 - 0.5}{0.5} = 2.0$$

To find the cut-off value for the test, identify the point on the ROC curve where a tangent to the curve has a slope of 2.0, as shown in Figure 5.17. The slope of the tangent to the ROC curve at any point on the curve is dy/dx, the instantaneous change along the *y* axis (true-positive rate) for a given change along the *x* axis (false-positive rate).

Cut-off value for screening: Patients who are candidates for screening to detect this infectious agent face a somewhat different situation. The prevalence of this disease in asymptomatic persons is only 0.001 (1 case in 1000 asymptomatic persons). There is considerable benefit to disease detection because these individuals might inadvertently donate infectious blood. Since the treatment is so toxic, no one, by common agreement, starts treatment when the patient is asymptomatic. Therefore, the harms of treating patients who have positive tests but do not have disease is very low, although the patients have the psychological burden of knowing they may have a disease that could

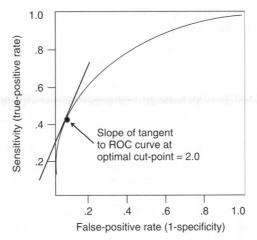

Figure 5.17 ROC curve for hypothetical test for antibodies to infectious agent causing serious disease.

later be fatal. On balance, the ratio of harms to benefit for disease detection is estimated to be 1 to 50. In this population, the test should be considered abnormal at the point on the ROC curve where its slope is

$$\text{slope of ROC curve} = \frac{H}{B} \times \frac{1 - P[D]}{P[D]} = \frac{1}{50} \times \frac{1 - 0.001}{0.001}$$

$$= \frac{1}{50} \times \frac{0.999}{0.001} = 20$$

To find the cut-off value for the test, identify the point on the ROC curve where a tangent to the curve has a slope of 20, which implies that for every increase of 0.01 in the false-positive rate, the true-positive rate will increase by 0.2. A test result corresponding to this steep slope of the ROC curve will occur somewhere close to the lower left hand corner of the ROC space plot where the false-positive rate is very low.

This example has an important lesson. Using a test to screen for disease in asymptomatic people requires a much lower false-positive rate than in symptomatic persons. The test must increase the probability of disease a great deal in order to justify trying to detect disease in asymptomatic persons, who have only 1 chance in 1000 of having the disease. To achieve a sufficiently low false-positive rate, the action threshold for the serum concentration of antibody should be set much higher than in symptomatic patients.

This example shows that choosing the definition of an abnormal test result requires attention to all facets of the clinical situation, including the clinical features of the patient and the consequences of detecting disease correctly or incorrectly.

5.8 Combining data from several studies of test performance

Replication of results is one of the most important sources of strength of the scientific method. To that end, the published literature typically contains several studies of the test performance of a diagnostic test. Their findings do not always agree, and the clinician will have difficulty choosing a value for the sensitivity and specificity or likelihood ratio of the test. In some instances, the clinician may choose one high quality study based on several criteria. The first criterion is the quality of the study design, as outlined earlier in this chapter. A second criterion is the similarity of the clinician's practice setting and the practice setting in which the study took place. Often several studies meet both of these criteria. If these studies obtained different values for the performance of the test, should the clinician pick one study or find some way to combine the results of the studies? The **systematic review** is the branch of science that deals with deriving conclusions from studies of the same subject. As applied to health care, a systematic review is a very powerful resource for setting clinical policy.

The systematic review has two basic components. The first is to perform a systematic search of the literature to find and evaluate all studies, published and unpublished, and display the results. This process requires defining inclusion and exclusion criteria, evaluating and grading study quality, and displaying test performance characteristics to illustrate important relationships. One way to display the results is to display the test performance from each study on a graph in ROC space, in which the horizontal axis is the false-positive rate (sensitivity) of the test (1 − specificity) and the vertical axis is the true-positive rate of the test (right hand panel of Figure 5.18). Each individual study of the test is one point in the space defined by the two axes. In the ROC plot, the position of the point represents the true-positive rate $(P[+|D])$ and

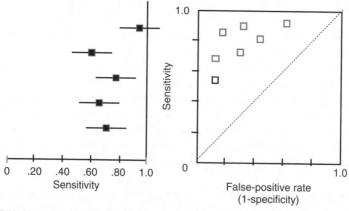

Figure 5.18 Several hypothetical studies of the accuracy of a diagnostic test plotted in ROC space (right hand panel) and as a forest plot of sensitivity (left hand panel). Each point represents a different study of test performance.

false-positive rate ($P[+|$no $D]$) of the test in that study (Figure 5.18). A second way to display the results is with a forest plot of sensitivity and, on another plot, specificity (left hand panel of Figure 5.18).

The ROC curve in Figure 5.18 will dishearten the reader who wants to decide upon a value for the test performance characteristics of this test. The points are distributed widely, indicating very poor agreement between the studies. Which point should the reader choose?

The second component of a systematic review is optional: to combine the results of the studies. This process is called **meta-analysis**. Combining studies increases the number of patients available to test the hypothesis that a difference is real rather than due to chance. However, combining a group of heterogeneous studies (as in Figure 5.18) is considered unsound practice.

Studies of test performance are an excellent case example of the need for caution when trying to combine results from a group of studies. The same test could perform quite differently in different studies for the following reasons, which underscores the complexity of the problem of analyzing a body of evidence about a test's performance:

- Different definitions of the cut-off value that defines an abnormal result.
- Different criteria for classifying an image into a defined category
- Different techniques for performing the test.
- Some studies have sicker patients, whose disease is easier to detect.
- Prospective studies that minimize test-review bias vs. retrospective studies in which test-review bias is severe.
- Different gold standard tests.

For these reasons, the first step in a systematic review of a group of studies of a diagnostic test is to do a qualitative analysis of the body of studies to decide if they are sufficiently alike to consider combining their results.

The last 25 years have seen substantial progress toward valid methods for combining the results of studies of diagnostic tests. All of them start with a plot of each study's results for sensitivity and 1 − specificity in ROC space (right hand panel of Figure 5.18). If the pattern of the points in space looks like a series of points on a typical ROC, it could mean that the studies were detecting the same thing but differed in the cut-point that defined a positive result. Moses *et al.* (1988) took the next step by log-transforming the points, fitting a straight line to them using regression techniques, transforming the points on the line back into logarithmic form, and finally connecting the points. The resulting "summary ROC curve" is the best fit to the collection of points in ROC space. The authors' approach had statistical shortcomings. Two newer approaches have overcome these shortcomings (the hierarchical summary ROC model and the bivariate random-effects model). Both models produce a valid summary ROC curve and an average value for sensitivity and specificity. Figure 5.19 shows a summary ROC curve and the average sensitivity and specificity with a 95% confidence interval. Summary likelihood ratios are not trustworthy for statistical reasons.

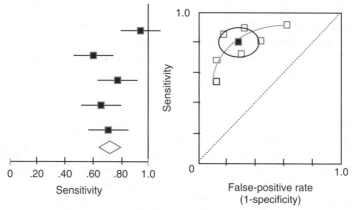

Figure 5.19 Two ways to summarize a collection of studies of the accuracy of a diagnostic test. The left hand panel is a forest plot of sensitivity. The diamond represents the average sensitivity. The right hand panel is a plot of several studies in ROC space. Each point represents a different study of test performance. The dark point represents the average sensitivity and false-positive rate. The curve represents a summary ROC curve. The oval represents the 95% confidence boundary. This illustration is a drawing, not a calculated plot. For an example with real-life data, see Figure 4 in the article by Leeflang *et al.* (2008).

Summary

1. The interpretation of new diagnostic information depends in part on the quality of the information.
2. The following expressions completely characterize diagnostic information:
   - $P[R|D]$: the likelihood of observing the finding in patients with the target condition.
   - $P[R|\text{no } D]$: the likelihood of the finding occurring in patients who do not have the target condition.
3. The predictive value of a test applies to the population in which it was measured. Applying it to other populations is unsound because the predictive value depends on the prevalence of disease in the study population.
4. Spectrum bias is the bane of studies of test performance. Ideally, one measures $P[R|D]$ and $P[R|\text{no } D]$ in patients who are typical of those subjected to the index test (the source population). In fact, the verified sample is usually a subgroup of the source population, chosen because the patients were sick enough to justify having the gold standard test or because of a positive index test result. Biased selection of study patients has several effects:
   - $P[R|D]$ is lower in the source population than in the verified sample.

- $P[R|\text{no } D]$ is lower in the source population (unless healthy volunteers comprised the verified sample).
5. The clinician should be prepared to adjust the true-positive rate and false-positive rate to take account of differences between the verified sample and the source population. Several techniques can make this adjustment, given appropriate data and valid assumptions.
6. Some tests have many possible results. Each result has a $P[R|D]$ and a $P[R|\text{no } D]$. The ROC curve is a plot of the $P[R|D]$ and $P[R|\text{no } D]$ of each test result. It is useful for comparing tests and for deciding on the right cut-point to define positive and negative results.
7. A test's cut-off value should be patient-specific. It depends on the patient's pre-test probability of disease and the harms of treating patients that do not have the target condition and the benefits of treating patients who do.

Problems

1. When testing for a fever (temperature greater than 99°F (37°C)), what is the true-positive rate for a thermometer which always reads 105°F (41°C)? What is the false-positive rate for this thermometer?
2. Consider a population consisting of 100 patients with coronary disease involving a single vessel, 50 patients with coronary disease involving two vessels, 30 patients with coronary disease involving three vessels, and 150 patients with no coronary disease. Suppose that the probability of a positive treadmill test in patients with single vessel disease is 0.4, the probability of a positive treadmill test in patients with double vessel disease is 0.6, and the probability of a positive treadmill test in patients with triple vessel disease is 0.8. What true-positive rate would be observed in this population if the treadmill test were used to detect coronary disease?
3. Suppose that you just completed the evaluation of a new test for lung cancer and much to your surprise you found that the probability of a positive result in patients with lung cancer is only 0.05 whereas the probability of a positive test in patients who do not have lung cancer is 0.85. Can you see any use for this test?
4. Suppose that I decide to call a patient diseased if a tossed coin lands "heads." What is the likelihood ratio for this peculiar test?

Appendix: Derivation of the method for using an ROC curve to choose the definition of an abnormal test result

The topic of the last section of this chapter is tests that can have many results. The serum concentration of an enzyme released from damaged heart muscle, such the serum troponin, can have any biologically reasonable value, ranging from 0–0,01 ng/ml in a normal person to 100 ng/ml in a patient with severe cardiac muscle damage. When a test has many possible results, the clinician must pick a result that defines the threshold for taking action as if the patient had the target condition. This appendix contains the derivation of the mathematical relationship for identifying the point on the ROC curve that corresponds to the preferred definition of an abnormal result. The decision to give or withhold treatment from a patient depends on whether the patient's test result is above or below this cut-point.

This derivation depends on concepts that first appear in the next few chapters. The reader should refer to these chapters as new concepts appear. The author has based this derivation on articles by Metz and by Swets (see Bibliography).

Our goal is to find the definition of an abnormal result that will maximize the net benefit of doing the test. Since the true state of the patient is unknown, we express the net benefit as an *expected value* (expected value decision making is introduced in Chapter 6). We will use the expected utility of the test (U[test]) as our measure of its worth (refer to Chapter 7 to learn about utility):

$$U[\text{test}] = EU(\text{test}) - EU(\text{no test}) \qquad (A5.1)$$

To calculate the expected utility of doing the test, we use a decision tree (Figure 5.20). See Chapter 6 for a description of decision trees. The first chance node on the tree represents the unknown true state of the patient ($D+ =$ diseased; $D- =$ not diseased). The second chance node (reading from left to right) represents the outcome of the test ($T+ =$ test positive; $T- =$ test negative). The probability of disease is $P(D)$. The probability of a positive test in a diseased patient is $P(+|D)$, which is the true-positive rate of the test.

Inspection shows four possible outcomes of the test (true-positive, false-negative, false-positive, and true-negative). If the patient's test result is above the optimum cut-point that defines an abnormal test result, the patient will receive treatment ($A+$). If the result is below this value, the patient will not receive treatment ($A-$). Thus, depending on the patient's true state ($D+$ or $D-$)

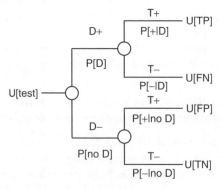

Figure 5.20 A decision tree.

and the outcome of the test, a patient will be in one of four states:

True-positive result : $D + A+$
False-negative result : $D + A-$

False-positive result : $D - A+$
True-negative result : $D - A-$

The patient's utility (or preference) for a true-positive result is $U(D+A+)$ or, in a more compact notation, U_{tp}. In this notation, tp refers to a true-positive test result. A true-positive result implies treatment of a diseased patient, which presumably is a better outcome than a false-negative result, which implies not treating a diseased patient. Thus, one would expect U_{tp} to be greater than U_{fn} the utility of a false-negative test result.

   To obtain the expected utility of the test and no test options, average out at the chance nodes in the tree shown in Figure 5.20, as described in Chapter 6. To do so, multiply the utility of each outcome by the probability that it will occur, which is the product of the probabilities along the path to the outcome (the path probability):

$$U(\text{test}) = [P(D) \times P(+|D) \times U_{tp}] + [P(\text{no } D) \times P(-|\text{no } D) \times U_{tn}]$$

$$+ [P(\text{no } D) \times P(+|\text{no } D) \times U_{fp}] + [P(D) \times P(-|D) \times U_{fn}] \qquad (A5.2)$$

but

$$P(-|\text{no } D) = 1 - P(+|\text{no } D) \quad \text{and} \quad P(-|D) = 1 - P(+|D)$$

Substituting these relationships and rearranging terms, we get

$$U(\text{test}) = [(U_{tp} - U_{fn}) \times P(D) \times P(+|D)] + [(U_{fp} - U_{tn}) \times P(\text{no } D)$$

$$\times P(+|\text{no } D)]$$

The ROC curve describes the relationship between the true-positive rates and false-positive rates for different cut-points of a diagnostic test. Let the function $R[\ ]$ denote this relationship. The relationship between the true-positive rate and the false-positive rate is given by this functional relationship:

$$P(+|D) = R[P(+|\text{no } D)]$$

Substituting this relationship in equation (A5.2),

$$U(\text{test}) = [(U_{tp} - U_{fn}) \times P(D) \times R[P(+|\text{no } D)]] + [(U_{fp} - U_{tn})$$

$$\times P(\text{no } D) \times P(+|\text{no } D)]$$

The next step is from differential calculus. Differentiate $U(\text{test})$ with respect to $P(+|\text{no } D)$ to find the point on the ROC curve where $U(\text{test})$, the patient's utility for testing, is a maximum. This step is an important reason to use this method for choosing the cut-point, because it maximizes the patient's best interests:

$$\frac{dU[\text{test}]}{d[p(+|\text{no } D)]} =$$

$$(U_{\text{tp}} - U_{\text{fn}}) \times P[D] \times \frac{d[R[P(+|\text{no } D)]]}{d[P(+|\text{no } D)]} + (U_{\text{fp}} - U_{\text{tn}}) \times P(\text{no } D)$$

Now set $dU[\text{test}]/d[P(+|\text{no } D)] = 0$ to find the point where U is a maximum

$$0 = (U_{\text{tp}} - U_{\text{fn}}) \times P[D] \times \frac{d[R[P(+|\text{no } D)]]}{d[P(+|\text{no } D)]} + (U_{\text{fp}} - U_{\text{tn}}) \times P(\text{no } D)$$

Solving this equation for $d[R[P(+|\text{no } D)]]/d[P(+|\text{no } D)]$, the slope of the ROC curve at the cut-point that maximizes the value of testing,

$$\frac{d[R[P(+|\text{no } D)]]}{d[P(+|\text{no } D)]} = \frac{P[\text{no } D]}{P[D]} \times \frac{(U_{\text{fp}} - U_{\text{tn}})}{(U_{\text{fn}} - U_{\text{tp}})} \tag{A5.3}$$

In Chapter 9, we refer to $(U_{\text{fp}} - U_{\text{tn}})$ as the "harm" of treating a non-diseased person (denoted as H), and $(U_{\text{fn}} - U_{\text{tp}})$ as the "benefit" of treating a diseased person (denoted as B). Thus, Equation A5.3 becomes

$$\frac{d[R[P(+|\text{no } D)]]}{d[P(+|\text{no } D)]} = \frac{P[\text{no } D]}{P[D]} \times \frac{H}{B} \tag{A5.4}$$

The left hand side of Equation A5.3 is the rate of change of the true-positive rate with respect to the false-positive rate of the test, which is the slope of the ROC curve:

- A test result corresponding to a point on the ROC curve to the right of the cut-point is defined as "positive" and leads to action consistent with the target condition being present.
- A test result corresponding to a point on the ROC curve to the left of the cut-point is defined as "negative" and leads to action consistent with the target condition being absent.

Equation A5.4, which is the same expression that appears in the last section of Chapter 5, indicates that the cut-off value that maximizes the patient's utility is where the slope of the ROC curve equals the odds that disease is absent times the ratio of harms to benefits of treatment.

Bibliography

Begg, C.B. and Greenes, R.A. (1984) Assessment of diagnostic tests when disease verification is subject to selection bias. *Biometrics*, **39**, 207–15.

Information about correcting for disease verification bias in selecting participants in studies of diagnostic test performance.

Bossyut, P.M., Reitsma, J.B., Bruns, D.E. *et al.* (2003) Standards for reporting of diagnostic accuracy. Towards complete and accurate reporting of studies of diagnostic accuracy: The STARD Initiative. *Annals of Internal Medicine*, **138**, 40–4.

A brief article describing the key elements of a study of diagnostic test accuracy and how to report them. An accompanying online-only article goes into much greater depth.

Diamond, G.A. and Forrester, J.S. (1979) Analysis of probability as an aid in the clinical diagnosis of coronary-artery disease. *New England Journal of Medicine*, 300, 1350–8.

A valuable source of data for ROC curves for cardiac tests.

Gray, R., Begg, C.B., and Greenes, R.A. (1984a) Construction of receiver operating characteristic curves when disease verification is subject to selection bias. *Medical Decision Making*, **4**, 151–64.

If selection for the verified sample depends on the results of the index test, the method described in this article can be used to correct the published true-positive rates and false-positive rates and obtain an improved estimate of these data in the source population.

Hanley, J.A. and McNeil, B.J. (1982) The meaning and use of the area under a receiver operating characteristic (ROC) curve. *Radiology*, **143**, 29–36.

A good article for those who wish to learn more about ROC curves and how they may be used to compare diagnostic tests.

Irwig, L., Tosteson, A.N.A., Gatsonis, C. *et al.* (1994) Guidelines for meta-analyses evaluating diagnostic tests. *Annals of Internal Medicine*, **120**,1 667–76.

An in-depth review.

Leeflang, M.M.G., Deeks, J.J., Gastsonis, C.G., and Bossyut, P.M.M. (2008) Systematic reviews of diagnostic test accuracy. *Annals of Internal Medicine*, **149**, 889–97.

An excellent up-to-date description of the key elements of a systematic review of diagnostic test accuracy, including reliable statistical methods for combining the results of studies.

McNeil, B.J., Keeler, E., and Adelstein, S.J. (1975) Primer on certain elements of medical decision making. *New England Journal of Medicine*, **293**, 211–15.

This classic article brought the principles of decision analysis to a wide medical audience.

Metz, C.E. (1978) Basic principles of ROC analysis. *Seminars in Nuclear Medicine*, **8**, 283–98.

This article is the acknowledged classic on ROC analysis. It contains a derivation of the method for choosing the optimum cut-off value for a diagnostic test.

Moses, L.E., Shapiro, D., and Littenberg, B. (1998a) Combining independent studies of a diagnostic test into a summary ROC curve: data-analytic approaches and some additional considerations. *Statistics in Medicine*, **12**, 1293–1316.

This article describes how to characterize the results of many studies of test performance by a summary ROC curve.

Philbrick, J.T., Horwitz, R.I., Feinstein, A.R., Langou, R.A., and Chandler, J.P. (1982a) The limited spectrum of patients studied in exercise test research: analyzing the tip of the iceberg. *Journal of the American Medical Association*, **248**, 2467–70.

The authors show how selection factors limit the number of patients in the source population who can participate in studies of the true-positive rate and false-positive rate of a test.

Ransohoff, D.F. and Feinstein, A.R. (1978) Problems of spectrum and bias in evaluating the efficacy of diagnostic tests. *New England Journal of Medicine*, **299**, 926–30.

The classic description of the effect of biased patient selection on the true-positive rate and false-positive rate.

Simel, D.L. and Rennie, D. (2008) *The Rational Clinical Examination: Evidence-based Clinical Diagnosis*, McGraw-Hill Medical, New York.

An excellent source of trustworthy information about the performance of many different diagnostic tests.

Swets, J.A., Tanner, W.P., and Birdsall, T.G. (1964) Decision processes in perception. In *Signal Detection and Recognition by Human Observers: Contemporary Readings*, Swets, J.A. (ed.), pp. 3–58. John Wiley & Sons, Inc., New York.

A classic book. The first chapter contains a derivation of the optimal operating point on the ROC curve.

Weiner, D.A., Ryan, T.J., McCabe, C.H. *et al.* (1979a) Exercise stress testing: correlation among history of angina, ST-segment response and prevalence of coronary artery disease in the Coronary Artery Surgery Study (CASS). *New England Journal of Medicine*, **301**, 230–5.

This study illustrates how measurement of the true-positive rate and false-positive rate in clinical and anatomic subgroups of patients can pay off in new insights. This study showed that the true-positive rate of the exercise electrocardiogram depends on the patient's history.

CHAPTER 6

Expected value decision making

So far this book has focused on diagnosis. We have seen how the tools of probability theory can quantify the uncertainty in clinical observation and test interpretation. The implicit assumption of the first five chapters is that expressing diagnostic uncertainty as a probability will lead to better decision making. This chapter justifies that assumption by showing how to use these tools to help clinicians rank their options when faced with decisions large and small.

A clinician makes many choices every working day by ordering a test, choosing a treatment, or hospitalizing a patient. The experienced clinician makes many decisions easily because the stakes are low or because the problem is familiar. The experienced clinician has standard operating procedures for these situations. Thoughtfully chosen heuristics, or clinical policies, are among the distinguishing features of the master clinician. This chapter provides a decision analytic framework for understanding the ingredients of good heuristics.

The methods described in this chapter are based on four related concepts:

1. A decision can lead to any one of several possible outcomes, as determined by the chance occurrence of subsequent events.
2. Each of those outcomes can be represented by a number, such as the corresponding length of the patient's life. We refer to that number as the *value* of the outcome.
3. Each outcome also has a probability, which measures the likelihood that the patient will experience that outcome.
4. Expected value is a summary measure of all the outcomes that can result from a decision. It is computed by multiplying the value for each outcome by its probability and summing the products. When the outcome value is the length of the patient's life, that sum of products is the patient's life expectancy.

The fundamental notion in this chapter is that a person can compare the alternatives in a decision by computing the expected value for each alternative. In this chapter, we assume that the best decision is the alternative with the greatest expected value. Or when the person measures value by length of life, we assume that the best choice is the alternative providing the greatest life expectancy for the patient.

Medical Decision Making, Second Edition. Harold C. Sox, Michael C. Higgins and Douglas K. Owens.
© 2013 John Wiley & Sons, Ltd. Published 2013 by John Wiley & Sons, Ltd.

For example, consider a decision between a surgical treatment and a drug-based treatment. Surgical treatments typically involve a risk of immediate death. A patient surviving the surgery then faces the risk of death at various times in the future. In other words, we can think of the surgical treatment as a gamble that has a non-zero probability of causing the patient's immediate death followed by probabilities for all of the other possible lengths of life following the surgery. The life expectancy for the surgical treatment, denoted LE_{Surgery}, is then

$$LE_{\text{Surgery}} = [p \times 0 \text{ years}] + [(1 - p) \times LE_{\text{Post-surgery}}]$$
$$= (1 - p) \times LE_{\text{Post-surgery}} \tag{6.1}$$

where p is the probability of death during surgery and $LE_{\text{Post-surgery}}$ is the patient's life expectancy if the patient survives the surgery. The drug-based treatment is a different gamble: the probability of immediate death is 0 and the probabilities of the other possible lengths of life may differ from the surgical treatment. If LE_{Drug} denotes the patient's life expectancy with the drug-based treatment, we can reduce the decision between the two alternatives to comparing the numbers $(1 - p) \times LE_{\text{Post-surgery}}$ and LE_{Drug}. The analysis described in this chapter assumes that the surgical treatment is the preferred alternative if the patient's life expectancy with this treatment is greater than the patient's life expectancy with the drug-based treatment. That is, $(1 - p) \times LE_{\text{Post-surgery}}$ is greater than LE_{Drug}.

This chapter shows how to use expected value calculations – or more specifically, life expectancy calculations – to analyze a clinical decision. In this chapter, we will assume that the preferred decision is the one that maximizes the patient's life expectancy. This assumption makes sense to us because we mostly prefer longer life to shorter life, but it has one major shortcoming: for many clinical decisions the length of the patient's life is only one of the concerns. Patients also might be concerned about the degree of disability, the time spent convalescing, the amount of suffering, and the out-of-pocket cost. Some people might prefer a shorter life free of suffering to a longer life filled with suffering. Chapter 8 shows how to measure outcomes by taking into account the multiple dimensions of an outcome. Therefore, the life expectancy analysis presented in this chapter is not the whole story, but it is a general framework for managing the complexities in clinical decisions. The content of Chapter 8 uses this same framework.

The discussion in this chapter begins by identifying the key issues underlying decision analysis. This includes an introduction to the decision tree, which is simply a way to represent a decision problem. We will describe how to use the decision tree to identify the optimal decision. We then describe sensitivity analysis, which is used to determine the robustness of a decision. The chapter concludes by describing the general algorithm used to compute expected value for arbitrarily complex decision trees.

6.1   An example

The patient's story

A clinical decision from real life will illustrate the material presented in this chapter. The person who faced this decision was a 60-year-old man we will call "Hank." Hank had a history of eczema. Because of this chronic condition, he was unconcerned when a rash first appeared near his anus. However, the persistent discomfort eventually led Hank to seek medical attention. His dermatologist performed a biopsy, which showed that a rare skin cancer, called perianal Paget's disease, was causing Hank's newly discovered rash. This disease starts in the epidermis but often will metastasize. Therefore, the dermatologist referred Hank to an oncologist for treatment.

First treatment alternative – traditional surgery

The first oncologist examining Hank concluded that the disease was still limited to the lesions visible on the surface of Hank's skin. This oncologist recommended that Hank undergo a commonly performed surgical procedure, which would remove the visible lesions and the surrounding epidermis. Figure 6.1 provides a schematic depiction of this treatment, which we will call "traditional." The borders of the rash on the surface of the skin can understate the full extent of the malignant tissue, which often extends below the epidermis beyond the visible boundaries on the surface of the skin. To increase the likelihood of removing all of the malignant tissue, the traditional surgical approach removes the visibly affected area and a 3 cm margin surrounding it. Because of the location of Hank's lesion, the extra margin would include the mucosa lining the rectum. Restorative surgery after this treatment can repair the mucosa and allow normal bowel movements to occur. However, this first oncologist warned that the restorative procedure was likely to fail. In this case the Hank would lose the function of his rectum and be forced to live the remainder of his life with a colostomy bag.

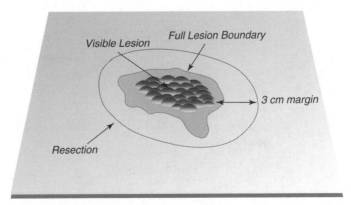

Figure 6.1 Traditional surgery for perianal Paget's disease.

Second treatment alternative – microscopically directed surgery

Hank sought the advice of a second oncologist who agreed that the disease was still localized to the perianal region. However, the second oncologist recommended a stepwise surgical procedure that would begin with a more limited resection. While the surgeons waited in the operating room, a pathologist would examine the edges of the removed tissue under a microscope to determine the location of any malignant cells. If Paget's cells were present, the surgeon would extend the margins of the excision, and tissue from the new margins would be examined under the microscope. The surgery ends when the margins of the excised tissue are free of Paget's cells. Figure 6.2 shows what the procedure might look like.

The advantage of this microscopically directed procedure is that the resections might stop short of the anal mucosa, thereby avoiding the risk of a colostomy. However, microscopically directed surgery has two disadvantages. First, the procedure could fail to remove all of the Paget's cells if the malignancy is not clustered together in a single connected lesion. If there are multiple malignant lesions the microscopically directed procedure could then stop at the end of one lesion while leaving in place the other lesions. Second, the microscopically directed procedure could lead to the same outcome as conventional surgery with a 3 cm margin of excised tissue around the visibly affected tissue if Paget's cells were present in the anal mucosa.

Therefore, the second oncologist also recommended collecting several samples of anal mucosa tissue prior to starting the microscopically directed surgery. These samples would be examined for the presence of Paget's cells. If Paget's cells were found, the surgeon would proceed with the more aggressive conventional treatment. The biopsies, as a sample of tissue, would be an imperfect test since a negative finding would not rule out the possibility that the microscopically directed surgery still might lead to the removal of the anal mucosa.

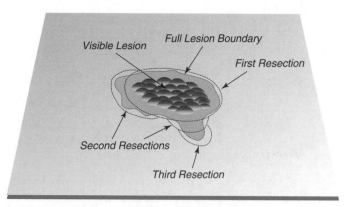

Figure 6.2 Microscopically directed surgery for perianal Paget's disease.

Third treatment alternative – do nothing

Hank recognized that his third treatment alternative was to do nothing about his disease. This alternative would leave him with untreated local disease, which ultimately could result in an invasive cancer, metastases, and death. Furthermore, without treatment, Hank would continue to experience the discomfort caused by the rash. Still, choosing to forgo treatment might avoid a colostomy unless the untreated malignancy progressed to the point of interfering with normal bowel movements.

Analyzing the alternatives

The relative merits of each alternative depend on a number of considerations. For example, the *do nothing* alternative avoids the colostomy, at least temporarily. However, the possibility that untreated local disease could become a life-threatening problem offsets this advantage. The *traditional surgery* alternative removes the local disease but is likely to require a colostomy. The outcome of the *microscopically directed surgery* alternative depends on the skill of the pathologist and the extent of Hank's disease.

Length of life: Hank's choice of treatment would affect the *length* of his life:
- Doing nothing would leave in place a disease which could grow to the point of causing his death.
- Stepwise surgery might fail to remove all of the disease if the pathologist overlooked Paget's cell in the resected tissue or the lesion had satellites that were not directly connected to it. This would leave Hank with roughly the same prognosis as doing nothing.
- While Hank was confident that the traditional surgery with its aggressive removal of surrounding tissue would eliminate the disease and give the best survival, he did not like the prospect of living with a colostomy.
- The microscopically directed procedure could lead to a colostomy if the Paget's cells extended into the anal mucosa.

Quality of life: Hank's choice of a treatment could also affect the *long-term quality* of his life.
- The traditional surgery would remove the mucosa lining his rectum. Reconstructive surgery might be able to restore the mucosa; however, Hank would likely require a permanent colostomy and would use a colostomy bag for the rest of his life.
- The microscopically directed surgery has the advantage of avoiding a colostomy if the disease has not spread into Hank's anal canal.
- Forgoing treatment might avoid a colostomy unless it was subsequently required to deal with the consequences of untreated metastatic disease.

Table 6.1 summarizes the advantages and disadvantages for Hank's three treatment alternatives. In the interest of simplicity, this discussion assumes that Hank decided to ignore several short-term issues. For example, the surgeries are uncomfortable and, depending on the extent of the disease, the microscopically directed procedure will require a longer procedure. The

Table 6.1 Hank's treatment alternatives.

Alternative	Advantage	Disadvantage
Do nothing	Avoids colostomy in the short term	Left with untreated local disease that could spread and be fatal
Traditional surgery	Could be curative yet avoid colostomy	Colostomy is likely
Microscopically directed surgery	Could avoid colostomy	Could miss local disease that could spread and be fatal

greater discomfort will be ignored. The discussion also ignores cost, which would differ greatly for the three alternatives. This assumption is reasonable for Hank since his health care costs are covered by a third-party payer. However, ignoring cost also reflects the implicit assumption that we are considering this problem from Hank's perspective. In reality the issues excluded by this simplifying assumption could dominate the decision. Chapter 7 discusses methods for incorporating a more complex view of the outcomes.

6.2 Selecting the decision maker

We will present this problem from Hank's perspective, which means that we will cast Hank in the role of *decision maker*. In reality, several interested parties could be the decision maker. These include:

- Dermatologist making the initial diagnosis.
- Oncologist recommending traditional surgery.
- Oncologist recommending microscopically directed surgery.
- Hospital where the treatment will be performed.
- Insurance company paying for the treatment.

Each of these decision makers views this problem from a different perspective. For example, the insurance company would place more emphasis on balancing its payments to the health care providers with the survival of a premium-generating customer. This perspective would ignore Hank's quality of life and quite likely the insurance company would prefer a different treatment alternative than Hank would prefer. For example, expected value analysis for an insurance company probably would be based on cost and revenue rather than the patient's life expectancy.

The decision makers also may differ in the likelihood they assign to the possible outcomes. For example, the oncologist recommending the traditional surgery probably assigns a high likelihood to the possibility that the pathologist will fail to detect Paget's cells in the margins of the tissue removed during the stepwise surgery. Skepticism about the ability of the pathologists to detect Paget's cells is why this surgeon prefers traditional surgery. The oncologist recommending the microscopically directed procedure probably has more confidence that the pathologist will detect Paget's cells.

Deciding which decision maker's perspective to adopt is fundamental to formal decision analysis. While the methodology can produce a valid analysis from the perspective of any one of the possible decision makers, *it can only be applied to one decision maker's perspective at a time.* The probabilities and especially the values will depend on who is the decision maker, and the conclusions reached by the analysis will change accordingly. This methodology accommodates the subjective elements of decision making, which is one reason for its enduring appeal to people who must make high-stakes decisions. We will discuss these subjective elements in detail in this chapter and in Chapter 8.

6.3 Decision trees: structured representations for decision problems

The outcome of Hank's treatment decision will depend on a number of uncertainties such as:

- Extent of the Paget's disease.
- Ability of the pathologist to detect Paget's cells and provide valid advice to guide the microscopically directed procedure.
- Success of surgery to repair the anal mucosa after traditional surgery.

Decision analysts use a tree diagram to keep track of these considerations. The conventional decision tree uses a box (□) to depict a decision point, such as the choice of treatment, and a circle (○) to depict an event whose outcome is up to chance, such as the aftermath of a treatment. We will use a solid circle to denote an outcome (also known as a terminal node).

For example, Figure 6.3 shows the tree for a simple decision: whether or not to treat when the presence of disease is uncertain. This generic tree has one decision node, two chance nodes, and four possible outcomes corresponding to four combinations of treatment alternatives and disease states. The ordering of the nodes from left to right corresponds to the temporal order in which the uncertain events following the decision will resolve. For example, the problem

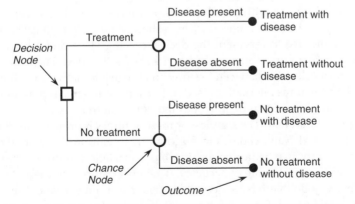

Figure 6.3 Generic decision tree for two disease states and two treatment alternatives.

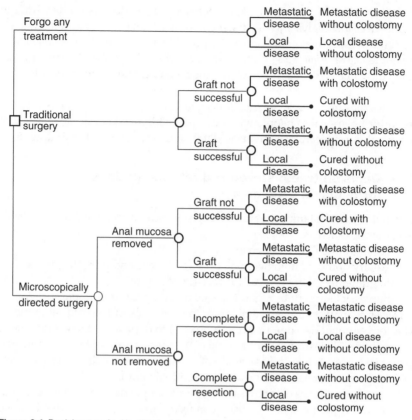

Figure 6.4 Decision tree for Hank's decision problem after negative punch biopsy.

assumes that the treatment decision must be made before the uncertainty about the disease state will be resolved.

For simplicity, we will start the decision process after Hank has had the punch biopsy of the anal mucosa, which showed no malignant cells, and we will draw the tree to represent the decision facing Hank and his physician after a negative punch biopsy. Figure 6.4 shows this tree. The initial node represents the decision between the three treatment alternatives. The branches for each of the three alternatives lead to portions of the tree representing the possible outcomes of that treatment (often called subtrees).

Forgoing treatment: The simplest of these subtrees represents the possible outcomes if Hank chooses to forgo all treatment. In this case, the only uncertainty is whether he already has metastatic cancer, which would likely shorten his life expectancy. This uncertainty is represented by a chance node that has two possible outcomes, (1) metastatic disease and (2) local disease. Figure 6.5 represents this simple problem.

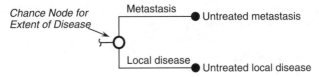

Figure 6.5 Possible outcomes for forgoing any treatment.

Traditional surgery: As shown in Figure 6.6, the possible outcomes for traditional surgery are slightly more complicated because of uncertainty about the outcome of the reconstructive surgery that will be performed afterward. That surgery will attempt to repair the anal mucosa that would be damaged by taking the large margin of tissue around the visible lesion. Hank will not require a colostomy if this procedure is successful. With traditional surgery Hank would still face the same uncertainty about the possibility that the surgery would not remove all of the malignant tissue. Note that Hank believed that traditional surgery would cure his local disease. The surgeons that he consulted supported this belief.

Microscopically directed surgery: Hank is more cautious about the possibility of cure with the microscopically directed procedure. Referring to Figure 6.7, he faces the risk that the resection is incomplete if the procedure stops short of excising the anal mucosa. In other words, he could be left with incomplete treatment of his local disease. The possible consequences for the microscopically directed surgery also include the risk that the surgeons will need to excise the anal mucosa because Paget's cells will be present in or just underneath the mucosa. In this case Hank would encounter the same risk of a colostomy that he faced with traditional surgery. Hank would also face the risk of metastasis regardless of the completeness of the procedure.

Because the punch biopsy was negative, the microscopically directed surgery probably will not extend into the anal mucosa, but it could have missed Paget's cells that were present in the sampled region. Therefore, the probability of the

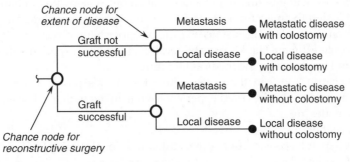

Figure 6.6 Possible outcomes for traditional surgery.

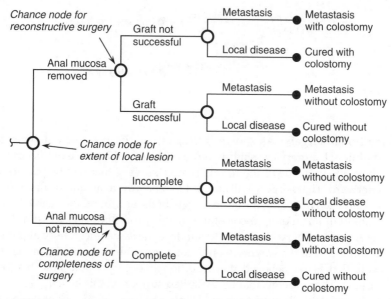

Figure 6.7 Possible outcomes for microscopically directed surgery.

upper branch in Figure 6.7 is not zero. In the next section, we will show how to use Bayes' theorem to compute this probability.

6.4 Quantifying uncertainty

Since Hank is the decision maker, we should base the analysis on his uncertainty about the possibilities he faces. The patient whose dilemma inspired Hank's example was a scientist who had spent his career working with data. He would have preferred to quantify his uncertainty using empirical observations. However, perianal Paget's disease is very rare. With only a handful of cases described in the literature, he had no empirical basis for thinking about the uncertainty in his decision. Hank was comfortable thinking about uncertainty in subjective terms, as described in Chapter 3. For Hank's decision problem, we will measure the likelihood of an outcome by the probability he would assign to an event. Since Hank was not a practicing clinician, he had to rely on the probabilities stated by the oncologists involved with his case, who would estimate Hank's risks by recalling their own experience of similar cases and by searching the medical literature.

The chance nodes in the decision tree for Hank's problem describe the uncertain events that he could experience while living with his disease. These chance nodes are:

- Extent of disease.
- Successful reconstructive surgery after traditional surgery (and avoidance of a colostomy).

- The need to remove anal mucosa during microscopically directed surgery.
- Complete removal of Paget's cells by microscopically directed surgery.

Diagnostic tests can reduce the uncertainty about these events by driving their probability toward 0 or 1. We will describe how to estimate their effect on Hank's uncertainty.

Extent of disease: The first oncologist performed a series of tests that showed no evidence of metastatic disease. However, these tests are not perfect, and their results leave some uncertainty. Failure to detect metastatic disease does not rule out the possibility that the cancer has already spread to other organs – a *false negative*. Similarly, the examination can mistake a benign condition for a life-threatening metastasis – a *false positive*. Nevertheless, the negative tests greatly reduced the probability of widespread disease. Based on these findings Hank believed that the likelihood of widely metastatic disease was about 5%.

Successful reconstructive surgery: To quantify the uncertainty about the outcome of the reconstructive surgery, Hank asked the two surgeons for their best guess. The surgeon favoring the traditional procedure claimed that the reconstructive surgery was successful in 90% of cases. The surgeon favoring the microscopically directed surgery placed the likelihood of success for the reconstructive procedure at around 30%. In the end, Hank split the difference and assessed his probability of successful reconstructive surgery to be 60%.

Paget's cells in the anal mucosa: In order to complete the analysis Hank needed to determine the likelihood that the disease had already spread to his anal mucosa. Before the punch biopsy of the skin, his doctors agreed that the probability of Paget's cells in Hank's anal mucosa was around 30%. How does this probability change after the negative punch biopsy?

Chapter 4 introduced Bayes' theorem as a method for determining the effect of a test result on the probability of disease. Specifically, Equation 4.7 showed that

$$P[D|-] = \frac{P[D] \times P[-|D]}{(P[D] \times P[-|D]) + (P[\text{no } D] \times P[-|\text{no } D])} \tag{6.2}$$

For Hank's problem (recall that $P[A|B]$ denotes the probability of event A given that event B is true)

$$P[D] = P[\text{Anal mucosa has Paget's cells}] \tag{6.3}$$

$$P[-|D] = P[\text{Negative punch biopsy} \mid \text{Anal mucosa has Paget's cells}] \tag{6.4}$$

$$P[-|\text{no } D] = P[\text{Negative punch biopsy} \mid \text{Anal mucosa is free of Paget's cells}] \tag{6.5}$$

$$P[D|-] = P[\text{Anal mucosa has Paget's cells} \mid \text{Negative punch biopsy}] \tag{6.6}$$

Therefore, we need to determine the true-positive and the false-positive rates for the punch biopsy as well as the pre-test probability for Paget's cells in Hank's anal mucosa. We will start with the false-positive rate.

Punch biopsy false-positive rate: After talking with his oncologist, Hank was confident that a pathologist would be unlikely to mistake normal tissue for a Paget's cell. Therefore, his false-positive rate for the punch biopsy is

P[Positive punch biopsy | Anal mucosa is free of Paget's cells] $= 0.01$ (6.7)

Punch biopsy true-positive rate: A punch biopsy is only a sample of the tissue that could contain Paget's cells, so affected cells might not be included in the punch biopsy. Moreover, the pathologist could overlook a Paget's cell that was present in the sample. Therefore, two things are required for a true-positive punch biopsy: Paget's cells are included in the biopsy sample and the pathologist recognizes that they are Paget's cells. That is,

P[Positive punch biopsy | Anal mucosa has Paget's cells]

$\quad = P$[Paget's cells included in sample | Anal mucosa has Paget's cells]

$\quad \times P$[Positive punch biopsy | Paget's cells present in sample] (6.8)

Hank believed that the punch biopsy had a 50% chance of including Paget's cells if Paget's cells were present in the anal mucosa. That is, he believed that the first term on the right hand side of Equation 6.8 is 0.50. Hank doubted that the pathologist would fail to identify Paget's cells if they were present in the biopsy. Therefore, he believed that the second term in Equation 6.8 was 0.95. Therefore,

P[Positive punch biopsy | Anal mucosa has Paget's cells]

$$= 0.50 \times 0.95 = 0.48 \qquad (6.9)$$

Pre-test probability: Finally, Hank's pre-test probability for the presence of Paget's cells in his anal mucosa was 30%.

Post-test probability: Inserting these probabilities into Bayes' theorem determines Hank's post-test probability for Paget's cells in his anal mucosa after a negative punch biopsy:

P[Anal mucosa has Paget's cells | Negative punch biopsy]

$$= \frac{0.3 \times 0.52}{(0.3 \times 0.52) + (0.7 \times 0.99)} = 0.19 \qquad (6.10)$$

Therefore, the negative punch biopsy reduced Hank's uncertainty about whether Paget's cells were in the anal mucosa from 30% to about 19%. Figure 6.8 shows how the post-test probability after a negative punch biopsy varies with Hank's pre-test probability that Paget's cells were in the anal mucosa.

Anal mucosa removed by microscopically directed surgery: There are two ways that the microscopically directed surgery could lead to removal of part of the anal mucosa. First, the pathologist examining the excised tissue

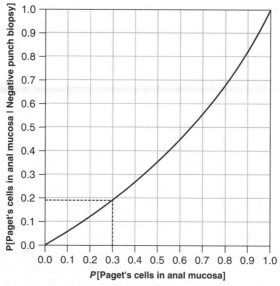

Figure 6.8 Probability of Paget's cells in anal mucosa.

detects Paget's cells in the anal mucosa – a true positive. Second, Paget's cells may be absent from the anal mucosa but the pathologist mistakenly identifies a normal cell as a Paget's cell – a false positive. Either event could lead to removal of the anal mucosa, so the probability that anal mucosa will be removed is the sum of the two probabilities. Symbolically,

P[Anal mucosa removed]

$\quad = P$[Paget's cells present and recognized by pathologist]

$\quad + P$[Paget's cells absent and pathologist makes a mistake] (6.11)

Recall the definition of conditional probability in Equation 4.1:

$$P[A|B] = \frac{P[A \text{ and } B]}{P[B]} \tag{6.12}$$

Therefore, we can write the two right hand terms of Equation 6.11 as

P(Anal mucosa removed) $= P$(Pathologist correct | Paget's cells present

$\quad \times$ Paget's cells present)

$\quad + P$(Pathologist wrong | Paget's cells absent

$\quad \times$ Paget's cells absent) (6.13)

In the previous section, we learned that the probability of Paget's cells in Hank's anal mucosa after the negative punch biopsy was 19%. In that discussion we noted that Hank was confident that the pathologist would not mistake a normal cell for a Paget's cell. That is, he believed

$$P[\text{Pathologist wrong} \mid \text{Paget's cells absent}] = 0.01 \tag{6.14}$$

Similarly he believed that

$$P[\text{Pathologist correct} \mid \text{Paget's cells present}] = 0.95 \tag{6.15}$$

Therefore, from Equation 6.13,

$$P[\text{Anal mucosa removed}] = 0.95 \times 0.19 + 0.01 \times 0.81 = 0.18 \tag{6.16}$$

which is more or less the same as the probability that Paget's cells are present in Hank's anal mucosa because Hank assigned such a low probability to the pathologist making a false-positive error (Equation 6.14).

Complete removal of Paget's cells by microscopically directed surgery: Finally, the microscopically directed surgery will remove the Paget's cells as long as the pathologist detects Paget's cells that are present in the resected tissue, which is the pathologist's true-positive rate. As noted above, Hank believes that the pathologist's true-positive rate for finding Paget's cells in a sample is 95%. Therefore

$$P[\text{Complete resection with microscopically directed surgery}] = 0.95 \tag{6.17}$$

6.5 Probabilistic analysis of decision trees

Figure 6.9 shows Hank's decision tree after adding the probabilities determined in the previous sections. This tree can be used to compute the probability of any single outcome by multiplying the probabilities at each chance node on the branches leading to that outcome (often called the *path probabilities*). For example, the probability that Hank will be cured without a colostomy if he chooses traditional surgery is

$$P[\text{Cured without colostomy} \mid \text{Traditional surgery}] = 0.60 \times 0.95 = 0.57 \tag{6.18}$$

Two paths involving microscopically directed surgery lead to the outcome *Cured without colostomy*, one with and the other without removal of anal mucosa. Since a person can travel only one of these paths, the probability of this outcome is the sum of the path probabilities

$$P[\text{Cured without colostomy} \mid \text{Microscopically directed surgery}]$$

$$= (0.19 \times 0.60 \times 0.95) + (0.81 \times 0.60 \times 0.95) = 0.84 \tag{6.19}$$

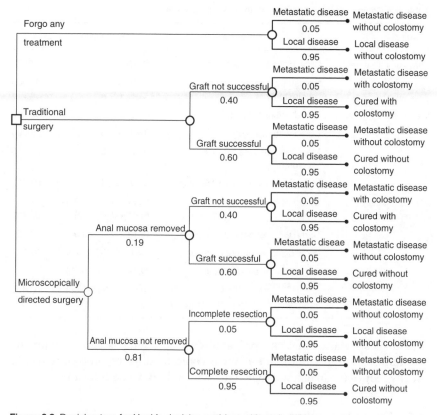

Figure 6.9 Decision tree for Hank's decision problem with probabilities.

Table 6.2 lists all of the probabilities for all of the possible outcomes in Hank's decision problem. These probabilities can provide a quantitative meaning to several of the statements made earlier about Hank's treatment alternatives. For example, the probability of cure for traditional surgery is

$$0.57 + 0.38 = 0.95 \tag{6.20}$$

whereas the probability of cure for the microscopically directed procedure is

$$0.84 + 0.07 = 0.91 \tag{6.21}$$

Therefore, Hank should believe that the more complicated surgery is slightly less likely to cure his disease. At the same time, the probability that Hank will end up with a colostomy with the traditional treatment is

$$0.38 + 0.02 = 0.40 \tag{6.22}$$

whereas the same probability for microscopically directed surgery is

$$0.07 + 0.01 = 0.08 \tag{6.23}$$

Table 6.2 Computing the outcome probabilities for hank's decision.

Alternative	Outcome	Probability	
Forgo any treatment	Local disease without colostomy	*By direct assessment*	0.0500
	Metastatic disease without colostomy	$1.00 \times 0.05 =$	0.9500
Traditional surgery	Cured without colostomy	$0.60 \times 0.95 =$	0.5700
	Cured with colostomy	$0.40 \times 0.95 =$	0.3800
	Metastatic disease without colostomy	$0.60 \times 0.05 =$	0.0300
	Metastatic disease with colostomy	$0.40 \times 0.05 =$	0.0200
Microscopically directed surgery	Cured without colostomy	$(0.19 \times 0.60 \times 0.95) +$ $(0.81 \times 0.95 \times 0.95) =$	0.8409
	Cured with colostomy	$0.19 \times 0.40 \times 0.95 =$	0.0704
	Local disease without colostomy	$0.81 \times 0.05 \times 0.95 =$	0.0387
	Metastatic disease without colostomy	$(0.19 \times 0.60 \times 0.05) +$ $(0.81 \times 0.05 \times 0.05) =$	0.0462
	Metastatic disease with colostomy	$(0.19 \times 0.40 \times 0.05) =$	0.0038

This analysis shows that the probability of surviving is similar with the two forms of surgery but that the microscopically directed procedure would greatly reduce the likelihood that Hank will end up with a colostomy.

6.6 Expected value calculations

Because Hank is the decision maker, he must decide whether or not the reduction in the likelihood of a colostomy justifies the slight reduction in the probability of a cure. His perspective shows up in the probabilities used in these calculations, since they are what he chooses to believe. However, his perspective should also shape the values he places on the possible outcomes of a decision. In Chapter 8, we describe a method for assessing a patient's preferences for outcomes. In this introductory chapter, we choose length of life as the measure of outcome and compute an expected value for length of life, for each of the outcomes.

Length of life was only one of several outcome measures that we could have chosen. It was a reasonable choice since Hank wanted to live a long time. However, we could have used several other measures. Hank would be concerned about how long he would be unable to work or the time spent in treatment and rehabilitation. And Hank did not want to live with a colostomy. Furthermore, each of the outcomes will incur costs, which would have been especially interesting to the insurance company if it had been the decision maker, whereas Hank was not especially concerned about costs because he had health insurance.

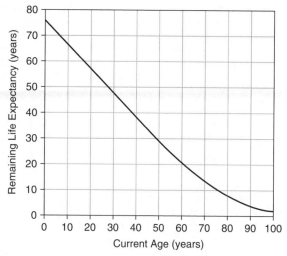

Figure 6.10 US life expectancy for white males (2997 data).

Life expectancy is the average length of life remaining at a stated aged. How do we estimate it? We start with average figures in the population. Figure 6.10 shows the life expectancy for white males in the US, based on 2007 data. At age 60, Hank could expect to live about 20 more years if he could regain his health after cure of his perianal Paget's disease.

Hank would face lower life expectancies for the other possible outcomes that he could experience. For example, he would only expect to live another two years if his Paget's disease had already metastasized. With untreated local disease Hank believed that his life expectancy would be five years, based on the survival rates reported for malignant melanoma. The impact of having a colostomy on life expectancy was less clear to Hank. Based on conversations with his doctors and patients with colostomies, he expected that a colostomy would not affect the length of his life.

Table 6.3 lists Hank's probabilities and life expectancies for each of the possible outcomes. Later in this chapter we will discuss how to estimate the life expectancies associated with outcomes. For now, we will take Hank's estimates as a given. We can use the numbers in this table to compute the life expectancy associated with each treatment alternative.

For example, 95% of patients forgoing treatment will live the five years expected for a patient with untreated local disease. The remaining 5% of these patients will live the two years expected by a patient with metastatic disease. Therefore, if Hank forgoes treatment, his life expectancy is

$$(0.95 \times 5 \text{ years}) + (0.05 \times 2 \text{ years}) = 4.9 \text{ years} \tag{6.24}$$

In general, the life expectancy for an alternative is the sum of the products obtained by multiplying the length of life for each outcome by the probability

Table 6.3 Outcome probabilities and life expectancies for Hank's possible outcomes.

Alternative	Outcome	Probability	Life expectancy
Forgo any treatment	Local disease without colostomy	0.95	5 years
	Metastatic disease without colostomy	0.05	2 years
Traditional surgery	Cured without colostomy	0.57	20 years
	Cured with colostomy	0.38	20 years
	Metastatic disease without colostomy	0.03	2 years
	Metastatic disease with colostomy	0.02	2 years
Microscopically directed surgery	Cured without colostomy	0.84	20 years
	Cured with colostomy	0.07	20 years
	Local disease without colostomy	0.04	5 years
	Metastatic disease without colostomy	0.04	2 years
	Metastatic disease with colostomy	0.01	2 years

of that outcome. This can be expressed by the following equation:

$$LE[\text{Alternative}] = (P[\text{Outcome 1}|\text{Alternative}] \times LE[\text{Outcome 1}])$$
$$+ (P[\text{Outcome 2}|\text{Alternative}] \times LE[\text{Outcome 2}]) + \cdots$$
$$+ (P[\text{Outcome } N \mid \text{Alternative}] \times LE[\text{Outcome } N]) \quad (6.25)$$

Table 6.4 shows the life expectancy calculations for each of Hank's treatment alternatives.

Forgoing any treatment has the lowest life expectancy for Hank. It is clear why none of his doctors recommended this alternative. The traditional surgical approach would maximize Hank's life expectancy because it is most likely to cure his perianal Paget's disease. However, his life expectancy with microscopically directed surgery is only about half a year shorter than his life expectancy with traditional surgery.

Table 6.4 Life expectancy calculations.

Alternative	Life expectancy
Forgo any treatment	0.95 × 5 years + 0.05 × 2 years = 4.9 years
Traditional surgery	0.57 × 20 years + 0.38 × 20 years + 0.03 × 2 years + 0.02 × 2 years = 19.1 years
Microscopically directed surgery	0.84 × 20 years + 0.07 × 20 years + 0.04 × 5 years + 0.04 × 2 years + 0.01 × 2 years = 18.6 years

Table 6.5 Comparison of Hank's alternatives.

Alternative	P[Colostomy]	Life expectancy
Forgo any treatment	0.00	04.9 years
Traditional surgery	0.40	19.1 years
Microscopically directed surgery	0.08	18.6 years

Table 6.5 summarizes the probability and life expectancy calculations shown earlier in this chapter. The probability that each alternative will result in a colostomy was computed in Equations 6.21 and 6.22. The life expectancies are copied from Table 6.4. Notice the following: Hank's decision problem originally had three different alternatives, four different uncertain events, and eleven possible outcomes. The analysis summarized in Table 6.5 has reduced that complex problem to a relatively simple comparison between a six-month reduction in life expectancy and a reduction in the risk of colostomy from 40% to roughly 8%. Hank still has a decision to make, but it is far less complex than the decision as it was originally framed.

Table 6.5 illustrates both the strength and weakness of using expected values to analyze a decision. An expected value does combine both the likelihood of the possible outcomes and the benefit to the patient – the length of life. The life expectancies in the table clearly indicate why Hank should prefer one of the surgical procedures over no treatment. However, expected value analysis only captures that single aspect of what can happen to Hank – the length of his life. It ignores the impact of the decision on other factors, such as his quality of life. Methods for incorporating quality of life in an outcome state are the subject of Chapter 8.

6.7   Sensitivity analysis

The validity of the analysis presented in this chapter depends on the validity of the numbers it uses. Of course, given Hank's subjective approach to estimating the probabilities in this analysis, validity is harder to judge than if we had relied on data from published studies. If Hank believes that his risk of metastatic disease is 5%, who can say that he should believe otherwise? But then Hank may have doubts about his subjective probabilities. He may wonder if he should believe that the risk of metastatic disease is 10% or even 1%. The subjective assessment techniques discussed in Chapter 3 can minimize the distortions caused by cognitive biases. However, Hank might still wonder if his responses to the assessment process accurately represent how he feels about the risks he faces.

Sensitivity analysis is the systematic exploration of how the value of one or more parameters will affect the decision-making implications of a model. This tool can support the validity of decision analysis by revealing how changes in

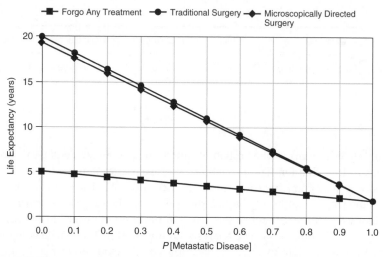

Figure 6.11 Life expectancy for alternatives versus P[Metastatic disease].

the probabilities will affect the conclusions of the analysis. The explicit nature of decision analysis makes this possible.

For example, Figure 6.11 shows that the life expectancies for the three alternatives vary as Hank's risk of metastatic disease changes. From this figure it is clear that forgoing treatment always results in a shorter life expectancy. Moreover, irrespective of the probability of metastatic disease, life expectancy with traditional surgery is similar to the microscopically directed procedure. This simple analysis shows that Hank should not worry about how accurately he has assessed his uncertainty about metastatic disease because it is not important to the choice he must make. Performing a sensitivity analysis on the other probabilities in the decision tree in Figure 6.9 leads to the same conclusion about them as well.

We can do sensitivity analysis on the other factors in the model, such as the life expectancy for the possible outcomes. Figure 6.12 shows that life expectancy for the treatment alternatives varies with changes in life expectancy for untreated perianal Paget's disease. In this figure, we vary the possible values for life expectancy with untreated disease from the worst case (metastatic disease) to the best case (being disease-free). Note that the life expectancy for the two surgical procedures is roughly the same for this range of values. Forgoing treatment does not become a credible option unless Hank believes that his life expectancy with untreated disease is virtually the same as his life expectancy without the disease (20 years).

The point of sensitivity analysis is to determine if the conclusions drawn from the model change when any of the model parameters change. When

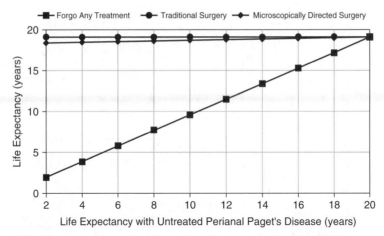

Figure 6.12 Life expectancy for alternatives versus life expectancy for untreated disease.

the conclusion is sensitive to a parameter, it is a signal to pay more attention to determining the value of that parameter accurately. The examples in this section vary one parameter at a time (so-called "one-way sensitivity analysis"). However, we can apply the same method to explore the sensitivity of the analysis to changes in two or more variables. The graphs are more difficult to draw; however, the principle of the method is the same. Examples in the next chapter will demonstrate multivariate sensitivity analysis.

6.8 Folding back decision trees

This final section of Chapter 6 describes an algorithm for computing the expected values for a decision tree when the problem includes more than one decision node. For example, suppose that the decision maker first must decide whether to perform a test. The treatment decision can be based on the result of the test or the decision maker can select the treatment alternative without first performing the test.

Figure 6.13 shows a decision tree for this type of problem. Node 1 in the depicted tree represents the initial decision about the test. Node 2 represents the result of the test. Node 3 represents the treatment decision if the test is not performed. Nodes 4 and 5 represent the treatment decision based on the test result. Nodes 6 through 11 represent the outcome of the treatment. Arbitrary probabilities have been assigned to the chance node branches. Similarly, arbitrary life lengths have been assigned to each of the possible outcomes. How shall we compute the life expectancy for this more complicated tree?

The algorithm, called "Folding Back," uses a reduction process based on two observations. First, expected value decision making chooses between

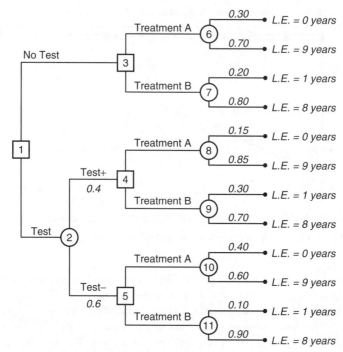

Figure 6.13 Example used to illustrate the basic algorithm.

alternatives based on the corresponding expected values. Therefore, the expected value of a decision node is the maximum of the expected values for the alternatives faced by that decision node. Therefore, we can replace a decision node by an outcome with value equal to the expected value of the decision alternative with the highest expected value (i.e., the maximum of the expected values). That is,

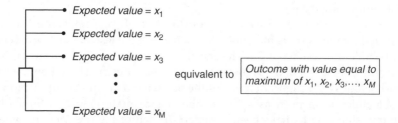

Second, because we choose between alternatives based on their expected values, a chance node, with several possible outcomes, is equivalent to a single outcome whose value is equal to the expected value for that chance node. In other words,

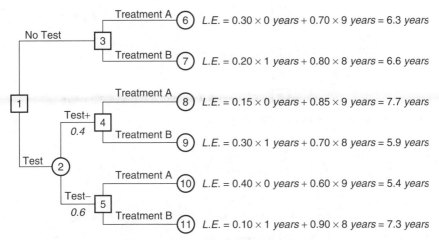

Figure 6.14 Reducing the treatment outcome chance nodes.

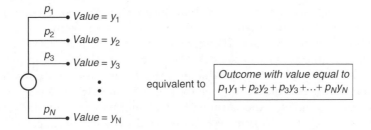

For example, Figure 6.14 has replaced the treatment outcome chance nodes (Nodes 6 to 11) in Figure 6.13 with their expected values. Doing so has not changed the tree in the sense that a chance node is equivalent to its expected value. For example, the expected value for Node 6 is

$$LE \text{ for Node } 6 = 0.3 \ 0 \text{ years } + 0.7 \ 9 \text{ years } = 6.3 \text{ years} \qquad (6.26)$$

In expected value analysis, 6.3 years for certain are equivalent to the gamble represented by Node 6 in Figure 6.13.

Figure 6.15 shows the next step in the process in which the decision nodes (Nodes 3 to 5) have been replaced by the alternative with the greatest expected value. For example, Node 3 is a choice between Node 6, which has an expected value of 6.3 years, and Node 7, which has an expected value of 6.6 years. Therefore, the expected value for Node 3 is

$$LE \text{ for Node } 3 = \max(6.3 \text{ years}, 6.6 \text{ years}) = 6.6 \text{ years} \qquad (6.27)$$

Figure 6.16 further simplifies the tree by replacing the remaining chance (Node 2) by its expected value:

$$LE \text{ for Node } 2 = 0.6 \ 7.7 \text{ years } + 0.4 \ 7.3 \text{ years } = 7.5 \text{ years} \qquad (6.28)$$

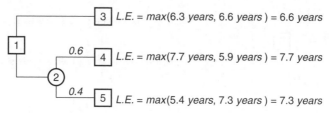

Figure 6.15 Reducing the treatment decision nodes.

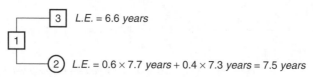

Figure 6.16 Reducing the test result chance node.

The decision tree has now been reduced to a simple choice between an alternative with an expected value of 6.3 years and an alternative with an expected value of 7.5 years. Therefore, expected value analysis of the tree shown in Figure 6.13 establishes that the preferred decision is to pick the treatment after having the test. Moreover, for Figure 16.4 we see that if the test is positive, Treatment A is preferred since its life expectancy (7.7 years) is greater than the life expectancy with Treatment B (5.9 years). Conversely, if the test is negative, Treatment B is preferred since its life expectancy (7.3 years) is greater than the life expectancy with Treatment A (5.4 years).

This process can be generalized to the following algorithm:

Algorithm for folding back a decision tree

1. Start with the most distal nodes.
2. Replace each chance node with its expected value

$$p_1 y_1 + p_2 y_2 + p_3 y_3 + \cdots + p_N y_N$$

where

$$p_1, p_2, p_3, \cdots, p_N$$

are the probabilities for the possible outcomes and

$$y_1, y_2, y_3, \cdots, y_N$$

are the corresponding values associated with the outcomes.

3. Replace each decision node with the maximum expected value for the possible alternatives

Maximum of $x_1, x_2, x_3, \ldots, x_M$

where

$x_1, x_2, x_3, \ldots, x_M$

are the expected values for the possible alternatives.
4. Repeat until the initial node is reached.

Summary

This chapter has described a method for analyzing clinical decisions based on expected value calculations. This method uses a decision tree to represent the structure of the decision problem. The nodes in the decision tree correspond to the decision alternatives (e.g., choice of treatment) and the chance events (e.g., treatment outcome) in the problem.

Decision analysis calculates a number that reflects the value of each decision alternative. Therefore, the analyst must use numbers to characterize the uncertainties and outcomes faced by the decision maker. The first step in this method is to identify this person or institution, because the numbers assigned to the parameters of a decision model often depend on a personal (e.g., the patient) or institutional (e.g., the insurance company) perspective. Moreover, the goal of the analysis is to determine the expected values for each alternative from the perspective of the person making the decision.

We illustrate this method with an extended example in which the decision maker – in this case, a patient – provides the subjective viewpoint for assigning probabilities to the uncertainties in the problem. To simplify the presentation, we do not incorporate the decision maker's perspective when placing a numerical value on the outcomes that he may experience. Instead our illustrative example uses the patient's length of life as the outcome measure rather than his feelings about that length of life and the health states that he may experience. The following chapter takes the next step and uses the decision maker's point of view to quantify the measures assigned to the possible outcomes.

The explicit nature of the method enables the analyst to see if the conclusions of the analysis change when subjected to different assumptions about the numbers assigned to the model parameters. Those parameters that affect the results of the analysis can be the focus of further exploration in order to increase the decision maker's confidence that the analysis has identified the alternative that truly aligns with the decision maker's point of view.

Problems

1. Determine if Hank's life expectancy with microscopically directed surgery would still be greater than his life expectancy with traditional surgery if the punch biopsy is not performed.
2. Extend the decision tree for Hank's decision problem shown in Figure 6.4 to include the decision whether or not perform the punch biopsy.
3. Redraw the decision tree in Figure 6.13 for the case when the optional test has a 10% mortality rate. Determine if undergoing the test would still be the preferred alternative.
4. Draw the decision tree for working up a patient for chest pain for coronary artery disease using the following assumptions:
   - The decision begins after completion of the history and physical. Based on the history and physical the decision maker believes that the probability of coronary artery disease in the patient is 20%.
   - The decision maker can subject the patient to a treadmill test. Treat the treadmill test as a binary test with a true-positive rate of 0.60 and a false-positive rate of 0.10. Assume that the treadmill test carries no risk to the patient's survival.
   - The decision maker also can order arteriography for the patient. Treat this procedure as a binary test with a true-positive rate of 0.90 and a false-positive rate of 0.01. Assume that undergoing arteriography has a fatal complication rate of 0.1% (i.e., 1 in 1000 results in death).
   - Assume that surgical treatment of coronary artery disease has a fatal complication rate of 1% (i.e., 1 in 100 procedures results in death).
   - Assume the following life expectancies for the patient:

Life expectancy without CAD	20 years
Life expectancy with untreated CAD	5 years
Life expectancy with treated CAD	10 years

Bibliography

Holloway, C.A. (1979) *Decision Making Under Uncertainty: Models and Choices*, Prentice Hall, Englewood Cliffs, NJ.

Chapter 3 covers the same material as the Raffia book mentioned below. Holloway's book was written for business school students; however, the writing is very clear.

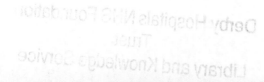

Raffia, H. (1968) *Decision Analysis Introductory Lectures on Choices under Uncertainty*, Addison-Wesley, Reading, MA.

What many consider to be the standard reference for the mathematical analysis of decision making under uncertainty. Chapter 2 of this book provides a thorough introduction to the topic of expected value decision making.

Weinstein, M.C. and Fineberg, H.V. (1980) *Clinical Decision Analysis*, W.B. Saunders, Philadelphia.

Chapter 2 includes several examples of decision trees for clinical problems.

CHAPTER 7

Markov models and time-varying outcomes

This chapter describes alternatives to the basic decision tree that can be used to represent problems in which the outcomes unfold over time. Time complicates most medical decisions. Occasionally a treatment decision leads to an immediate outcome, such as death during a surgical procedure. However, most outcomes emerge over time during that process we call "life." We touched on this aspect of medical decisions in Chapter 6 when we described a decision problem in which the patient had a choice whose expected outcomes spanned a range of possible lengths of life. In that example, we used the patient's life expectancy as the outcome measure, recognizing that life expectancy – defined as the average length of life remaining – only summarizes the distribution for the possible years of life remaining for the patient. The actual length of the patient's life remains uncertain. This chapter presents a method for representing the uncertainty in the outcomes of processes that play out over time. We will use a model first described in the nineteenth century by the Russian mathematician, Andrey Markov.

We will start with Markov models – a standard tool for representing gambles that unfold over time. We will see that analysts use Markov models when a decision problem is too complex to be represented accurately by a decision tree. Then, we will build on the insights provided by the Markov model to present a mathematical model of survival known as the *exponential survival model*.

7.1 Markov model basics

Markov models represent the patient's future as a series of transitions between health states. Each health state represents a well-defined stage in the progression of the patient's condition. For example, a Markov model of breast cancer treatment might include health states labeled "Symptom Free" and "Systemic Relapse." Two health states can be connected by a link corresponding to the possibility that the patient's condition will progress from one state to the other. A fixed time period, such as a month or year, is picked for the model. The probability associated with a link measures the likelihood that the corresponding health state transition will have occurred by the end of that time period.

Medical Decision Making, Second Edition. Harold C. Sox, Michael C. Higgins and Douglas K. Owens.
© 2013 John Wiley & Sons, Ltd. Published 2013 by John Wiley & Sons, Ltd.

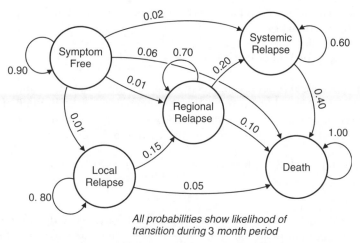

All probabilities show likelihood of
transition during 3 month period

Figure 7.1 Simplified Markov model of postoperative breast cancer survival.

Figure 7.1 shows a simplified Markov model of postoperative survival after breast cancer surgery.[1] This model assumes that the patient is symptom free after completion of her operation. This means that the patient starts in the state labeled "Symptom Free." The transition probabilities shown in Figure 7.1 are based on a three-month time period. For example, the probability of 0.02 on the link between the "Symptom Free" state and the "Systemic Relapse" state indicates that during a three-month period 2% of the asymptomatic patients will develop a systemic relapse. Techniques for determining the transition probabilities used in a Markov model are discussed later in this section.

It is important to note that when we talk about life expectancy for the patient in a Markov model, we mean the patient's life expectancy starting with the patient's entry into the situation represented by the model. As noted earlier, a Markov model represents what happens to the patient in the future. Therefore, the life expectancy equals the patient's age when entering the model plus the average time spent in the model before reaching the final health state. In this chapter we focus on determining the life expectancy for the remainder of the patient's life with the understanding that the true life expectancy is the patient's age plus the life expectancy implied by the model.

Notice that the Markov model in Figure 7.1 includes links representing the possibility that a patient will remain in the same health state. For example, the probability is 0.90 that an asymptomatic patient will still be asymptomatic at the end of a three-month period. This is called the *survival probability* for the "Symptom Free" state since it measures the likelihood of remaining in

---

[1] The probabilities shown in Figure 7.1 are not derived from the medical literature. They are chosen to illustrate the methodology rather than describe the actual disease.

that state. The survival probabilities are particularly important because of the following relationship:

$$\text{average time spent in health state} = \frac{1}{1 - \text{survival probability}} \qquad (7.1)$$

(the mathematical proof for this relationship can be found in the appendix to this chapter). Note that since the average time is expressed in units of time, the survival probability is expressed as 1 over that time unit. For example, in Figure 7.1, the average time spent in the "Symptom Free" state is

$$\text{average time spent Symptom Free} = \frac{1}{0.1/\text{quarter}} = 10.0 \text{ quarters}$$

$$= 30 \text{ months} \qquad (7.2)$$

Later in this section we will see that Equation 7.1 is useful for determining the patient's overall life expectancy and for estimating the transition probabilities.

Notice that for any given health state, the sum of the transition probabilities leading away from that health state, plus the survival probability, equals 1. This is because the patient obviously must either move to another health state or else stay in the same in the health state. Also notice that death appears in this model as a health state for which the "survival" probability is 1. In other words, Markov models represent death as a trapping state from which there is no exit.

The simple Markov model shown in Figure 7.1 focuses on prognosis following the treatment of breast cancer. The recurrence of the cancer as a local, regional, or systemic relapse corresponds to transitions to health states with reduced survival probabilities. For example, the survival probability for the "Systemic Relapse" health state is 0.60 compared to a survival probability of 0.90 for the "Symptom Free" health state. The model also represents the progression of a local relapse to a regional relapse and the progression of a regional relapse into a systemic release.

The survival probability for the "Symptom Free" health state in Figure 7.1 quantifies the effectiveness of the treatment initially used to make the patient symptom free. The value of the survival probability increases with the effectiveness of the treatment. Therefore, the model could be used to analyze the impact of the initial treatment on the patient's life expectancy. However, this simple model ignores the treatments that might be used to manage a relapse.

The model has been revised in Figure 7.2 to show a revision that includes the management of a local relapse. This revision assumes that treatment of the local relapse lasts one time period (three months) and concludes with the patient either entering a "Controlled Local Relapse" health state or else progressing to the "Regional Relapse" health state. In other words, the probability of remaining in the "Local Relapse Treatment" health state for more than one time period is 0. The Markov model in Figure 7.2 assumes that a controlled local relapse will not progress to a regional relapse. If this assumption was not correct then a link would be added that would represent the possibility that the patient could change from the "Controlled Local

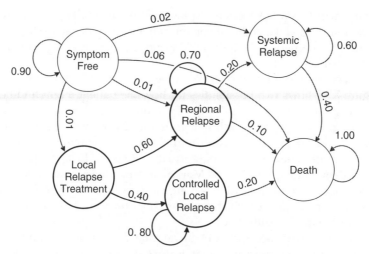

All probabilities show likelihood of
transition during 3 month period

Figure 7.2 Markov model of breast cancer with local relapse management.

Relapse" state to the "Regional Relapse" state. The point is that Markov models can be easily extended to represent a wide variety of assumptions about the patient's future. Markov modeling is a very flexible method for representing the dynamic nature of health care outcomes.

7.1.1 Markov Independence

Markov models are based on an independence assumption. We need to introduce some notation in order to fully describe this assumption. Let $S(k)$ denote the patient's health state at the beginning of time period k. For example, in the breast cancer model depicted in Figure 7.1, $S(1)$ is the "Symptom Free" health state because patients are assumed to start out symptom free. Suppose that the patient stayed symptom free for two time periods and then developed a local relapse. The values for $S(1)$, $S(2)$, and $S(3)$ would then be

$S(1) = $ Symptom Free

$S(2) = $ Symptom Free

$S(3) = $ Local Relapse

Given this notation, *Markov independence* can be stated formally as:

Markov independence

The process governing the transitions between health states has Markov independence if

$P[S(k)|S(1), \dots , S(k-1)] = P[S(k)|S(k-1)]$

In other words, Markov models assume that the patient's health state during the next time period depends only on the patient's current health state during the current time period. It does not depend on the path that brought the person to her current health state.

For example, notice that the Markov model in Figure 7.1 (and reproduced in Figure 7.3) shows two possibilities for how the patient might find herself in the "Regional Relapse" health state. First, the patient can progress directly to the "Regional Relapse" health state from the "Symptom Free" health state (labeled Path 1 in Figure 7.3). Second, the patient can first progress to the "Local Relapse" health state and then progress to the "Regional Relapse" health state (labeled Path 2 in Figure 7.3). The Markov independence assumption is that the probabilities for the transition leaving the "Regional Relapse" health state are the same regardless of which path describes how the patient reached the "Regional Relapse" health state.

Markov independence may not always be a realistic assumption. For example, breast cancer relapse that is first detected as a regional recurrence could be more aggressive than a relapse that is first detected as a local recurrence. In the former case, the survival probability once in the "Regional Relapse" health state would be lower than if the patient reached this health state after first being in the local recurrence state.

Fortunately, departures from Markov independence often can be addressed by adding health states to the model. Figure 7.4 shows how this can be done. Regional relapse is now represented by two health states: "Direct Regional Relapse" for progression directly from the "Symptom Free" health state and "Indirect Regional Relapse" for progression through the "Local Relapse" health state. Notice that the survival probability for the "Direct Regional

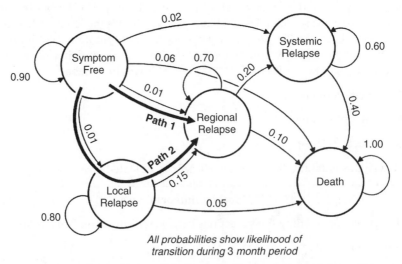

All probabilities show likelihood of transition during 3 month period

Figure 7.3 Paths to "Regional Relapse" health state in the breast cancer Markov model.

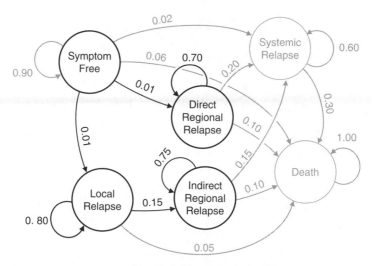

All probabilities show likelihood of
transition during 3 month period

Figure 7.4 Breast cancer model revised to assure Markov independence.

Relapse" health state (0.70) is less than the survival probability for the "Indirect
Regional Relapse" (0.75), indicating that the former has less favorable implications for the patient's prognosis. A similar refinement of the model would
be required if survival in the "Systemic Relapse" health state depends on how
the patient reached this health state. The resulting model is more complicated
to draw but the methods used to analyze Markov models still apply.

7.1.2 Estimating transition probabilities

While we can use the subjective assessment techniques discussed in Chapter 3
to estimate transition probabilities, this section will focus on estimating
probabilities from empirical observations. In a properly designed Markov
model, a transition probability quantifies the likelihood of an observable
event during a specified interval of time, such as the detection of a disease,
relapse after treatment, transition to greater disability, or death itself. As these
events occur in a cohort of patients, clinical observation provides an empirical
basis for estimating transition probabilities.

Perhaps the simplest empirical approaches are based on the relation between
the survival probability and the average time spent in a health state. Recalling
Equation 7.1,

$$\text{average time spent in health state} = \frac{1}{1 - \text{survival probability}} \qquad (7.3)$$

From this relationship, one can estimate the survival probability for a health
state by measuring the average time patients spend in that health state.

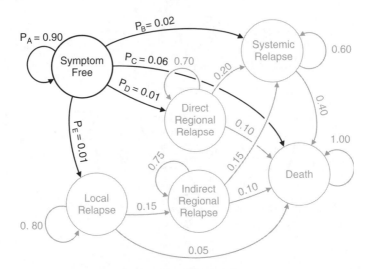

All probabilities show likelihood of
transition during 3 month period

Figure 7.5 Survival and transition probabilities for "Symptom Free" health state.

The other transition probabilities can be determined by recalling that for any given health state the survival probability plus the sum of the transition probabilities equals 1. That is,

$$\text{survival probability} + \sum \text{transition probabilities from health state} = 1 \quad (7.4)$$

For example, referring to the labels that we assign to the probabilities associated with the "Symptom Free" state in Figure 7.5, we can write

$$P_A + P_B + P_C + P_D + P_E = 1 \quad (7.5)$$

Knowing the survival probability (P_A) from measuring the average time spent in the "Symptom Free" health state and rearranging terms, we form an equation that will help us to estimate an unknown transition probability:

$$P_B + P_C + P_D + P_E = 1 - P_A \quad (7.6)$$

By definition, the sum on the left in Equation 7.6 measures the probability that the patient will leave the "Symptom Free" state during a three-month period. Ascertaining each of the transition probabilities is the problem of apportioning that sum between the four links leaving the "Symptom Free" health state. Picking one of the links, such as the link from the "Symptom Free" health state to the "Death" health state, we note that

$P[\text{Death} \mid \text{Patient leaves Symptom Free health state}]$

$$= \frac{P_C}{P_B + P_C + P_D + P_E} \quad (7.7)$$

For example, suppose the average postoperative breast cancer patient remains symptom free for 2.5 years, or 10 quarters. Using the labeling in Figure 6.21, this would imply that the survival probability is

$$P_A = 1 - \frac{1}{10} = 0.90 \qquad (7.8)$$

Suppose also that 60% of postoperative breast cancer patients die from other causes without ever experiencing a relapse of their breast cancer. Then from Equation 6.31 we can write

$$0.60 = \frac{P_C}{P_B + P_C + P_D + P_E} = \frac{P_C}{1 - P_A} = \frac{P_C}{0.10} \qquad (7.9)$$

Or, rearranging terms, the survival probability for the "Symptom Free" health state is

$$P_C = 0.60 \times 0.10 = 0.06 \qquad (7.10)$$

Similar calculation-based observations about the relative frequencies of systemic, regional, and local relapses would be used to determine the other transition probabilities.

7.1.3 Age-adjusted survival probabilities

One of the challenges in determining survival probabilities is the usual age mismatch between the patient of interest and the patients included in a study reporting survival statistics. We can use the simple two-state Markov model shown in Figure 7.6 to correct for age differences.

As an example, consider the problem of modeling the progression of leukemia in a 50-year-old male patient and suppose that we have access to a large study in which the average age of male leukemia patients is 33 years. Assume that the annual survival rate in that population is 0.550. We could use this survival rate as the value for p in Figure 7.6, except that it is the survival rate for 30-year-old males rather than 50-year-old males. Patients with the diagnosis of leukemia may face roughly the same annual mortality rates from leukemia regardless of age. However, the annual mortality rates from other causes do vary significantly with age, as shown in Figure 7.7.

We can use the survival rate from the hypothetical leukemia study of 33-year-old men and the age-adjusted annual mortality rates (Figure 7.7) to draw the three-state Markov model for 30-year-old patients shown in Figure 7.8. The survival probability of 0.550 for the "Alive" health state is taken from

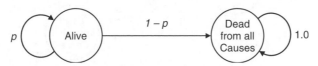

Figure 7.6 Simple two-state Markov model.

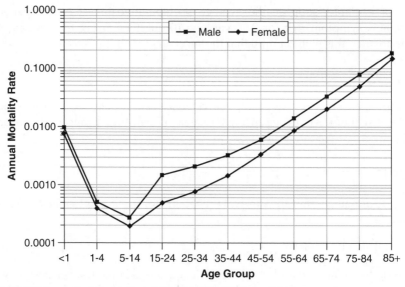

Figure 7.7 Age-adjusted annual mortality rate (1993 US Census data).

the hypothetical study. The transition probability (0.002) for the link between the "Alive" health state and the "Dead from other Causes" health state is taken from the curve in Figure 7.7. As noted in Equation 7.4, the survival probability and the transition probabilities must sum to 1. Therefore, the transition probability (0.448) for the link between the "Alive" health state and the "Dead from Leukemia" health state is given by

$$0.448 = 1 - 0.550 - 0.002 \tag{7.11}$$

Figure 7.9 shows the same three-state model for the 50-year-old male patient. We assume that patients with the diagnosis of leukemia face roughly the same annual mortality rate from leukemia regardless of age. Therefore,

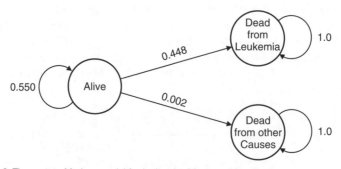

Figure 7.8 Three-state Markov model for leukemia, 30-year-old patient.

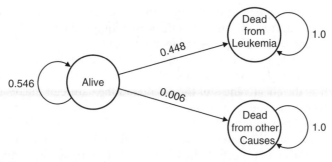

Figure 7.9 Three-state Markov model for leukemia, 50-year-old patient.

the transition probability (0.448) for the link from the "Alive" health state to the "Dead from Leukemia" health state is unchanged. The higher transition probability of 0.006 for the link between the "Alive" health state and the "Dead from other Causes" health state is taken from the curve in Figure 7.7. Finally, the survival probability (0.546) is determined by the applying the relationship in Equation 7.4:

$$0.546 = 1 - 0.448 - 0.006 \tag{7.12}$$

We must observe two caveats when using this approach to compute age-adjusted mortality rates. The first is actuarial. The annual mortality rates shown in Figure 7.7 include deaths from leukemia. Therefore, the transition probabilities in Figures 7.8 and 7.9 for the link to the "Dead from other Causes" actually include leukemia deaths. However, leukemia is a relatively rare cause of death, accounting for less than 0.5% of the deaths recorded by the Centers for Disease Control (CDC). Therefore, leukemia deaths have a negligible effect on the transition probabilities shown in Figures 7.8 and 7.9. The effect would not be negligible if the disease in question were more common. For example, cardiovascular disease causes almost 30% of the deaths recorded in the United States. Determining the age-adjusted mortality rates for more common diseases requires mortality rates that exclude the disease in question. Actuarial data from sources like the CDC usually allows the exclusion of specific diseases when computing mortality rates.

The second caveat is medical in nature and more difficult to address. Our age adjustment method assumes that the effect of age on total mortality is entirely contained in the risk of death from other causes. In other words, the models in Figures 7.8 and 7.9 assume that a 30-year-old leukemia patient faces the same risk of dying from leukemia during the next year as the 50-year-old leukemia patient. This assumption may be reasonable when comparing 30 year olds and 50 year olds, but it would not be reasonable when comparing 30 years olds and 90 year olds. Advanced age often changes how patients react to a disease like leukemia; they are more likely to die of complications of treatment, for example, because they are simply more fragile. The changes of advanced age can translate into different age-adjusted mortality rates from the disease itself. Age adjustment in this case requires data from studies that include patients with ages in the range of interest.

Markov models are valuable to clinical decision analysis because they can reveal the relationship between the patient's life expectancy and considerations such as the effectiveness of treatment and the nature of the disease as it evolves over time. The next two sections describe how life expectancies are computed for Markov models.

We describe two different approaches. The first applies to relatively simple models like those that illustrate this chapter. This approach is similar to the tree folding algorithm discussed in Section 6.9. We use the second approach for larger and more complicated Markov models. For example, later chapters in this book use Markov models to analyze policy questions. These models involve large numbers of health states and use complex processes to determine the transition probabilities. The second method uses an algorithm called Monte Carlo simulation to determine the life expectancy for a patient faced with the clinical situation represented in a Markov model.

7.1.4 Determining life expectancy for time-invariant acyclic Markov models

The Markov models that illustrate the following discussion have two properties that allow us to determine life expectancy directly from the model. First, the transition probabilities remain constant over time. For example, referring to Figure 7.10, we assume that the survival probability for asymptomatic patients (0.90) remains constant for the rest of the patients' life. We call Markov models with this property *time invariant*. Second, once the patient leaves a health state she will never return to that health state (Figure 7.10). We call Markov models with this property, *acyclic*.

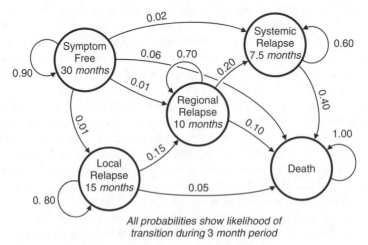

All probabilities show likelihood of
transition during 3 month period

Figure 7.10 Breast cancer Markov model showing average stay in each health state.

Life expectancy can be determined for time-invariant acyclic Markov models by determining two properties of the model: (1) the average time a patient will spend in each health state once the patient enters that health state; and (2) the probabilities that the patient enters each of the health states. As we noted in Equation 7.1, the average time spent in a health state can be determined from the survival probability for that health state:

$$\text{average time spent in health state} = \frac{1}{1 - \text{survival probability}} \qquad (7.13)$$

For example, the average stay in the "Regional Relapse" health state in Figure 7.10 is

$$\text{average stay in Regional Relapse} = \frac{1}{0.3/\text{quarter}} = 3.3 \text{ quarters}$$
$$= 10 \text{ months} \qquad (7.14)$$

The average stay for each of the health states has been added to the simple breast cancer Markov model in Figure 7.10.

Now we will compute the patient's overall life expectancy for each of the relapse health states. For example, as shown in Figure 7.11, once the "Systemic Relapse" health state is reached, the patient's life expectancy for the remainder of her life is determined entirely by how long she remains in this health state. Therefore, the life expectancy for the "Systemic Relapse" health state is simply 7.5 years. This is because the model assumes that the patient only leaves the "System Relapse" health state when she dies.

The same is not true for the "Regional Relapse" health state. Referring to Figure 7.12, some of the patients leave this health state by dying. However,

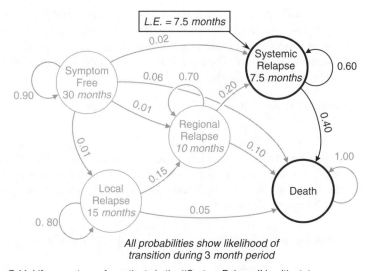

All probabilities show likelihood of transition during 3 month period

Figure 7.11 Life expectancy for patients in the "System Relapse" health state.

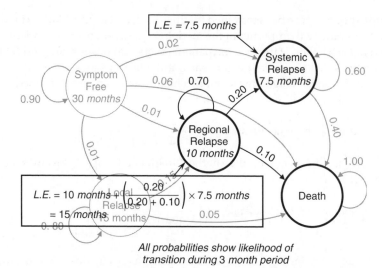

Figure 7.12 Life expectancy for patients in the "Regional Relapse" health state.

others leave it by developing a systemic relapse. According to the Markov model, in each time period 30% of the patients leave this state, either by dying or by progressing to a systemic relapse. Moreover, twice as many of those patients will develop a systemic relapse as will die. Therefore,

$$P[\text{Systemic Relapse} \mid \text{Patient leaves Regional Relapse}] = \frac{0.20}{0.10 + 0.20}$$

$$= 0.67 \qquad (7.15)$$

Therefore, the probability is 0.67 that a patient in the "Regional Relapse" health state will reach the "Systemic Relapse" health state. Once in the "Systemic Relapse" health state the patient has a life expectancy of 7.5 months, as we determined earlier. Therefore, the overall life expectancy for a patient in the "Regional Relapse" health state is

$$LE \text{ for Regional Relapse} = 10 \text{ months} + 0.67 \times 7.5 \text{ months}$$

$$= 15 \text{ months} \qquad (7.16)$$

Figure 7.13 shows the life expectancy calculation for the "Local Relapse" health state. The model assumes that patients leave this state either by dying or by developing a regional relapse. Therefore, the life expectancy for a patient in the "Local Relapse" health state is

$$LE \text{ for Local Relapse} = 15 \text{ months} + \left(\frac{0.15}{0.15 + 0.05} \right) \times 15 \text{ months}$$

$$= 26.3 \text{ months} \qquad (7.17)$$

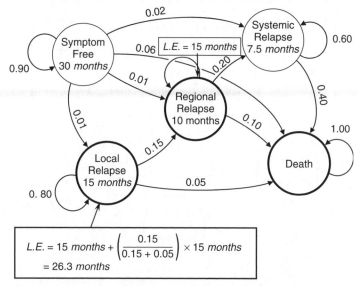

Figure 7.13 Life expectancy for patients in the "Local Relapse" health state.

Finally, Figure 7.14 shows the life expectancy calculation for the "Symptom Free" health state. For this health state, the patient can move to three possible health states other than death: "Local Relapse," "Regional Relapse," and "Systemic Relapse." Therefore, life expectancy is given by the following calculation:

LE for Symptom Free = 30 months

$$+ \left(\frac{0.02}{0.01 + 0.01 + 0.06 + 0.02} \right) \times 7.5 \text{ months}$$

$$+ \left(\frac{0.01}{0.01 + 0.01 + 0.06 + 0.02} \right) \times 15.0 \text{ months}$$

$$+ \left(\frac{0.01}{0.01 + 0.01 + 0.06 + 0.02} \right) \times 26.3 \text{ months}$$

$$= 35.6 \text{ months} \tag{7.18}$$

The method illustrated for this simple Markov model can be extended to more complicated models provided that probabilities remain constant and no paths are added that would return the patient to a health state after it has been left. The requirement that the Markov model be acyclic often can be satisfied by adding health states, like we did in Section 7.2.1, in order to satisfy the Markov independence assumption. Time invariance can be a more difficult requirement to satisfy. When assuming that the transition probabilities are constant is not reasonable, the following method can be used to determine the life expectancy for a Markov model.

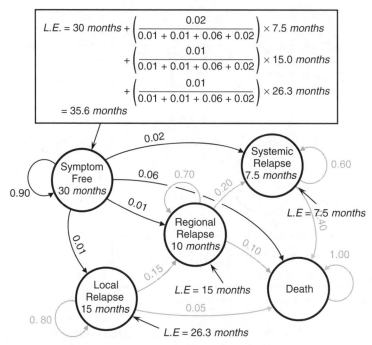

$$L.E. = 30 \text{ months} + \left(\frac{0.02}{0.01 + 0.01 + 0.06 + 0.02} \right) \times 7.5 \text{ months}$$

$$+ \left(\frac{0.01}{0.01 + 0.01 + 0.06 + 0.02} \right) \times 15.0 \text{ months}$$

$$+ \left(\frac{0.01}{0.01 + 0.01 + 0.06 + 0.02} \right) \times 26.3 \text{ months}$$

$$= 35.6 \text{ months}$$

Figure 7.14 Life expectancy for patients in the "Symptom Free" health state.

7.1.5   Determining life expectancy by Monte Carlo simulation

Complicated Markov models typically are analyzed using an algorithm called Monte Carlo simulation. The mathematician John von Neumann was the first person to describe this algorithm (we will see another of von Neumann's contributions in the next chapter). Monte Carlo simulation uses the transition probabilities in a Markov model to randomly generate a large sample of possible paths through the model, each ending with death. Because the algorithm uses the transition probabilities to generate these paths, the prevalence of a particular path in the sample is proportional to the probability that the patient will experience that path in the clinical situation represented by the Markov model. Therefore, averaging the length of the generated paths produces an estimate for the patient's life expectancy. As with any sampling method, the accuracy and precision of the estimate increases with the number of generated paths. However, unlike the challenges in increasing the sample size for a clinical trial, increasing the sample size for a Monte Carlo simulation only requires that a computer program runs longer.

We will use our simplified Markov model for breast cancer to illustrate this process. This Markov model has been redrawn in Figure 7.15. Our assumption is that the patient begins in the "Symptom Free" health state, which is labeled "A" for "Asymptomatic" in Figure 7.15. Therefore, the first step in the algorithm is to determine the patient's health state at the end of the first time period. The algorithm does this by generating a uniformly distributed random number between 0 and 1. By "uniformly distributed" we mean that

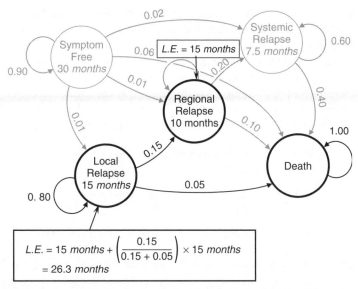

Figure 7.15 Breast cancer Markov model used to illustrate Monte Carlo simulation.

all possible values between 0 and 1 are equally likely. Let X_1 denote this first random number. Because we defined the range of the distribution to lie between 0 and 1, the probability is 1 that X_1 is between 0 and 1. Since X_1 is uniformly distributed, for some number p that is greater than 0 and less than 1, the probability that the value for X_1 falls between 0 and P also equals p. In particular, if p is the survival probability (0.90) for the "Symptom Free" health state, the probability that the random number X_1 is between 0 and X_1 equals the probability that the patient remains in the "Symptom Free" health state. Therefore, the Monte Carlo simulation algorithm decides that the patient remains in the "Symptom Free" health state according to the following rule:

If $0.00 \leq X_1 \leq 0.90$ then health state for first time period is Symtom Free

(7.19)

Similarly, the algorithm decides if the patient moves to one of the other health states according to the rules

If $0.90 < X_1 \leq 0.91$ then health state for first time period is *Local Relapse*

(7.20)

If $0.91 < X_1 \leq 0.92$ then health state for first time period is
Regional Relapse (7.21)

If $0.92 < X_1 \leq 0.94$ then health state for first time period is
Systemic Relapse (7.22)

If $0.94 < X_1 \leq 1.00$ then health state for first time period is *Death* (7.23)

Suppose, for example, that X_1 is equal to 0.915 802 693 732 358. The algorithm would decide that the patient is in the "Regional Relapse" health state for the first time period.

The first time period is now over, and the patient is in the "Regional Relapse" health state. What will happen in the second time period? The algorithm then picks a second random number X_2, also uniformly distributed between 0 and 1, and applies the same logic as above, except that the algorithm would use the transition probabilities for the "Regional Relapse" health state:

If $0.00 \leq X_2 \leq 0.70$ then health state for second time period is
$$\text{Regional Relapse} \tag{7.24}$$

If $0.70 < X_2 \leq 0.90$ then health state for second time period is
$$\text{Systemic Relapse} \tag{7.25}$$

If $0.90 < X_2 \leq 1.00$ then health state for second time period is Death $\quad$ (7.26)

For example, the algorithm would decide that the patient remains in the "Regional Relapse" health state for the second time period if X_2 is equal to 0.492 226 024 091 847. The second time period is over, and the patient is still in the "Regional Relapse" health state. To represent what happens in the third time period, the algorithm chooses a third random number X_3 using the same criteria as shown in Equations 7.24 to 7.26 (because the patient is still in the "Regional Relapse" health state). If X_3 equals 0.946 212 071 913 374, the patient would enter the "Death" health state, and the path would conclude. The entire path for this example would then be

Period 1 : Regional Relapse

Period 2 : Regional Relapse

A Monte Carlo simulation uses this approach to generate a large number of paths for the Markov model. Table 7.1 lists 10 of the paths generated by a Monte Carlo simulation of the example used in this section. The health states occupied during a time period are represented by the letters assigned to each state in Figure 7.15.

Continuing the simulation for 100 paths through the model yields a sample for which the average length of life is 11.92 quarters (or 35.8 months), with a 95% confidence interval of ± 0.12 quarters (or 0.35 months). This result agrees with a life expectancy of 12 quarters (or 36 months) that we calculated in the previous section for this Markov model.

Monte Carlo simulation is a powerful method because it can be applied to models with large numbers of health states. Monte Carlo simulation also can be used to analyze models that have cyclic paths. Figure 7.16 is an example of a cyclic model. It shows a simple three-state Markov model for a hypothetical disease in which the patient alternates between a "Well" health state and a "Sick" health state. Notice that the chance of death is 10 times as high when

Table 7.1 Ten paths generated by Monte Carlo simulation of Markov model in Figure 7.15.

	Path*	Length of life
1	AAAAAAAAAAAAAAAAAAAA	20 quarters
2	AAAAAAAAAAAAAAAAAAAAAAAAAAAAAAAAAAASS	37 quarters
3	AAAAAAAAAAAAAAAA	16 quarters
4	AA	2 quarters
5	SSS	3 quarters
6	AAAAAALLRRRRRSSSS	18 quarters
7	AALRRRS	7 quarters
8	AAAAAAAAAAAAAAAAAAAAAAAAAAAAAA	30 quarters
9	AAAAAAAAAAA	11 quarters
10	AAAAAAAAARS	11 quarters

*"A" = Symptom Free, "L" = Local Relapse, "R" = Regional Relapse, "S" = Systemic Relapse.

the patient is in the "Sick" health state (0.20 versus 0.02). The model assumes that a patient in the "Sick" health state continues to face this elevated risk until the patient recovers and returns to the "Well" health state. A Monte Carlo simulation generating 1000 paths estimates the patient's average length of life (life expectancy) to be 13.8 time periods, with a 95% interval of ±0.05 time periods.

The simple three-state model in Figure 7.16 can be used to explore different management strategies for this hypothetical disease. For example, suppose that a preventive strategy (say stopping smoking) could halve the probability of changing from "Well" to "Sick" – that is, changing from 0.20 to 0.10. A Monte Carlo simulation of this preventive strategy estimates that the patient's life expectancy would increase to 20.2 time periods – an increase of 6.4 time periods. Another strategy might be to use a treatment that would increase the probability that a patient in the "Sick" health state will change back to the

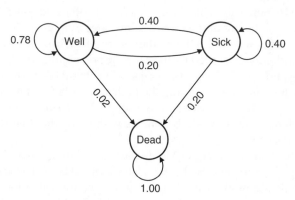

Figure 7.16 Three-state Markov model.

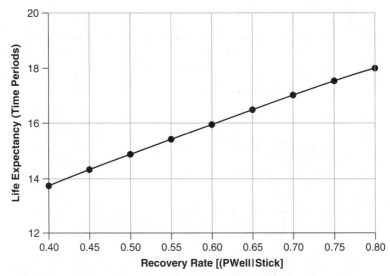

Figure 7.17 Life expectancy versus recovery rate for the three-state Markov model.

"Well" health state in a time period – what we might call the *recovery rate*. In Figure 7.16 this transition probability is 0.40. By using Monte Carlo simulation for models with different values for the transition probability from "Sick" to "Well", we can see the possible impact of this second strategy. The results are shown in Figure 7.17.

This chapter focuses on life expectancy. Accordingly the discussion of Markov models and Monte Carlo simulation has been limited to the use of these tools in determining this single measure of the patient's outcome. In reality these powerful tools can answer a broader range of questions since the paths generated by the Monte Carlo simulation represent the *type* of outcomes that the patient will experience as well as the length of time that the patient spends in a health state.

For example, notice in Table 7.1 that paths 1, 3, 4, 8, and 9 end without the patient moving into any of the three health states involving a relapse. These represent patients who die without the return of their breast cancer. In the 100 paths randomly generated by the Monte Carlo simulation, 59 (or 59%) of the paths did not involve any of the relapse health states. Some of the paths were only a few time periods long; the patient died before her cancer could relapse. This observation illustrates the concept of *competing causes of mortality*. In effect, different causes of death compete with each other to be the cause of an individual's death.

Finally, the other advantage of Monte Carlo simulation is that the transition probabilities do not have to be held constant. The analyst can use any suitable prediction model (see Chapter 3) to vary the value for a transition probability during a simulation. For example, holding the survival probability for the "Symptom Free" health state constant is equivalent to assuming that mortality rates do not change as the patient changes. However, as was clearly evident back in Figure 7.7, mortality rates do increase with age. Therefore, a more realistic Markov model would vary the survival probabilities as the patient's age increases during a generated path. The power of Monte Carlo simulation is that it allows the analyst to incorporate details like this into the model, which increases the fidelity of the simulation accordingly.

7.2 Exponential survival model and life expectancy

The analysis of life expectancy ultimately is the study of factors that put the patient's life at risk. In the decision tree analysis of Hank's decision problem, those factors are represented by the chance nodes for the risks resulting from the extent of his disease and the effectiveness of his treatments. Markov models represent risks by the probabilities for the transitions that move the patient toward that final trapping state we call death. This section describes another widely used method for representing risk based on what is called the *exponential survival model*. The following is a formal definition of the exponential survival model:

Exponential survival model

The remaining length of a patient's life (x) can be described by the exponential survival model if

$P[\text{Remaining length of life} > x] = e^{-\lambda x}$

where the parameter λ is such that $1/\lambda$ is the expected value for the remaining length of life.

(7.27)

Note that the units for λ are 1/time. The graph in Figure 7.18 shows the exponential survival model when $1/\lambda$ equals 1.5 years.

Figure 7.'8 Exponential survival model with $1/\lambda = 1.5$ years.

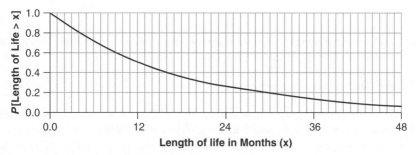

Figure 7.18 Exponential Survival Model with $1/\lambda = 1.5$ years.

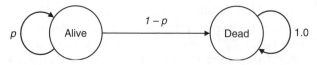

Figure 7.19 Simple two-state Markov model with constant survival probability.

We will now use the simple two-state Markov model shown in Figure 7.19 to understand the properties of the exponential survival model. In the case of the Markov model, the likelihood that the patient survives a fixed-length time period is represented by the constant survival probability, denoted p in the simple two-state Markov model shown in Figure 7.19. We will see that the exponential survival model implies a constant survival probability except that we allow the length of the time period in the Markov model in Figure 7.19 to be arbitrarily short. In other words, the exponential survival model is a Markov model with a continuous rather than discrete view of time.

We will start this demonstration by deriving the survival function for the Markov model in Figure 7.19. This survival function will determine the probability that the patient is still alive after a given number of time periods. Note that in order for the patient to be alive at the beginning of the nth time period, the patient must be alive at the beginning of the $(n-1)$st time period and not die during this time period. That is,

$$P[\text{Length of life} > n \text{ time periods}]$$
$$= p \times P[\text{Length of life} > n - 1 \text{ time periods}] \tag{7.28}$$

Since the patient starts out alive we have that

$$P[\text{Length of life} > 0 \text{ time periods}] = 1 \tag{7.29}$$

Combining Equations 7.28 and 7.29 we can then write

$$P[\text{Length of life} > 1 \text{ time period}] = p \times 1 = p \tag{7.30}$$
$$P[\text{Length of life} > 2 \text{ time periods}] = p \times p = p^2 \tag{7.31}$$

$$\vdots$$

and so forth. In general, the probability of surviving at least n time periods in the two-state Markov model is given by

$$P[\text{Length of life} > n \text{ time periods}] = p^n \tag{7.32}$$

In the top graph in Figure 7.20, we have plotted this relationship when we set the time period to be one year and the survival probability p to be 0.33/year. The other graphs in Figure 7.20 show the same relationship for models with the same life expectancy but shorter time periods. By holding the life

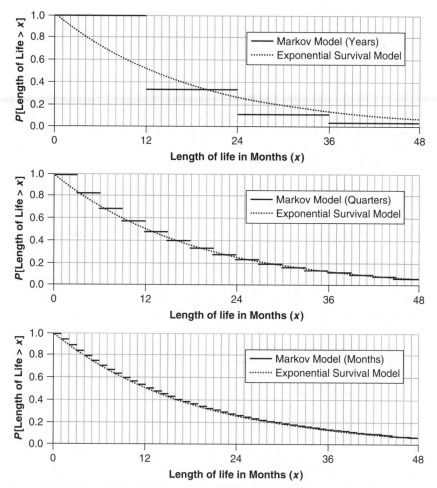

Figure 7.20 Markov model with different time periods and exponential survival model.

expectancy constant we are using Markov models that are equivalent from the patient's perspective.

Recall from Equation 7.1 that

$$\text{life expectancy in two-state model} = \frac{1}{1 - \text{survival probability}} \tag{7.33}$$

Therefore, the top graph in Figure 7.20 plots the survival curve for a Markov model with a life expectancy of

$$\text{life expectancy in two-state model} = \frac{1}{1 - 0.33/\text{year}} = 1.5 \text{ years} \tag{7.34}$$

The middle graph in Figure 7.20 plots the survival curve for a similar Markov model in which the patient faces the same life expectancy of 1.5 years except that now the time period has been shortened from one year to one quarter. Solving for the survival probability in Equation 7.33, we see that for this second Markov model the survival probability (p in Figure 7.19) is given by

$$\text{survival probability} = 1 - \frac{1}{1.5 \text{ years}} = 1 - \frac{1}{6 \text{ quarters}} = 0.83/\text{quarter} \quad (7.35)$$

Similarly the bottom graph in Figure 7.20 plots the survival curve for a Markov model in which the patient still faces a life expectancy of 1.5 years except that now the time period has been shortened to one month. The survival probability for this third Markov model is

$$\text{survival probability} = 1 - \frac{1}{1.5 \text{ years}} = 1 - \frac{1}{18 \text{ months}} = 0.94/\text{month} \quad (7.36)$$

Therefore, the survival curves in Figure 7.20 describe three Markov models that are equivalent in that they all correspond to the same life expectancy of 1.5 years for the patient. The reason for drawing these three curves is to note that they converge toward the same smooth curve as the length of the time period decreases. In fact, the Markov model survival curves converge to an exponential survival model with the same life expectancy of 1.5 years. That exponential survival model is shown as a dotted line that plots Equation 7.27 for $1/\lambda$ equal to 1.5 years in each of the three graphs.

So the exponential survival model can be thought of as a type of Markov model. This means that some of the same types of analysis demonstrated for Markov models earlier in this chapter can also be performed with the exponential survival model.

For example, recall the discussion of age-adjusted survival probabilities in Section 7.2.3. Figure 7.21 reproduces one of the figures used in that discussion of how different causes of death contribute to the life expectancy of a 50-year-old patient with leukemia.

Using the same hypothetical transition probabilities as before, let

$$P[\text{Death from leukemia}] = p_{\text{Leukemia}} = 0.448/\text{year} \quad (7.37)$$

$$P[\text{Death from other causes}] = p_{\text{Other}} = 0.006/\text{year} \quad (7.38)$$

From the definition of the Markov model in Figure 7.21 we have that

$$\text{survival probability} + p_{\text{Leukemia}} + p_{\text{Other}} = 1 \quad (7.39)$$

Therefore, from Equation 7.33,

$$\text{life expectancy} = \frac{1}{1 - \text{survival probability}} = \frac{1}{p_{\text{Leukemia}} + p_{\text{Other}}} \quad (7.40)$$

In other words, in the Markov model, the transition probabilities $p_{\text{Leukemia}} + p_{\text{Other}}$ can be combined to determine the patient's life expectancy.

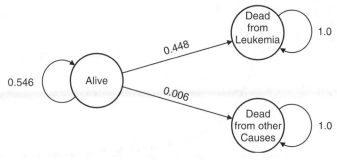

Figure 7.21 Three-state Markov model for leukemia, 50-year-old patient.

The important relationship demonstrated in Equation 7.40 has an equally important parallel in the exponential model. In order to see this parallel let $\lambda_{\text{Leukemia}}$ denote the parameter for an exponential survival model in a population of patients who eventually die from leukemia. Similarly, let λ_{Other} denote the parameter for an exponential survival model in a population of patients who eventually die from other causes. The exponential survival model for patients dying from all causes is

$$P[\text{Remaining length of life} > x] = e^{-(\lambda_{\text{Leukemia}} + \lambda_{\text{Other}})x} \tag{7.41}$$

The life expectancy for patients facing the risk described by the model in Equation 7.41 is given by

$$\text{life expectancy} = \frac{1}{\lambda_{\text{Leukemia}} + \lambda_{\text{Other}}} \tag{7.42}$$

In other words, the model parameters in the exponential survival model can be summed to determine the life expectancy, just as the probabilities of deaths from various causes can be summed in the Markov model to determine life expectancy. The useful relationship illustrated in Equation 7.42 was given the name *Declining Exponential Approximation for Life Expectancy* or DEALE when J. Robert Beck, Jerome P. Kassirer, and Stephen G. Pauker introduced it to the medical decision-making community.

As the letter "A" in the name acknowledges, DEALE analysis is based on an approximation. It is an approximation because DEALE applies only if the patient's mortality rate is constant (i.e., does not change for the remainder of the patient's life). Recalling the annual mortality rate curves in Figure 7.7, this assumption is not true when viewed over the entire span of a normal lifetime. However, in the context of cancers and other aggressive threats to the patient's survival, the changes in the age-dependent mortality rate over time usually can be ignored. The grim reality is that patients with aggressive fatal diseases seldom live long enough to face the age-dependent changes in their mortality rates. For example, referring to the transition probabilities shown

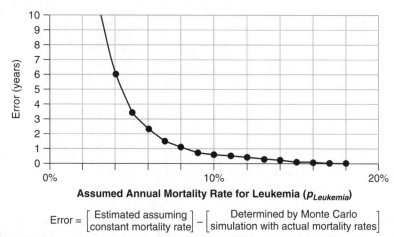

$$\text{Error} = \begin{bmatrix} \text{Estimated assuming} \\ \text{constant mortality rate} \end{bmatrix} - \begin{bmatrix} \text{Determined by Monte Carlo} \\ \text{simulation with actual mortality rates} \end{bmatrix}$$

Figure 7.22 Error for exponential survival model of leukemia, 50-year-old male patient.

in Figure 7.21, the risk to the patient's survival due to leukemia is 100 times greater than the risk from other causes.

Figure 7.22 graphs the error resulting from holding the mortality rate for other causes (p_{Other}) constant as the patient ages, given different assumed mortality rates for leukemia (p_{Leukemia}). Error for the constant mortality rate model is measured relative to a model that varies the mortality rate from other causes according to the values shown in Figure 7.7, starting with the annual mortality rate for 50-year-old males. Both models were evaluated using Monte Carlo simulation. Note that the constant mortality rate model overestimates life expectancy because it ignores the increased mortality rate faced as the patient ages. On the other hand, the error is less than a year once the annual mortality rate for leukemia is greater than 10%. The error is too small to be represented by Monte Carlo simulation, once the annual mortality rate for leukemia reaches 20%.

Indeed, the exponential survival model often provides a good fit to actual survival data. The comparison shown in Figure 7.23 is a typical example. This graph compares the exponential survival model and observed survival rates for 1103 Stage IV prostate cancer patients, as published by the Veterans Administration Cooperative Urological Research Group (1968).

The data in Figure 7.23 can be used to illustrate how to fit an exponential survival model to survival rate data. The goal is to determine the parameter λ so that the following equation matches the data:

$$P[\text{Survive until time } x] = e^{-\lambda x} \tag{7.43}$$

Taking the natural logarithm of both sides of Equation 7.43 yields

$$\ln(P[\text{Survive until time } x]) = \ln(e^{-\lambda x}) = -\lambda x \tag{7.44}$$

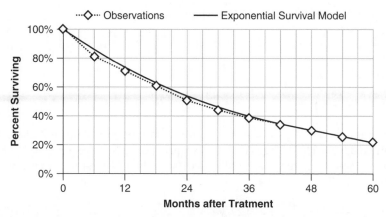

Figure 7.23 Exponential survival model fit to Stage IV prostate cancer data.

Therefore, the natural logarithm of the observed survival rate varies in proportion to the length of life (x). The constant of proportionality is $-\lambda$. Figure 7.24 illustrates this approach by graphing the logarithm of the survival rates shown in Figure 7.23.

Equation 7.44 provides a simple approach to determining the parameter λ from observational data. Suppose that a study lasting x years started with s_0 patients and reported that s_N patients were alive at the end of the study. The survival probability would then be

$$P[\text{Survive until time } x] = \frac{s_N}{s_0} \tag{7.45}$$

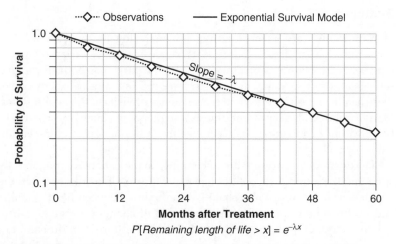

$$P[\text{Remaining length of life} > x] = e^{-\lambda x}$$

Figure 7.24 Fitting exponential survival model to survival data shown in Figure 7.23.

Therefore, from Equation 7.44 we have that

$$\ln\left(\frac{s_N}{s_0}\right) = -\lambda x \qquad (7.46)$$

Or solving for λ

$$\lambda = -\frac{1}{x}\ln\left(\frac{s_N}{s_0}\right) \qquad (7.47)$$

For example, the VA Cooperative Study data plotted in Figure 7.23 started with 1103 ($s_0 = 1103$) Stage IV prostate cancer patients. At year 5 ($x = 5$ years), 259 of those patients were still alive ($s_N = 259$). Therefore, according to Equation 7.47,

$$\lambda = -\frac{1}{5\ \text{years}}\ln\left(\frac{259}{1103}\right) = 0.29/\text{year} \qquad (7.48)$$

The shortcoming of Equation 7.47 is its sensitivity to any statistical anomalies that might have occurred at year 5 of the study. For example, suppose that the fifth anniversary coincided with the peak of the flu season. That coincidence would artificially reduce the observed survival rate, which, in turn, would distort the estimation of λ.

A more reliable method for estimating the parameter λ is based on linear regression techniques, applied to all of the data, rather just a single data point like the final survival rate. As we saw in Equation 7.44, the exponential survival curve becomes a straight line when the natural logarithms of the survival rates are plotted. Moreover, Equation 7.44 shows that the slope of that straight line is $-\lambda$. Linear regression techniques can be used to determine the straight line that best fits the logarithmic plot of the survival data. Figure 7.24 illustrates this approach. The details are described in the appendix to this chapter.

Summary

Markov models are a versatile tool for analyzing the uncertainty in a process, such as an illness, that runs its course over time. A Markov model represents the possible outcomes faced by the patient as paths through a set of health states. At any moment in time, the patient is in exactly one of these health states. An outcome is a sequence of visits to the health states. Markov models also represent time as a sequence of equal-length periods. By convention, transitions between health states only occur at the end of a time period.

Markov models represent the uncertainty in the patient's experience by assigning transition probabilities to each of the possible links between the health states. A transition probability on the link between health state A and health state B quantifies the likelihood of changing from A to B in a time period. One minus the sum of all possible transition probabilities from a health state equals the probability that the patient will remain in that health state at the end of a time period. The probability of remaining in a health state is called the *survival probability* for that health state. Survival probabilities are particularly interesting because 1 divided by the survival probability for a health state equals the average length of stay in that health state.

The fundamental assumption of Markov modeling is that the probability of a transition to any given health state at the end of a time period depends only on the current health state – and not on the sequence of health states experienced prior to reaching the current health state. This assumption is called *Markov independence*.

This chapter described an algorithm that calculates the patient's life expectancy when the Markov model is acyclic, meaning that the patient cannot return to a health state after once leaving that health state. This algorithm determines life expectancy by combining the average length of stays for each health state with the probabilities for visiting each health state.

We described a more general approach to analyzing Markov models, based on an approach called Monte Carlo simulation. This method requires computer software to create the model, store the model's parameters, run the simulations, and compute results. The software randomly generates a large number of paths through the model, starting at the initial health state and concluding with death. The paths differ according to which state-to-state transitions occur and the number of time periods in a state before a transition from it occurs. The likelihood that a transition will happen in one of the simulated paths is determined by the corresponding transition probability in the model. Therefore, the likelihood that a path will be generated in the simulation matches the likelihood that the patient would experience the corresponding sequence of health states in real life. Life expectancy is the average length of the generated paths.

This chapter concluded with a discussion of exponential survival models. We can think of the exponential survival model as a Markov model with a very short time period. This model has a single parameter λ that measures the likelihood of death at any point in time. The important property of the exponential survival model is that life expectancy equals 1 over the model parameter. Moreover, the outcome for a patient facing multiple potential causes of death can be described in terms of separate exponential survival models for each possible cause of death. That patient's overall survival is then described by an exponential survival model with a parameter that is the sum of the parameters for those separate exponential survival models. Moreover, the model can describe the outcome for a patient facing multiple potential causes of death in terms of separate exponential survival models for each possible cause of death. The exponential survival model describes that patient's overall survival by a parameter that is the sum of the parameters for each of the exponential survival models for the causes of death. Moreover, the patient's life expectancy equals 1 over the sum of the model parameters for the individual possible causes of death. The name of this approach to estimating life expectancy is *Declining Exponential Approximation of Life Expectancy* or DEALE.

Problems

1. Figure 7.25 (copied from Figure 7.4 in Section 7.2.1) shows how to construct and modify the breast cancer Markov model in order to satisfy the Markov independence assumption when the survival rate for the "Regional Relapse" health state depends on whether or not the patient first experienced a local relapse. Draw a Markov model by modifying the model shown in Figure 7.25 so that the Markov independence assumption is still satisfied if the survival probability for the "Systemic Relapse" health state depends on whether or not the patient first experienced either a local or regional relapse. Assume that the survival probability for the "Indirect Local Relapse" health state is 0.65/quarter if the patient first experiences either a local or regional relapse. Assume that the survival probability for the "Direct Systemic Relapse" is 0.60/quarter.

2. Use the algorithm described in Section 7.2.4 to determine the life expectancy for the remainder of the patient's life if she faces the uncertainty represented

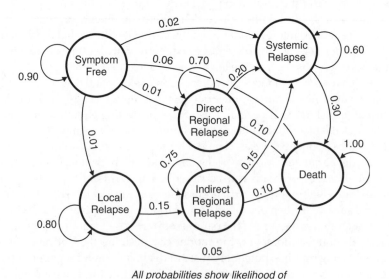

All probabilities show likelihood of
transition during 3 month period

Figure 7.25 Markov model for Problems 1 and 2.

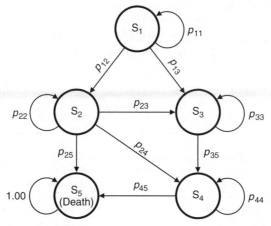

Figure 7.26 Markov model for Problem 3.

by the Markov model shown in Figure 7.25. Do the same for the Markov model you developed for your answer to Problem 1.

3. Figure 7.26 shows an abstract Markov model with five health states denoted S_1 to S_5. The transition probability from health state S_i to S_j is denoted p_{ij}. Assuming that the patient starts in health state S_1, what is the patient's life expectancy?

4. Figure 7.27 summarizes the life expectancies for each of the health states in the simplified breast cancer Markov model discussed in this chapter. Suppose that the patient's initial health state is uncertain and described by

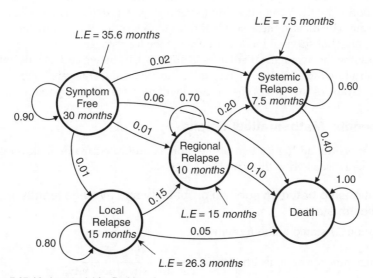

Figure 7.27 Markov model for Problem 4.

Table 7.2 Survival rates reported for prostate cancer patients, by stage.

Stage	Percentage of patients alive by month										
	0	**6**	**12**	**18**	**24**	**30**	**36**	**42**	**48**	**54**	**60**
I	100	89	85	81	79	77	75	72	68	64	64
II	100	90	87	83	77	75	72	70	66	63	62
III	100	87	81	75	69	65	60	55	54	52	48
IV	100	81	71	61	51	44	39	34	30	25	22

Table 7.3 Assumed average age, by stage.

Stage	Average age
I	50 years
II	60 years
III	70 years
IV	80 years

the following probabilities:

P[Symptom Free] $= 0.70$
P[Local Relapse] $= 0.15$
P[Regional Relapse] $= 0.10$
P[Systemic Relapse] $= 0.05$

Given the transition probabilities shown in Figure 7.27, what is the patient's life expectancy?

5. The survival rates shown in Table 7.2 are taken from the survival data reported by the Veterans Administration Cooperative Urological Research Group (1968). Use these survival rates to determine the parameter for the exponential survival models for each of the four stages.

Assume the average patient ages in Table 7.3, by stage, and use the annual mortality rates shown in Figure 7.7 to determine the age-adjusted life expectancies for each of the cancer stages for a 65-year-old patient.

Appendix: Mathematical details

This appendix addresses two of the more complicated mathematical results that were discussed in this chapter.

Relationship between survival probability and average length of stay for health states

Equation 7.1 stated without proof that

$$\text{average time spent in health state} = \frac{1}{1 - \text{survival probability}} \tag{A7.1}$$

Let p denote the sum of the probabilities for transitions leaving the health state and note that the probability that the patient stays for at least k time periods is $(1 - p)^k$. Therefore, the probability that the patient stays in the health state for exactly k time periods is

$$P[\text{Stay for exactly } k \text{ time periods}] = p \times (1 - p)^{k-1} \tag{A7.2}$$

That is, in order to stay exactly k time periods the patient must stay for $k - 1$ time periods, an event which has probability $(1 - p)^{k-1}$, and then leave, an event which has probability p. Under the Markovian assumption these two events are independent. Therefore, the probability that both events occur equals the product of the probabilities for each event.

The average time spent in the health state is then given by the following infinite sum:

$$\text{life expectancy} = \sum_{i=1}^{\infty} ip(1 - p)^{i-1} = p \times \sum_{i=1}^{\infty} i(1 - p)^{i-1} \tag{A7.3}$$

The following algebraic manipulations can be used to solve this infinite sum. The basic idea is to determine the limit for the partial sum. Let q equal the complement of the probability p. The partial sum can then be written as follows:

$$\text{partial sum of first } n \text{ terms} = (1 - q) \times \sum_{i=0}^{n} (i + 1) \times q^i$$

$$= \sum_{i=0}^{n} (i + 1)q^i - \sum_{i=0}^{n} (i + 1)q^{i+1}$$

$$= \sum_{i=0}^{n} (i + 1)q^i - \sum_{i=1}^{n+1} i \times q^{i+1}$$

$$= \sum_{i=0}^{n} q^i + \sum_{i=0}^{n} iq^i - \sum_{i=i}^{n+1} iq^i \tag{A7.4}$$

However, the terms in the second sum and third sum cancel except for the first term in the second sum and the last term in the third sum. Therefore,

$$\text{partial sum of first } n \text{ terms} = \left(\sum_{i=0}^{n} q^i \right) + 0 \times q^0 - (n + 1)q^{n+1}$$

$$= \left(\sum_{i=0}^{n} q^i \right) - (n + 1)q^{n+1} \tag{A7.5}$$

Therefore, the life expectancy for a patient faced with the simple two-state Markov model equals the limit of this partial sum as n approaches infinity. But notice that since q is less than 1,

$$(n+1)\,q^{n+1} \to 0 \text{ as } n \to \infty \tag{A7.6}$$

So life expectancy is given by the following infinite sum:

$$\text{life expectancy} = \sum_{i=0}^{\infty} q^i \tag{A7.7}$$

This simpler infinite sum is evaluated by repeating the same approach used above. Notice that

$$(1-q) \times \sum_{i=0}^{n} q^i = \sum_{i=0}^{n} q^i - \sum_{i=0}^{n} q^{i+1} = \sum_{i=0}^{n} q^i - \sum_{i=1}^{n+1} q^i \tag{A7.8}$$

All of the terms cancel except for the first term in the first sum and the last term in the second sum. Therefore, dividing by $1-q$ and replacing q by $1-p$ reduces the partial sum to the following simple expression:

$$\text{partial sum of first } n \text{ terms} = \frac{1-(1-p)^{n+1}}{p} \to \frac{1}{p} \text{ as } n \to \infty \tag{A7.9}$$

This completes the proof.

Fitting exponential survival model to survival data

Determining the exponential survival model parameter λ by fitting a straight line to a logarithmic graph of the survival rates takes advantage of the entire set of survival observations. This is done using standard linear regression techniques.

For example, suppose that survival rates $r_1, \dots, r_N$ are reported for the N times $t_1, \dots, t_N$. That is,

$$r_i = P[\text{Survive until time } t_i] \tag{A7.10}$$

The estimate for parameter λ that minimizes the squared error is given by the relationship

$$\lambda = \frac{N \sum_{i=1}^{N} (t_i \ln(r_i)) - \left(\sum_{i=1}^{N} t_i \right) \left(\sum_{i=1}^{N} \ln(r_i) \right)}{N \sum_{i=1}^{N} (t_i t_i) - \left(\sum_{i=1}^{N} t_i \right) \left(\sum_{i=1}^{N} t_i \right)} \tag{A7.11}$$

Bibliography

Beck, J.R., Kassirer, J.P., and Pauker, S.G. (1982) A convenient approximation of life expectancy (the "DEALE"), I. Validation of the method. *American Journal of Medicine*, **73**, 883–888.

This paper introduced the power of exponential survival models to the medical community.

Howard, R.A. (1971) *Dynamic Probabilistic Systems Volume I: Markov Models*, John Wiley & Sons, Inc., New York.

A mathematically oriented discussion of Markov models that provides a thorough introduction to this fascinating topic.

Veterans Administration Cooperative Urological Research Group (1968) Factors in the prognosis of carcinoma of the prostate: a cooperative study. *Journal of Urology*, **100**, 59–65.

CHAPTER 8

Measuring the outcome of care – expected utility analysis

Chapters 6 and 7 presented a method for computing the expected values for the choices available to a decision maker. The motivation behind expected value analysis is the assumption that decision makers prefer the alternative that maximizes expected value. For example, when value is measured by the length of the patient's life, expected value analysis identifies the alternative that maximizes the patient's life expectancy – a commonly used approach to medical decision making. The methods presented in Chapters 6 and 7 are highly scalable and can be applied to very complicated problems. The resulting arithmetic calculations may require a computer as the number of nodes or health states increases. However, the concepts underlying expected value analysis apply just a well to complicated problems as to simple ones.

This chapter shows how to extend the power of expected value analysis by introducing a more comprehensive approach to assigning values to outcomes. By necessity, expected value analysis uses a single dimension, such as length of life, to represent the relative merits of the outcomes that can result from the decision maker's choice. But then, many medical decisions are inherently multidimensional as illustrated by the example in Chapter 6. Hank, the decision maker in that example, wanted a decision that would take into account both the quality of his life and the length. Expected value analysis fails to capture the multidimensionality that is inherent to Hank's decision problem.

Expected value analysis also fails to account for *risk attitudes*. A simple monetary example illustrates this concept. Suppose that a business offers for sale a gamble that awards a prize according to the outcome of a coin toss. The buyer wins the prize if the coin lands heads and wins nothing if the coin lands tails. The prize in this case is a doubling of the buyer's income for one year. How much should a buyer be willing to pay for this unusual gamble? Expected value analysis would conclude that an individual should be willing to pay his or her entire annual income for this gamble. But then, few of us would be willing to pay that much for the gamble. Doubling your income for a year would be wonderful but the risk of losing all income for a year more than outweighs that attractive possibility. In other words, most of us are *risk*

Medical Decision Making, Second Edition. Harold C. Sox, Michael C. Higgins and Douglas K. Owens.
© 2013 John Wiley & Sons, Ltd. Published 2013 by John Wiley & Sons, Ltd.

averse in the sense that a large positive outcome is more than offset by the disadvantage of an equally large negative outcome.

The expected value analysis presented in Chapter 6 ignores risk aversion. Therefore, this chapter shows how to assign measures to outcomes that capture both risk attitudes as well as the multidimensionality found in most medical decision problems. These outcome measures are called *utilities*. They are the basis for a method called *utility analysis*. The mathematics of expected value analysis and of utility analysis are similar. Both compare alternatives based on the sum of outcome measures, weighted according to the outcome probabilities. Utility analysis differs in how it assigns measures to outcomes.

8.1 Basic concept – direct utility assessment

The fundamental approach of utility analysis is to determine a measure for each outcome, called the *outcome utility*, so that the alternative with the highest expected utility is the alternative most preferred by the decision maker. The method for calculating expected *utility* is the same as the method described in Chapter 6 for calculating expected *value*. The difference is that the utility assigned to the outcomes reflects the decision maker's concerns about all aspects of the outcome rather than a single dimension, such as the length of life. Of course, the key step is the assignment of outcome utilities so that the calculation produces an expected utility that reflects the decision maker's preferences.

This chapter starts with a formal approach to assessing a decision maker's outcome utilities. The method described is called *direct assessment*. The remainder of the chapter presents alternative approaches to determining a decision maker's outcome utilities, each based on simplifying assumptions about the decision maker's preferences.

Direct utility assessment is based on a formalism introduced by John von Neumann and Oskar Morgenstern back in 1947. They established a method for determining outcome utility based on five core assumptions about an individual's preferences when choosing between uncertain outcomes. Discussing the details of these assumptions, or axioms, would divert us from the pragmatic intent of this book. Therefore, we moved that theoretical discussion to an appendix to this chapter. Nevertheless, these assumptions are not magical or unreasonable. For example, von Neumann and Morgenstern assumed that preferences are transitive: if outcome A is preferred to outcome B and outcome B is preferred to outcome C then outcome A must also be preferred to outcome C. In short, utility analysis is based on a reasonable set of assumptions about how decision makers think about the outcomes they face in a decision problem with uncertainty.

Given these five assumptions, the direct assessment process goes as follows. Let $X_1, \ldots, X_N$ denote the N possible outcomes for a decision problem. Assume that these outcomes are numbered so that the least preferred outcome is X_1 and the most preferred outcome is X_N. Then the utility for X_1 is 0, the utility for X_N is 1, and any intermediate outcome X_i is the probability π_i such that the decision maker is indifferent between outcome X_i and a gamble that awards outcome X_N with probability π_i and outcome X_1 with probability $1 - \pi_i$. Symbolically, we depict this equivalence as

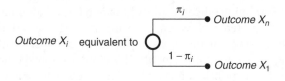

This equivalence is called the *standard reference gamble* or *standard gamble*. The decision maker would prefer the gamble on the right if the probability of the best outcome is close to 1 since the gamble would then be almost certain to yield the best possible outcome. Conversely the decision maker would prefer the intermediate outcome on the left if the probability of the best outcome is close to 0 since the gamble would then be almost certain to yield the worst possible outcome. By changing the value of the probability for outcome X_N, the gamble can be adjusted so that the decision maker is exactly indifferent between the intermediate outcome and the gamble. This value for π_i is called the *indifference probability* for the intermediate outcome relative to the best and worse outcomes.

Direct assessment process

Let $X_1, \ldots, X_N$ denote the N possible outcomes for a decision problem. Assume that these outcomes are numbered so that the least preferred outcome is X_1 and the most preferred outcome is X_N. Then

- Utility for X_1 is 0.0.
- Utility for X_N is 1.0.
- Utility for X_i is the value of π_i such that the following equivalence is true:

Outcome X_i equivalent to — π_i → Outcome X_n ; $1 - \pi_i$ → Outcome X_1

The equivalence between the gamble on the right and the outcome on the left means that both have the same expected utility. That is,

$$Utility\ (X_i) = [\pi_i \times Utility\ (X_N)] + [(1 - \pi_i) \times Utility\ (X_1)]$$

$$= [\pi_i \times 1] + [(1 - \pi_i) \times 0] = \pi_i \qquad (8.1)$$

Therefore, direct assessment assigns utilities to the intermediate outcomes based on the indifference probabilities for gambles between the best and worst possible outcomes. If the utility of X_1 is 0 and the utility of X_N is 1, the indifference probability is the utility of the intermediate outcome.

For example, recall the five possible outcomes faced by Hank in the decision problem analyzed in Chapter 6. Hank must choose between three treatment alternatives. Listed in order of decreasing preference for Hank, the possible outcomes he faced are:
- Cured without colostomy.
- Cured with colostomy.
- Local disease without colostomy.
- Metastatic disease without colostomy.
- Metastatic disease with colostomy.

In other words, from Hank's perspective the best possible outcome would be "Cured without colostomy" and the worse possible outcome would be "Metastatic disease with colostomy." Therefore,

$$Utility \text{ (Cured without colostomy)} = 1.0 \qquad (8.2)$$

$$Utility \text{ (Metastatic disease with colostomy)} = 0.0 \qquad (8.3)$$

Hank's utility for one of the intermediate outcomes, such as "Cured with colostomy," would then be the probability π such that the following equivalence is true:

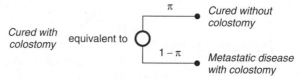

The indifference probability in this comparison would be very close to 1 if Hank considers the outcome "Cured with colostomy" to be almost as good as the outcome "Cured without colostomy." Conversely, the indifference probability would be close to 0 if Hank considers the outcome "Cured with colostomy" to be almost as bad as the outcome "*Metastatic* disease with colostomy." In other words, the indifference probability measures the value Hank places on avoiding a colostomy relative to his concerns about metastatic disease.

For Hank the indifference probability was 90%, meaning that he would accept up to a 10% chance of having metastatic disease if it meant that he could avoid a colostomy. Table 8.1 shows Hank's utilities for all of the outcomes he faced in his decision problem.

Table 8.1 Hank's utilities for the possible outcomes he faced.

Outcome	Utility
Cured without colostomy	1.0
Cured with colostomy	0.9
Local disease without colostomy	0.8
Metastatic disease without colostomy	0.1
Metastatic disease with colostomy	0.0

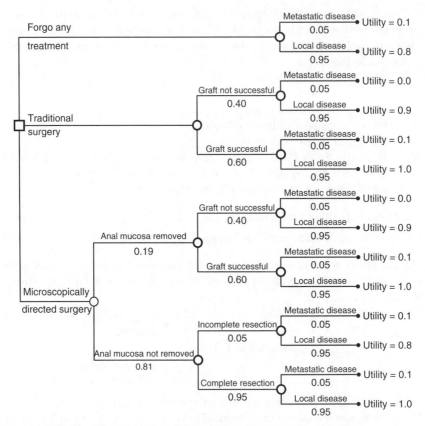

Figure 8.1 Decision tree for Hank's decision problem with probabilities and utilities.

These utilities have been added to Hank's decision tree in Figure 8.1. The methods presented in Chapter 6 for computing life expectancy can now be used to compute Hank's expected utility for his treatment alternatives. The calculations are shown in Table 8.2. The results indicate that Hank slightly prefers microscopically directed surgery, because this alternative balances the life-shortening risk of untreated disease with the chance of avoiding a colostomy, which would improve his quality of life.

Table 8.2 Expected utility calculations.

Alternative	Expected utility
Forgo any treatment	$(0.95 \times 0.8) + (0.05 \times 0.1) = \mathbf{0.77}$
Traditional surgery	$(0.57 \times 1.0) + (0.38 \times 0.9) + (0.03 \times 0.1) + (0.02 \times 0.0) = \mathbf{0.92}$
Microscopically directed surgery	$(0.84 \times 1.0) + (0.07 \times 0.9) + (0.04 \times 0.8) + (0.05 \times 0.1) + (0.00 \times 0.0) = \mathbf{0.94}$

Constructing the decision tree and assessing Hank's utility has reduced the complexity of what he must consider as the decision maker. Hank initially faced a complicated choice between three treatment alternatives involving uncertainties about the extent of his disease, the success of reconstructive surgery, and the possibility that he would have a colostomy for the remainder of his life. The combination of his decision and the subsequent uncertainty would lead to outcomes ranging from complete cure to metastatic disease. Constructing the decision tree divided that complex problem into a small collection of possible outcomes. Direct assessment presents the decision maker with relatively simple comparisons between those outcomes. The resolution of a complicated problem has been reduced to three direct assessment questions based on the standard reference gamble. The analysis uses straightforward mathematics to assemble the answers to those assessment questions into a final result that resolves the original problem.

Utility assessment requires input from the decision maker. After all, the goal is a set of outcome measures that capture that individual's preferences. Direct utility assessment provides a systematic way of collecting that input. Different decision makers typically will provide very different responses to the same assessment questions. Like subjective probability assessment, which we discussed in Chapter 3, the cognitive heuristics we use when we think about uncertainty can distort utility assessment. Therefore, the techniques discussed in Chapter 3 for avoiding the bias caused by these heuristics apply to the utility assessment process.

For example, consider the standard reference gamble used to assess Hank's utility for the outcome "Local disease without colostomy":

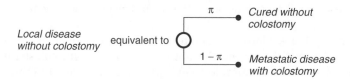

Referring to Table 8.3, suppose that the assessment process has already determined that the utility for "Metastatic disease without colostomy" is 0.1 and the utility for "Cured with colostomy" is 0.9. Since Hank's preferences rank "Local disease without colostomy" between these outcomes, we know that its utility is between 0.1 and 0.9. Therefore, the assessment process might begin with π equal to 0.1. We would expect that Hank would prefer "Local disease without colostomy" to the gamble in this first question.

Next we would pose the standard reference gamble with π equal to 0.9. Now we would expect Hank to prefer the gamble, verifying that the utility for the outcome is between 0.1 and 0.9. The third step would ask Hank to consider the standard reference gamble with π equal to 0.2. Assuming that Hank once again preferred "Local disease without colostomy" to the gamble, we would have narrowed the range for the utility of the outcome in question to 0.2 and 0.9.

Table 8.3 Hank's utilities for the possible outcomes he faced.

Outcome	Utility
Cured without colostomy	1.0
Cured with colostomy	0.9
Local disease without colostomy	**0.8**
Metastatic disease without colostomy	0.1
Metastatic disease with colostomy	0.0

The process continues by alternating between the two extremes, steadily narrowing the range of possible values for the indifference probability until Hank cannot decide between "Local disease without colostomy" and the gamble. In Hank's case the point of indifference was reached when π equals 0.8.

8.2 Sensitivity analysis – testing the robustness of utility analysis

Sensitivity analysis, described in Section 6.7 for probability analysis, can be applied to utility as well. Sensitivity analysis of the assessed utilities can strengthen the credibility of decision analysis based by determining if there are possible values for a utility that would change the recommended treatment alternative.

For example, consider Hank's utilities for the outcomes he faces. The utilities assessed for these five outcomes are shown in Table 8.3. We will use sensitivity analysis to determine if there are possible values for the outcome "Local disease without colostomy" that would change the conclusions of the analysis.

As noted above, Hank's preferences rank the outcome "Local disease without colostomy" between the outcomes "Cured with colostomy" and "Metastatic disease without colostomy". Therefore, referring to Table 8.3, the range of possible values for the utility of "Local disease without colostomy" is between 0.1 and 0.9. Figure 8.2 shows how the expected utility for the three treatment alternatives varies with the utility for the outcome "Local disease without colostomy" over this range. Note that the expected utility for microscopically directed surgery exceeds the expected utility for the other two alternatives, except when the utility for local disease without colostomy is close to 0.1.

Figure 8.3 focuses on the region in Figure 8.2 where the expected utility for Hank's two surgical alternatives is close together. We can see in Figure 8.3 that microscopically directed surgery has the greater expected utility, provided that Hank's utility for the outcome "Local disease without colostomy" is greater than 0.16. Therefore, the conclusion that microscopically directed surgery is the preferred alternative can be confirmed by asking Hank to consider the following assessment question:

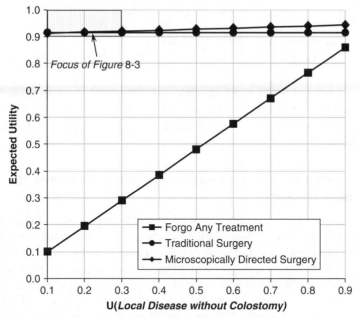

Figure 8.2 Sensitivity analysis for U(Local disease without colostomy).

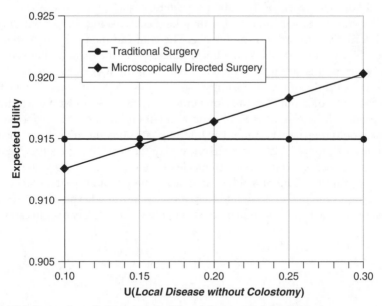

Figure 8.3 Focused sensitivity analysis for U(Local disease without colostomy).

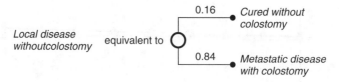

Hank's utility for "Local disease without colostomy" is greater than 0.16 if he prefers the outcome on the left side of this comparison, which confirms the conclusion that microscopically directed surgery is his preferred treatment alternative.

8.3 Shortcut – using a linear scale to express strength of preference

Utility assessment based on the standard gamble questions asks the decision maker to think about preferences in terms of gambles. But what if the patient has asked the physician to be the decision maker because the patient is confused by the notion of comparing gambles with intermediate outcomes? The physician would want to make a decision that incorporates the patient's preferences. However, using direct assessment sometimes is impossible because the patient lacks the cognitive ability needed to participate. Direct scaling is an alternative that lacks the theoretical foundations of direct utility assessment but still brings aspects of the patient's preferences into the analysis.

Like utility assessment, direct scaling begins by asking the patient to rank the alternatives in order of preference. The clinician then asks the patient to place the various outcomes on a linear scale so that the distance between the marks represents strength of preference (see Figure 8.4). For example, Hank ranked "Cured without colostomy" as the best outcome and "Metastatic disease with colostomy" as the worst outcome. These two outcomes would be represented by marks at the right end and left end of the scale, respectively. Hank would then be asked about an intermediate outcome, like "Local disease without colostomy": "Is it closer to one end of the scale than the other? Which end? Is it closer to the middle of the scale or the right end of the scale?"

By offering the patient a series of choices, the position on the scale corresponding to the patient's preferences can be determined. The process can be repeated for each possible outcome. This method is relatively easy to carry out

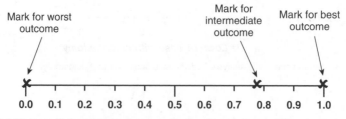

Figure 8.4 Linear scale for capturing the strength of preference for possible outcomes.

and measures the strength of the patient's preferences for the outcomes the patient faces. In effect, the positions of the marks on the linear scale approximate the indifference probabilities determined in the assessment process.

8.4   Exponential utility – a parametric model

This section describes an efficient method for measuring a decision maker's utility for length of life. The method is limited to outcomes that differ according to a single dimension – length of life. Therefore, this method has the shortcoming of being one dimensional. However, with this method we will be able to capture the decision maker's risk attitudes through the answer to a single assessment question. Later in this chapter we will see how to extend the method to outcomes with multiple quality states.

The utility model described in this section is similar to the exponential survival model discussed in Chapter 7. That discussion showed how the exponential survival model can represent the uncertainty in the remaining years of life for a patient. Because of the mathematical properties of the exponential survival model, life expectancy for the patient is simply $1/\lambda$, where λ is the annual mortality rate. The validity of an analysis based on this model depends on the annual mortality rate from a disease remaining constant for the rest of the patient's life. Although this assumption may not be valid as a chronic disease progresses and death approaches, this convenient model simplifies the comparison of two outcomes based on the corresponding mortality rates.

As with the exponential survival model, suppose that the outcomes in a decision problem only differ according to the length of the patient's life. The decision maker's utility for the possible outcomes can then be thought of as the function $U(x)$, which determines the utility for a life of x years. The exponential survival model is called a *parametric* model of survival since it can be completely described by the single parameter λ that measures the level of risk faced by the patient. Holding the parameter λ constant and varying the value of x determines the likelihood of surviving x years given that level of risk. The goal of this section is to establish a similar parametric model for utility.

The model we will consider is called the "exponential *utility* model" and has the form

$$U(x) = 1 - e^{-\gamma x} \tag{8.4}$$

Figure 8.5 graphs $U(x)$ for several possible values of γ when the maximum possible survival is 20 years. The exponential survival model captures the probability of a length of survival based on the single parameter λ. Similarly, the exponential utility model captures an individual's utility for a length of survival based on the parameter γ. We will see that γ measures the strength of the decision maker's risk aversion. Therefore, knowing the curve in Figure 8.5 that matches an individual's preferences will tell us that individual's utility for lengths of survival from 0 to 20 years for a given level of risk aversion. We

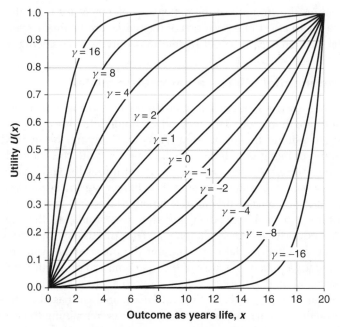

Figure 8.5 Exponential utility model $U(x) = 1 - e^{-\gamma x}$ scaled so that $U(20) = 1$.

determine the matching curve – in other words, the parameter γ – through a simple assessment process.

8.4.1 Exponential utility assessment

The single parameter γ greatly simplifies the assessment process for exponential utility. With direct assessment, determining the utility for survival requires assessment questions for several representative survival values. With exponential utility the assessment process is reduced to determination of that single parameter.

The following example shows how to fit an exponential utility function to outcomes that range from 0 to 20 years of survival. By convention, the utility of 20 years is 1.0 and the utility for 0 years is 0.0. The parameter γ is determined by assessing the decision maker's utility for an intermediate outcome, such as six years of survival. Therefore, suppose that the decision maker's indifference probability for the following assessment question is 0.7:

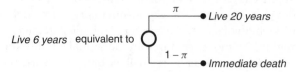

The decision maker's utility for six years is 0.7. Referring to Figure 8.5, the exponential utility function that assigns a value of 0.7 to six years has a value of 4 for the parameter γ. Therefore, this decision maker's utility function is

$$U(x) = 1 - e^{-4x} \tag{8.5}$$

Of course, nothing in the assessment process requires asking only one assessment question. In fact, if the decision maker's responses to multiple assessment questions all gave the same value of γ, one would have more confidence in the parameter γ chosen for the corresponding exponential utility model. Alternatively, multiple assessments implying different values for γ would suggest that the exponential utility model is not a good fit to that decision maker's preferences. The next section formalizes this notion.

8.4.2 Assumption underlying the exponential utility model

The applicability of the exponential utility model to a decision problem depends on a testable assumption about the decision maker's risk attitudes. In order to understand this assumption, consider monetary gambles involving prizes between $0 and $100. First suppose that the decision maker's indifference probability π in the following assessment question is 0.75:

```
                                        π
                                   ┌────────● Win $50
        Win $25   equivalent to    ○
                                   └────────● Win $0
                                     1 − π
```

That is, the decision maker is indifferent between $25 for sure and a gamble that has a 75% chance of awarding $50. Now suppose that the decision maker is asked to consider the following gamble in which all of the possible outcomes have been increased by $50:

```
                                        π
                                   ┌────────● Win $100
        Win $75   equivalent to    ○
                                   └────────● Win $50
                                     1 − π
```

Would the decision maker's indifference probability for this second assessment question still be 0.75? If so, then the decision maker's preferences are said to satisfy the *delta property*. Stated formally:

Delta property

The delta property holds if for any outcomes A, B, and C the following equivalence

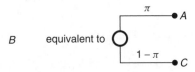

---

implies the following equivalence for the same indifference probability π for all values of Δ,

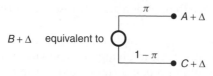

The importance of the delta property is that it holds for all decision makers with preferences that match the exponential utility model. Therefore, the delta property provides an easy test for determining if a decision maker's preference can be represented by the exponential utility model. The mathematically inclined reader can find a derivation of this important result in the appendix to this chapter.

8.4.3 Exponential utility and risk attitudes

Figure 8.6 shows three exponential utility curves that illustrate different types of risk attitudes. First, focus on the curve for $\gamma = 4$. For this curve the biggest increases in utility occur when the length of survival is close to 0. For example, changing survival from 0 to 2 years increases the utility from 0 to 0.34, whereas changing survival from 18 to 20 years has almost no change in utility. In other words, individuals with preferences described by this curve will place more importance on changes in near-term survival than changes in long-term survival. To varying degrees, this holds for all of the utility curves in Figure 8.6 with positive values for γ.

These individuals are *risk averse* because they would rather have X years for certain than a gamble that has an expected value of X years. To see this, consider how they respond to the following assessment question:

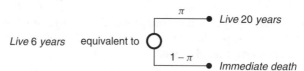

Following the dashed lines in Figure 8.6, the curve with $\gamma = 4$ implies that the individual's indifference probability would be approximately 0.7 for this assessment question. The expected value for the gamble in the assessment question is then

$$\text{expected value} = (0.7 \times 20 \text{ years}) + (0.3 \times 0 \text{ years}) = 14 \text{ years} \tag{8.6}$$

This individual would avoid a risky gamble even if the gamble, on the average, could result in a substantial increase in survival.

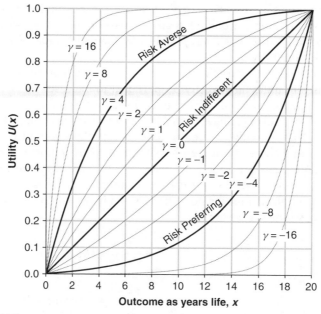

Figure 8.6 Utility curves illustrating risk-averse, risk-indifferent, and risk-preferring preferences.

Now consider the curve in Figure 8.6 with $\gamma = -4$. For this utility curve the biggest increases in utility occur when survival is close to the maximum possible value. For example, changing survival from 18 to 20 years increases the utility from 0.66 to 1.0. Conversely, utility changes very little for changes in near-term survival, for example, when survival increases from 0 to 2 years corresponds to almost no increase in utility. Individuals with preferences described by these curves place more importance on changes in long-term survival than changes in short-term survival. To varying degrees, this holds for all of the utility curves in Figure 8.6 with negative values for γ.

These individuals are *risk preferring* because they prefer a gamble that has an expected value of X years to X years for certain. To see this, consider how they would respond to the following assessment question.:

Live 14 years   equivalent to   ⃝ ⟨
π ● *Live 20 years*
$1 - \pi$ ● *Immediate death*

According to the curve in Figure 8.6, the individual's indifference probability would be approximately 0.3 for this assessment question. The expected value for the gamble in the assessment question is then

$$\text{expected value} = (0.3 \times 20 \text{ years}) + (0.7 \times 0 \text{ years}) = 6 \text{ years} \tag{8.7}$$

These individuals prefer the gamble because the possibility of surviving 20 years seems more important than the risk of immediate death, even if the expected value was considerably less than the value of the certain outcome – living 14 years.

Finally, consider the curve in Figure 8.6 with $\gamma = 0$. For this utility curve the increases in utility are exactly proportional to increases in survival. For example, changing survival from 18 to 20 years increases the utility from 0.8 to 1.0. Similarly, utility changes from 0 to 0.2 when survival changes from 0 to 2 years. Individuals with preferences described by this curve place the same importance on changes in long-term survival as changes in short-term survival.

These individuals are called *risk indifferent* because they are indifferent between a gamble that has an expected value of X years and X years for certain. To see this, consider how these individuals would respond to the following assessment question:

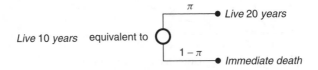

According to the corresponding curve in Figure 8.6, that individual's indifference probability would be 0.5 for this assessment question. The expected value for the gamble in the assessment question is then

$$\text{expected value} = (0.5 \times 20 \text{ years}) + (0.5 \times 0 \text{ years}) = 10 \text{ years} \tag{8.8}$$

These individuals prefer the gamble because the possibility of surviving 20 years seems more important than the risk of immediate death, even if the expected value is considerably less than the value of the certain outcome – living 14 years. These are the expected value decision makers discussed in Chapter 6.

8.5 Exponential utility with exponential survival

We will now show how to incorporate risk attitudes into the comparison of gambles based on the exponential survival model. The exponential model assumes that probabilities for possible lengths of life can be represented by the following function:

$$f(x) = \lambda e^{-\lambda x} \tag{8.9}$$

The mathematical integration of $f(x)$ with the exponential utility model determines the corresponding expected utility. This operation requires a working familiarity with calculus, knowledge that we do not assume that all of our readers have. However, the result is very simple. If the decision maker's utility

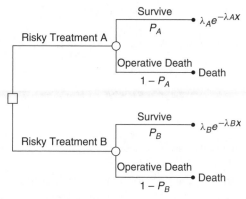

Figure 8.7 Choice between two risky treatments.

is exponential with parameter γ and survival is exponential with parameter λ, then the expected utility for the gamble is

$$\text{utility for exponential survival} = \frac{\gamma}{\gamma + \lambda} \tag{8.10}$$

Note that Equation 8.10 uses γ, the parameter for the exponential utility model, to incorporate the decision maker's risk attitudes into the comparison of outcomes.

For example, consider the simple decision problem shown in Figure 8.7 involving a choice between two treatments with uncertain outcomes. The lengths of the patient's life after surviving the chosen treatment will be distributed according to an exponential survival model. Denote the short-term probability of surviving Treatment A and Treatment B by P_A and P_B, respectively. Similarly, denote patient's life expectancy after surviving Treatment A or Treatment B by $1/\lambda_A$ or $1/\lambda_B$, respectively.

The life expectancy for Treatment A is

$$\text{life expectancy for Treatment A} = \left[P_A \times \frac{1}{\lambda_A} \right] + [(1 - P_A) \times 0] = \frac{P_A}{\lambda_A} \tag{8.11}$$

Similarly,

$$\text{life expectancy for Treatment B} = \frac{P_B}{\lambda_B} \tag{8.12}$$

Therefore, according to life expectancy analysis, Treatment A is preferred to Treatment B only if the following is true:

$$\frac{P_A}{\lambda_A} > \frac{P_B}{\lambda_B} \tag{8.13}$$

However, suppose that the decision maker's risk attitudes are described by an exponential utility model with coefficient γ. Using Equation 8.10, we compute the expected *utility* for Treatment A as follows:

$$\text{expected utility for Treatment A} = \left[P_A \times \frac{\gamma}{\gamma + \lambda_A} \right] + [(1 - P_A) \times 0]$$

$$= \frac{P_A \gamma}{\gamma + \lambda_A} \tag{8.14}$$

Similarly,

$$\text{expected utility for Treatment B} = \frac{P_B \gamma}{\gamma + \lambda_B} \tag{8.15}$$

Therefore, if we consider the decision maker's risk attitudes, Treatment A is preferred to Treatment B only if the following is true:

$$\frac{P_A \gamma}{\gamma + \lambda_A} > \frac{P_B \gamma}{\gamma + \lambda_B} \tag{8.16}$$

Notice that as long as γ is positive – meaning that the patient is risk averse – the inequality holds if we cancel γ from the numerator on both sides of Equation 8.16. That is, for the risk-averse decision maker Treatment A is preferred to Treatment B only if the following is true:

$$\frac{P_A}{\gamma + \lambda_A} > \frac{P_B}{\gamma + \lambda_B} \tag{8.17}$$

Also notice that this relationship is the same as Equation 8.13 – the relationship based on life expectancy analysis – if γ is 0. In other words, life expectancy analysis and the exponential utility models both reach the same conclusion when the decision maker is risk indifferent.

In summary, the exponential utility model is a useful tool for reflecting the decision maker's risk attitudes in a decision analysis. The assessment process requires only the answer to a single question. The mathematical structure of the exponential utility function allows it to be combined with the exponential survival model to more fully represent the concerns of a decision maker faced with uncertain outcomes that will unfold over time.

8.6 Multidimensional outcomes – direct assessment

Hank's example demonstrates a principal challenge in medical decision making, which is balancing concerns about both the quality and length of his life. We have just learned that the exponential utility function captures the decision maker's attitudes toward the risk of dying in the near term and later on in life. In this section, we extend those methods to incorporate the decision maker's concerns about the quality of life.

The goal is to capture how a decision maker's utility for length of life changes when the quality of life is taken into account. Figure 8.8 illustrates this goal. Suppose that a decision problem can result in outcomes with different life expectancies in two possible quality states, denoted Q_A and Q_B. For example, Q_A might be symptom-free life and Q_B is life with a side effect of a treatment, such as a colostomy. The curves in Figure 8.8 depict the decision maker's utility for the possible outcomes. The curve labeled $U(x, Q_A)$ is the decision maker's utility for length of life in quality state Q_A. The curve labeled $U(x, Q_B)$ is the same for Q_B.

Therefore, the challenge is how to determine the two curves in Figure 8.8 since they define the decision maker's utility. Direct assessment is one approach. First, we would select representative lengths of life, such as 10 years, 9 years, and so forth, down to immediate death. The assessment process would then consist of three steps.

Step 1: The first step involves assessment questions that determine the decision maker's risk attitudes toward length of life in quality state Q_A. The following would be a typical example:

Live 3 years in quality state Q_A equivalent to

$\pi_A(3)$ Live 10 years in quality state Q_A

$1 - \pi_A(3)$ Immediate death

For instance, notice that

$$Utility\,(3\text{ years}, Q_A) = [\pi_A(3) \times Utility\,(10\text{ years}, Q_A)]$$

$$+ [(1 - \pi_A(3)) \times U(\text{Death})]$$

$$= [\pi_A(3) \times 1] + [(1 - \pi_A(3)) \times 0]$$

$$= \pi_A(3) \tag{8.18}$$

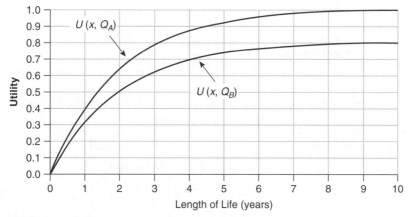

Figure 8.8 Utility for length of life with two quality states.

By repeating this assessment question for several lengths of survival in state Q_A (the left hand side of Equation 8.18) we establish several points on the curve. Connecting these points determines the shape of the top curve in Figure 8.8. In general, let $\pi_A(x)$ denote the indifference probability established by direct assessment of the decision maker's utility for x years in quality state Q_A. Step 1 determines that

$$Utility\ (x\ years, Q_A) = \pi_A(x) \tag{8.19}$$

Step 2: The second step poses the same assessment questions except that the quality state is now Q_B. The following would be a typical example:

Live 3 years in quality state Q_B equivalent to

- $\pi_B(3)$ → Live 10 years in quality state Q_A
- $1 - \pi_B(3)$ → Immediate death

Let $\pi_B(x)$ denote the indifference probability for one of these assessment questions and notice that

$$Utility\ (x\ years, Q_B) = [\pi_B(x) \times Utility\ (10\ years, Q_B)]$$
$$+ [(1 - \pi_B(x)) \times U(Death)]$$
$$= [\pi_B(x) \times Utility\ (10\ years, Q_B)] + [(1 - \pi_B(x)) \times 0]$$
$$= \pi_B(x) \times Utility\ (10\ years, Q_B) \tag{8.20}$$

These assessment questions determine the decision maker's utility for x years in quality state Q_B relative to a gamble for 10 years in quality state Q_B or immediate death. In order to complete the process, we must determine the decision maker's utility for 10 years of life in quality state Q_B. This is done in the third step.

Step 3: The third step requires a single assessment question:

Live 10 years in quality state Q_B equivalent to

- θ_B → Live 10 years in quality state Q_A
- $1 - \theta_B$ → Immediate death

The indifference probability θ_B for this last assessment question completes the process since we now can write

$$Utility\ (10\ years, Q_B) = [\theta_B \times Utility\ (10\ years, Q_A)]$$
$$+ [(1 - \theta_B) \times U(Death)]$$
$$= [\theta_B \times 1] + [(1 - \theta_B) \times 0]$$
$$= \theta_B \tag{8.21}$$

By combining Equations 8.20 and 8.21 we find that

$$Utility\ (x\ years, Q_B) = \pi_B(x) \times Utility\ (10\ years, Q_B)$$

$$= \pi_B(x) \times \theta_B \tag{8.22}$$

Or, in general,

$$Utility\ (x\ years, Q_i)\ = \pi_i(x) \times \theta_i \tag{8.23}$$

where θ_A is by definition equal to 1 since it measures the quality for the preferred quality state Q_A. Equation 8.23 fully captures the decision maker's utility for survival in the two quality states Q_A and Q_B. The indifference probabilities $\pi_A(x)$ and $\pi_B(x)$ capture the risk attitudes about the length of life x in the two quality states. The probability θ_B captures how the decision maker feels about quality state Q_B relative to quality state Q_A. We now have a general measure for outcomes that captures both the duration of survival as well as the quality of life. Expected utility analysis based on this measure will take into account the full significance of each possible outcome.

8.7 Multidimensional outcomes – simplifications

We can generalize the three-step process described in the previous section to solve more complicated decision problems with any number of health states. This process involves repeating Step 2 and Step 3 for each of the additional quality states. However, the number of questions required by this approach can be very large.

Let M denote the number of time points needed to define the curve that represents the patient's utility for the duration of life and let N denote the number of quality states. We can then calculate the required number of assessment questions by the following expression:

$$number\ of\ assessment\ questions = (M \times N) + (N - 1) \tag{8.24}$$

For example, suppose that assessing the length of life for each quality state requires five questions ($M = 5$) and there are three quality states ($N = 3$). Then the total assessment process would require 17 assessment questions:

$$number\ of\ assessment\ questions = (5 \times 3) + (3 - 1) = 17 \tag{8.25}$$

Seventeen questions would try the patience of almost anyone. Perhaps this process is impractical in the real world. To simplify it, we now consider several assumptions about the decision maker's preferences.

8.7.1 Simplification: assume independence between preferences for length and quality of life

Reasonable assumptions about the decision maker's preferences can eliminate several of the assessment questions. For example, consider the assessment questions in Step 2 of the process described above. These questions determine the decision maker's risk attitudes about length of life while experiencing quality state Q_B. The following is a typical assessment question used during this step in the process:

Live 3 years in quality state Q_B equivalent to

$\pi_B(3)$ — Live 10 years in quality state Q_B

$1 - \pi_B(3)$ — Immediate death

One possible assumption is to assume that the decision maker's indifference probability in this assessment question does not depend on the quality state Q_B. In other words, assume that

$$\pi_A(3) = \pi_B(3) \tag{8.26}$$

where $\pi_A(3)$ is the decision maker's indifference probability in the assessment question:

Live 3 years in quality state Q_A equivalent to

$\pi_A(3)$ — Live 10 years in quality state Q_A

$1 - \pi_A(3)$ — Immediate death

In other words, we assume that the decision maker's risk attitudes about length of life do not depend on the quality of life experienced during the remainder of the patient's life. This assumption is not the same as ignoring quality of life. We are only assuming that for any given quality state, the decision maker would accept the same risky tradeoffs in the length of life.

Under this assumption, if x denotes the length of life on the left side of the assessment question, we can drop the subscript from the indifference probability and write:

$$Utility\ (x\ years, Q_i) = \theta_i \times \pi(x) \tag{8.27}$$

The indifference probability $\pi(x)$ captures the risk attitudes about the length of life x in either of the two quality states. As before, the probability θ_B captures how the decision maker feels about quality state Q_B relative to quality state Q_A. The result is a general expression for the decision maker's utility for outcomes in the two quality states.

Eliminating the Step 2 assessment questions reduces the number of required assessment questions to

$$\text{number of assessment questions} = M + N - 1 \qquad (8.28)$$

For example, assessing the length of life for each quality state requires five questions ($M = 5$) and there are three quality states ($N = 3$). Then the total assessment process would require 7 assessment questions instead of 17:

$$\text{number of assessment questions} = 5 + 3 - 1 = 7 \qquad (8.29)$$

8.7.2 Simplification: assume the delta property

The delta property is the second assumption we will make about the decision maker's risk attitudes. Recall the discussion in Section 8.5.2, which showed that the decision maker's utility for length of life can be represented by the exponential utility function if we assume the delta property. Therefore, we can replace the direct assessment questions in Step 1 by a single assessment question. This one assessment question determines the parameter γ in the exponential utility function. This simplified version of Step 1 determines an exponential utility function for survival in quality state Q_A:

$$Utility\ (x\ \text{years}, Q_A) = 1 - e^{-\gamma x} \qquad (8.30)$$

The independence assumption discussed in the previous section means than we would assess the same value for γ if the questions were asked for quality state Q_B. The remaining step is to assess the value for θ_B, which compares life in quality state Q_B to life in quality state Q_A. This is done by asking the same assessment question as before:

The utility for x years in state Q_B is then

$$Utility\ (x\ \text{years}, Q_B) = \theta_B \times (1 - e^{-\gamma x}) \qquad (8.31)$$

When the exponential survival model represents the uncertainty for the length of life, the utility for an outcome then is:

$$\text{utility for exponential survival in quality state } i = \frac{\theta_i\,\gamma}{\gamma + \lambda} \qquad (8.32)$$

where $1/\lambda$ is the patient's life expectancy.

For example, Hank faced a decision problem that had three possible quality states:
- Q_A Symptom free and no colostomy
- Q_B Local perianal rash
- Q_C Colostomy

His indifference probability for the following assessment question is 0.95:

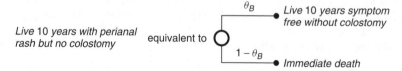

Similarly Hank's indifference probability for the following assessment question is 0.90:

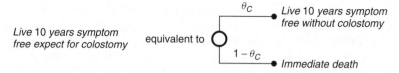

Based on the expression in Equation 8.32, Table 8.4 uses the values assessed for θ_B and θ_C (as before θ_A equals 1) to determine the utility for the various possible outcomes.

Using the approach described in Section 8.2, we calculate the expected utility for each of Hank's treatment alternatives. These calculations are shown in Table 8.5.

Therefore, incorporating Hank's concerns about quality into the analysis results in a conclusion that clearly favors microscopically directed surgery.

Sensitivity analysis of this example provides insight into how Hank's risk attitudes affect his choice of treatment. Figure 8.9 shows how the expected

Table 8.4 Probabilities, life expectancies, and utilities for quality and length of life.

Alternative	Outcome	Probability	$1/\lambda$	θ_i	Utility
Forgo any treatment	Local disease without colostomy	0.9500	5 years	0.95	0.9048
	Metastatic disease without colostomy	0.0500	2 years	0.95	0.8000
Traditional surgery	Cured without colostomy	0.5700	20 years	1.00	0.9877
	Cured with colostomy	0.3800	20 years	0.90	0.8889
	Metastatic disease without colostomy	0.0300	2 years	1.00	0.8889
	Metastatic disease with colostomy	0.0200	2 years	0.90	0.8000
Microscopically directed surgery	Cured without colostomy	0.8409	20 years	1.00	0.9877
	Cured with colostomy	0.0704	20 years	0.90	0.8889
	Local disease without colostomy	0.0387	5 years	0.95	0.9048
	Metastatic disease without colostomy	0.0463	2 years	1.00	0.8889
	Metastatic disease with colostomy	0.0037	2 years	0.90	0.8000

Table 8.5 Expected utility calculations.

Alternative	Life expectancy
Forgo any treatment	$0.9500 \times 0.9048 + 0.0500 \times 0.8000 = \mathbf{0.9017}$
Traditional surgery	$0.5700 \times 0.9877 + 0.3800 \times 0.8889 + 0.0300 \times 0.8889$
	$+ 0.0200 \times 0.8000 = \mathbf{0.9434}$
Microscopically directed surgery	$0.8409 \times 0.9877 + 0.0704 \times 0.8889 + 0.0387 \times 0.9048 +$
	$0.0463 \times 0.8889 + 0.0037 \times 0.8000 = \mathbf{0.9722}$

utility for the three treatment alternatives varies with changes in the exponential utility model parameter γ. Recall that γ, which measures Hank's risk aversion for length of life, increases as he focuses more on near-term survival. None of the alternatives includes a risk of near-term death. Instead the survival differences for the three alternatives depend on events in the future where Hank faces the risk of possible metastatic disease, untreated local disease, or other potential causes of death. Therefore, the differences between the three treatment alternatives decrease as γ increases. Moreover, Hank's relative ranking of the three alternatives does not change over the range of possible values for γ. Hank's decision does not depend on his risk aversion about length of life because none of the alternatives differ in terms of near-term survival.

Figure 8.10 shows the sensitivity analysis for the indifference probability θ_C in the comparison of life with colostomy and symptom-free life. Recall that θ_C was determined by Hank's response to the following assessment question:

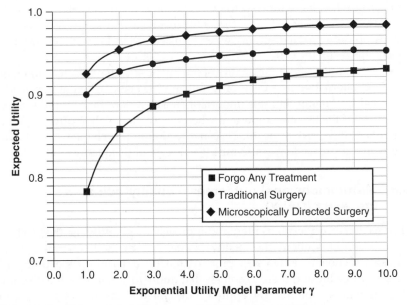

Figure 8.9 Sensitivity analysis for the exponential utility model parameter.

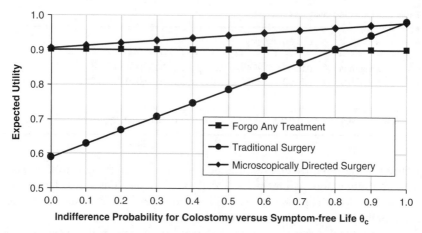

Figure 8.10 Sensitivity analysis for tradeoff between colostomy and symptom-free life.

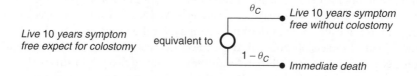

Microscopically directed surgery is the preferred alternative over the full range of possible values for θ_C. However, the strength of Hank's preference for this alternative varies with θ_C. The two surgical alternatives are roughly equivalent when life with colostomy is almost as good as symptom-free life ($\theta_C = 1$). At the other extreme, forgoing treatment is roughly equivalent to microscopically directed surgery when Hank considers life with colostomy to be as bad a death ($\theta_C = 0$).

So risk attitudes about the quality of life can be essential to determining the preferred alternative in a decision problem. The standard gamble provides a method for quantifying this important consideration. Risk attitudes about the length of life become important when the treatment alternatives differ in the timing of the risk of death. The final section to this chapter describes an alternative approach to quantifying attitudes about the quality of life.

8.8 Multidimensional outcomes – quality-adjusted life years (QALY)

This section considers an alternate approach to quantifying the decision maker's concerns about the quality of life. The method described in the previous section is a two-step process that (1) determines the utility for symptom-free life and then (2) adjusts that utility to account for the disutility of living with symptoms. The approach described in this section is based on the notion that life with a symptom is equivalent to fewer years of life that are symptom free. The utility of this quality-adjusted length of life equals the utility for years in the symptomatic state.

We will develop this new approach by first summarizing the method described in the previous section. Recall Equation 8.23, which determined the utility for x years of life in quality state Q_i:

$$\text{Utility } (x \text{ years}, Q_i) = \theta_i \times \pi_i(x) \tag{8.33}$$

The term θ_i in this expression captures the decision maker's risk attitudes about the *quality* of life in state Q_i and was determined by the response to the following assessment question:

The term $\pi_i(x)$ captures the decision maker's risk attitudes the *length* of life in state Q_i and was determined by the assessment question:

We made the simplifying assumption that risk attitudes about the length of life are independent of the quality of life. For example, given another quality state Q_j we assumed that

$$\pi_j(x) = \pi_i(x) = \pi(x) \quad \text{for all quality states } Q_i \text{ and } Q_j \tag{8.34}$$

This assumption is not the same as ignoring quality of life. We are only assuming that for any given quality state, the decision maker would accept the same risky tradeoffs in the length of life. With this assumption of independence, Equation 8.33 becomes

$$\text{Utility } (x \text{ years}, Q_i) = \theta_i \times \pi(x) \tag{8.35}$$

Notice that $\theta_i = 1$ if quality state Q_i is the same as symptom free. In this case Equation 8.35 becomes

$$\text{Utility } (x \text{ years, Symptom free}) = \pi(x) \tag{8.36}$$

Therefore, $\pi(x)$ equals the decision maker's utility for x symptom-free years and θ_i is the reduction in that utility needed to account for the disutility of living in quality state Q_i.

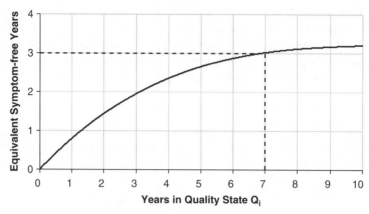

Figure 8.11 Tradeoff between years of symptom-free life for years in quality state Q_j.

Determining θ_i requires assessment based on the standard reference gamble – a process that can be difficult for some decision makers. The alternative described in this section is based on the relationship depicted in Figure 8.11. The curve in this figure shows how a decision maker would trade off years in symptomatic state Q_i for fewer symptom-free years. For example, this decision maker believes that seven years of life with the symptom are equivalent to three symptom-free years. In general, let $w_i(x)$ denote this relationship. That is, for this decision maker

$$\text{Utility } (x \text{ years in } Q_i) = \text{Utility } (w_i(x) \text{ symptom-free years}) \tag{8.37}$$

Or, using the notation in Equation 8.35, we can write

$$\text{Utility } (x \text{ years}, Q_i) = \pi (w_i(x)) \tag{8.38}$$

In other words, we determine the indifference probability $\pi(\ )$ for $w_i(x)$ rather than x. The relationship $w_i(x)$ is called the *quality-adjusted life years* or *QALY* relationship for Q_i.

Assessing the QALY relationship is the key step to using this method. Typically this is done by asking the decision maker to consider the following question for several values of x:

How many symptom-free years are equivalent to x years in quality state Q_i?

Plotting the answer to this question for the corresponding values of x determines the curve shown in Figure 8.11 for Q_i. This process would be repeated for each possible quality state. Determining the utility for symptom-free life then completely determines a utility function for the outcomes in the decision problem.

Asking the questions needed to fully draw the curve in Figure 8.11 can time consuming. Therefore, a linear approximation for the QALY relationship often is used. That linear approximation is determined by picking a representative value for the length of life x and then asking how many symptom-free years are equivalent to x years in quality state Q_i. Let y_i be the decision maker's response to this question. That is,

$$Utility\ (x\ years\ in\ Q_i) = Utility\ (y_i\ symptom\text{-}free\ years) \tag{8.39}$$

If ϕ_i denotes the ratio y_i/x, then ϕ_i is the slope of a linear approximation to the QALY relationship, as shown in Figure 8.12.

Assuming that the linear approximation matches the QALY relationship curve shown in Figure 8.12, we can write

$$Utility\ (x\ years\ in\ Q_i) = Utility\ (\phi_i x\ symptom\text{-}free\ years) \tag{8.40}$$

In other words, since $w_i(x) = \phi_i x$ we can use Equation 8.39 to write

$$Utility\ (x\ years, Q_i) = \pi\,(\phi_i x) \tag{8.41}$$

If we use the exponential utility model described in Section 8.5 to represent the decision maker's utility for symptom-free life, we then have

$$Utility\ (x\ years, Q_i) = 1 - e^{-\gamma \phi_i x} \tag{8.42}$$

Of course, the relationship in Equation 8.42 only holds over the range of values for x for which the straight line approximation is a good fit. However, like Equation 8.31, this simple relationship shows how the decision maker's risk aversion toward the length of life and the disutility assigned to life in quality state Q_i can be combined to determine the utility for an outcome. Therefore, this simple relationship provides a simple approach to taking into account the decision maker's preferences when analyzing a decision.

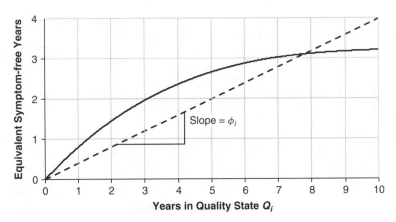

Figure 8.12 Linear approximation for the QALY relationship.

8.9 Comparison of the two models for outcomes with different length and quality

The two utility models described in the previous two sections represent different approaches determining an individual's utility for outcomes that differ according to length and quality. Each depends on different assumptions about the decision maker's preferences. This final section compares the implications for these underlying assumptions.

The first model, described in Section 8.8, assumes that the decision maker's *risk aversion* for length of life is the same for all quality states. The second model, based on QALY and described in Section 8.9, assumes that the decision maker's *time tradeoff* for different quality states is the same for all lengths of life. In this discussion we will call these the "constant risk aversion" model and the "constant time tradeoff" model, respectively. The goal in this section is to understand the consequences of these assumptions.

Figure 8.13 compares these models for an individual whose utility for life in quality state Q_A is described by the exponential utility model:

$$Utility\ (x\ years, Q_A) = 1 - e^{-\gamma x} \tag{8.43}$$

With the constant risk aversion model the same value for γ applies to both quality states. Therefore, this individual's utility for life in quality state Q_B can then be expressed as

$$Utility\ (x\ years, Q_B) = \theta_B \times (1 - e^{-\gamma x}) \tag{8.44}$$

where θ_B is the individual's indifference probability in the standard reference gamble comparing 10 years in quality state Q_A to 10 years in quality state Q_B:

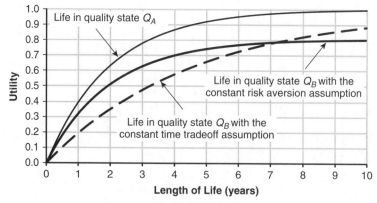

Figure 8.13 Constant time tradeoff and constant risk aversion utility models.

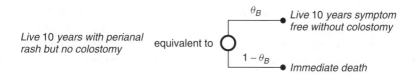

The utility function in Equation 8.44 is the lower solid curve in Figure 8.13.

With the constant time tradeoff model the decision maker's time tradeoff for different quality states is the same for all lengths of life. Therefore, the individual's utility for life in quality state Q_B can then be expressed:

$$Utility \ (x \ years, Q_B) = 1 - e^{-\gamma \phi_B x} \tag{8.45}$$

where ϕ_B is the QALY multiplier such that x years in Q_B is equivalent to $\phi_B x$ years in Q_A. The utility function in equation 8.45 is the dotted curve in Figure 8.13.

By definition, with the constant risk aversion model, the risk aversion for life in quality state Q_B is the same as the risk aversion for life in quality state Q_B. For example, if the following equivalence holds for x years in Q_A and probability π

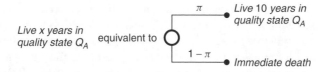

then the same equivalence must hold for x years in Q_B with the *same* value for probability π:

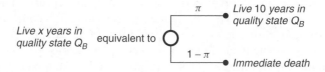

That is what it means to have constant risk aversion.

Look closely at Figure 8.13 and compare the two utility curves for life in Q_B. Compared to the constant risk aversion model (the solid curve), note that the constant time tradeoff model (the dashed curve) assigns lower utility to near-term survival and higher utility to long-term survival. Recalling the discussion in Section 8.5.3, this means that the constant time tradeoff model assumes that risk aversion is less when life will be lived in quality state Q_B. Mathematically, since the parameter in the exponential utility model γ measures risk aversion for life in quality state Q_A, the risk aversion for life in Q_B would be $\phi_B \gamma$. Keep in mind that ϕ_B is less than 1 since it is the amount the decision maker would be willing to shorten life in order to avoid the symptoms of quality state Q_B.

Therefore, with the constant time tradeoff model, the decision maker's risk aversion is assumed to be less for symptomatic life. In the extreme case of symptoms that are almost as bad a death (i.e., ϕ_B is almost 0) the decision maker is assumed to be virtually risk neutral in analysis based on the constant time tradeoff model of QALY analysis.

Whether or not this assumption accurately characterizes human behavior is a question that must be answered by the decision maker. The goal of utility analysis is to determine the alternative that best fits the decision maker's preferences. Decision makers who believe that their risk aversion decreases as symptoms worsen can find that best alternative using the constant time tradeoff assumption of QALY analysis. That is not true for decision makers who think of longevity and quality as independent contributors to their well-being. These individuals can be better represented by the constant risk aversion model. The power of these two models is that together they represent a utility assessment approach that can accommodate a broad range of risk attitudes.

Summary

This chapter has extended the analytic methods introduced in Chapters 6 and 7 by showing how to quantify the decision maker's preferences for the possible outcomes of a decision. The utility theory of John von Neumann and Oskar Morgenstern provides the foundation for this approach. The result is a generalizable method for capturing the value tradeoffs between the different dimensions of an outcome (length of life; quality of life) as well as the decision maker's attitudes toward risk.

The chapter describes several methods for applying the theory of von Neumann and Morgenstern, starting with an approach based on the direct assessment of a person's utility for each individual outcome. The shortcoming of direct assessment is the difficulty of staying focused on the task when doing it on a large scale for complex decision problems with large numbers of outcomes. Therefore, we described alternate methods, starting with a parametric model based on a testable assumption about the decision maker's preferences, called the delta property. When this property accurately describes the decision maker's preferences, the utility function has an exponential form whose shape is determined by a single parameter. This assumption reduces the assessment process to the relatively simple task of determining that single parameter. The exponential utility model can be combined with an exponential survival model to produce a compact expression for computing the expected utility for an outcome with a known life expectancy.

The remainder of the chapter presented methods for determining the decision maker's utility when the outcomes can involve several quality states. We described two methods, both starting with the decision maker's utility for length of life in one of the quality states – typically the symptom-free state. The two methods differ in how to adjust this utility function to reflect the decision maker's preferences for an alternate quality state. The first method determines a multiplier that adjusts that utility to account for the disutility of living with the symptom. The magnitude of the multiplier is assessed using a standard reference gamble that determines the risks of death the decision maker would accept in order to avoid the symptom. The second method, called quality-adjusted life years or QALY analysis, is based on the notion that people can express their attitude toward a quality state by adjusting the length of life without a symptom so that it is equivalent to the length of life with the symptom. The magnitude of the adjustment is assessed by asking time tradeoff questions that determine the reduction in the length of symptomatic life needed to have an equivalent length of life without symptoms.

In the end, both methods determine the decision maker's utility that incorporates both risk aversion toward the length of life as well as concerns about the quality of life. Therefore, these utility models support the purpose of a decision analysis, which is to identify the choice that best reflects the concerns of the decision maker.

Problems

1. Suppose that a patient with a toothache faces the decision tree shown in Figure 8.14. The patient can choose to have a root canal now or wait one month to see if the toothache stops on its own. If the toothache continues the patient will have the root canal. The patient also faces uncertainty about keeping the tooth. As shown in Figure 8.14, assume that delaying the root canal increases the chance that the patient will lose the tooth. Letting the toothache self-limit further increases the chances that the tooth will be lost. Use direct utility assessment to determine a friend's utility for the six possible outcomes. Determine if your friend would choose to delay the root canal, given the probabilities assumed in Figure 8.14.
2. Suppose that an individual told you that he or she was indifferent between the following two options:

What would this individual's indifference probability π be in the following assessment question if he or she had constant risk aversion?

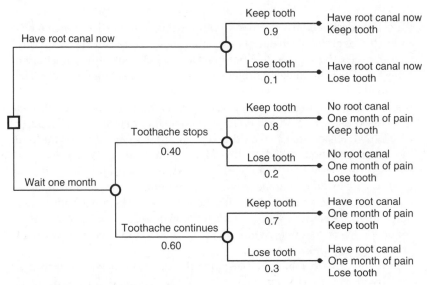

Figure 8.14 Decision tree for Problem 1.

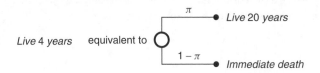

What is the value of the parameter γ for the exponential utility model describing this individual's preferences? Is this individual risk averse, risk preferring, or risk indifferent?

3. Assess a friend's utility for monetary prizes between $0 and $1000. Is your friend risk averse, risk preferring, or risk indifferent?

4. Assume that a patient facing the decision shown in Figure 8.15 has constant aversion for the length of his or her life. The decision is between Treatment A and Treatment B. The risk of immediate death is 0.10 for Treatment A; however, if the patient survives, the length of his or her life can be represented by an exponential survival model with parameter λ_A equal to 0.25. The risk of immediate death is 0.09 for Treatment B; however, if the patient survives, the length of his or her life can be represented by an exponential survival model with parameter λ_B equal to 0.20. Which treatment does the patient prefer if he or she is indifferent between the following two options?

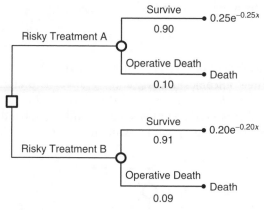

Figure 8.15 Decision tree for Problem 4.

5. Using the same decision problem described in Problem 4, assume that Treatment A involves an undesirable side effect that the patient will experience for the remainder of his or her life, if the patient survives the initial risk. Suppose that the patient's attitude is captured by the following equivalence:

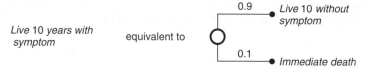

Assuming independence between preferences for length of life and quality of life, does this change your answer to problem 4?

Appendix: Mathematical details

This appendix covers some of the mathematical details that were skipped over in the early parts of this chapter. These details connect the methods described in this chapter to their origins in mathematical principles. We include this material for the reader who would like to understand these foundations.

Fundamental utility theorem

The fundamental result in von Neumann and Morgenstern's utility theory derives from five assumptions about the decision maker's preferences. These assumptions, or axioms, are as follows.

Axiom 1: Complete transitive ordering

The decision maker's preferences over the set of outcomes are such that for any two outcomes X_i and X_j one of the following is true:[1]

$$X_i \succ X_j \ \ or \ \ X_i \prec X_j \ \ or \ \ X_i \approx X_j \tag{A8.1}$$

---

[1] $X_i \succ X_j$ means that X_i is preferred to X_j; $X_i \approx X_j$ means that X_i is equivalent to X_j.

Moreover, for any three outcomes X_A, X_B, and X_C,

$$X_A \succ X_B \quad and \quad X_B \succ X_C \quad implies \quad X_A \succ X_C \tag{A8.2}$$

Axiom 2: Existence of indifference probabilities

For any three outcomes X_A, X_B, and X_C, if X_A is preferred to X_B and X_B is preferred to X_C then there exists a probability π such that the decision maker is indifferent between X_B and a gamble that awards X_A with probability π and X_C with probability $1 - \pi$:

$$X_B \approx \quad \overbrace{\quad}^{\pi \; \bullet X_A}_{1 - \pi \; \bullet X_C}$$

Axiom 3: Replacement with equivalence

Let outcomes X_A, X_B, and X_C and probability q be such that the decision maker is indifferent between X_B and a gamble that awards X_A with probability q and X_C with probability $1 - q$. Then X_B and the gamble between X_A and X_C can be interchanged without affecting the decision maker's preferences for a decision alternative. That is, for outcomes X_D and probability p the following equivalence holds:

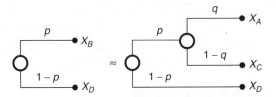

Axiom 4: Rules of probability apply

For any three outcomes X_A, X_B, and X_C and probabilities q and p, the following two gambles are equivalent:

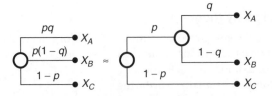

Axiom 5: Preference for dominant gambles

Let X_A and X_B be outcomes such that the decision maker prefers X_A over X_B. Then the decision maker prefers a gamble that yields X_A with probability p and X_B with probability $1 - p$ over a gamble that yields X_A

with probability q and X_B with probability $1 - q$ if and only if p is greater than q. That is, the following equivalence holds:

Von Neumann and Morgenstern's fundamental theorem guarantees the existence of a utility function which has the property that the expected utility is greatest for the most preferred alternative. This important result can be stated as follows:

Fundamental utility theorem

If the decision maker's preferences satisfy Axioms 1–5 for outcomes $X = \{X_1, \ldots, X_n\}$ then there exists a function $U(\ )$ over X such that for any alternatives A_j and A_k

$$\sum_{i=1}^{n} P[X_i | A_j] \times U(X_i) > \sum_{i=1}^{n} P[X_i | A_k] \times U(X_i) \qquad (A8.3)$$

if and only if the decision maker prefers A_j over A_k. That is,

$$E(U|A_j) > E(U|A_k) \text{ if and only if } A_j \succ A_k \qquad (A8.4)$$

The proof follows directly from the axioms. **Axiom 1** guarantees that the outcomes can be ranked according to the decision maker's preference. Therefore, all of the outcomes are preferred or equivalent to at least one of the outcomes. Denote this dominated outcome by X_1 and set $U(X_1) = 0$. Similarly, there exists at least one outcome that is preferred or equivalent to all of the other outcomes. Denote this dominating outcome by X_n and set $U(X_n) = 1$. For any outcome X_i, **Axiom 2** guarantees that there exists a probability π_i such that the decision maker is indifferent between X_i and a gamble that awards X_n with probability π_i and outcome X_1 with probability $1 - \pi_i$. That is,

Therefore, given alternatives A_j and A_k, with conditional probability density functions $P[X|A_j]$ and $P[X|A_k]$, respectively, note that these two alternatives can be represented by the tree structures:

Consider for a moment the tree corresponding to A_j. According to **Axiom 3**, this simple tree is equivalent to the compound tree formed by replacing each of the outcomes with the equivalent gamble between X_1 and X_n. That is,

Axiom 4 can then be used to combine the probabilities for the two outcomes resulting in an equivalent tree involving only X_1 and X_n:

In other words, A_j is equivalent to a lottery that awards X_n with probability $\sum_{i=1}^{n} P[X_i|A_j]\pi_i$ and X_1 with probability $1 - \sum_{i=1}^{n} P[X_i|A_j]\pi_i$. Similarly, A_k is equivalent to a lottery that awards X_n with probability $\sum_{i=1}^{n} P[X_i|A_k]\pi_i$ and X_1

with probability $1 - \sum_{i=1}^{n} P[X_i|A_k]\pi_i$. That is,

Since X_n is preferred to X_1 it follows from **Axiom 5** that A_j is preferred to A_k if and only if $\sum_{i=1}^{n} P[X_i|A_j]\pi_i$ is greater than $\sum_{i=1}^{n} P[X_i|A_k]\pi_i$. Setting $U(X_i) = \pi_i$ completes the proof.

Delta property and exponential utility

Proving the relationship between the delta property and exponential utility will not be fully reproduced here. The interested reader can find this proof in Chapter 4 of the book by Keeney and Raiffa (1976). Their proof starts with the definition of $R(\ )$, the *local risk aversion* function for utility function $U(\ )$:

$$R(x) = \frac{-\frac{d^2 U(x)}{dx^2}}{\frac{dU(x)}{dx}} \tag{A8.5}$$

Readers familiar with analytic geometry will recognize that $R(\ )$ measures the curvature of the corresponding utility function, which is why it is called the local risk aversion function. It turns out that $R(\ )$ also fully specifies a utility function in the sense that two utility functions are equivalent whenever they have the same local risk aversion functions. The proof that the delta property implies exponential utility follows from two intermediate results. First, the delta property implies that $R(x)$ is constant for all values of x. Second, from a straightforward calculus manipulation it can be shown that $R(\ )$ can only be constant if $U(\ )$ is exponential.

The elegance of the local risk aversion function is that it links preferences to a wide range of parametric utility modes that can be used when the delta property does not apply.

Computing expected utility for exponential survival and utility

Finally, the expected utility for an outcome measured by a continuous variable x is given by the integral

$$Expected\ Utility = \int_{x_{min}}^{x_{max}} f(x)u(x)dx \tag{A8.6}$$

where $f(x)$ is the probability density for x and $u(x)$ is the corresponding utility function. For the special case of exponential survival and exponential utility this integral becomes

$$Expected\ Utility = \int_{0}^{\infty} \lambda e^{-\lambda x}(1 - e^{-\gamma x})dx \tag{A8.7}$$

Expanding the integral yields

$$Expected\ Utility = \int_{0}^{\infty} \lambda e^{-\lambda x}dx - \int_{0}^{\infty} \lambda e^{-\lambda x}e^{-\gamma x}dx \tag{A8.8}$$

Or

$$Expected\ Utility = \int_{0}^{\infty} \lambda e^{-\lambda x}dx - \frac{\lambda}{\lambda + \gamma} \int_{0}^{\infty} (\lambda + \gamma)e^{-(\lambda+\gamma)x}dx \tag{A8.9}$$

But the two integrals in Equation A8.9 are both 1. Therefore

$$Expected\ Utility = 1 - \frac{\lambda}{\lambda + \gamma} = \frac{\gamma}{\lambda + \gamma} \tag{A8.10}$$

which is the result used in Equation 8.10.

Bibliography

Holloway, C.A. (1979) *Decision Making Under Uncertainty: Models and Choices*, Prentice Hall, Englewood Cliffs, NJ.

An overview of decision analysis.

Keeney, R.L. and Raffia, H. (1976) *Decisions with Multiple Objectives: Preferences and value tradeoffs*, John Wiley & Sons, Inc., New York.

Features a highly detailed description of utility models. Chapter 4 of this important book covers parametric models. Chapter 6 covers the utility independence concepts.

Raffia, H. (1968) *Decision Analysis: Introductory Lectures on Choices under Uncertainty*, Addison-Wesley, Reading, MA.

A general introduction to the use of the von Neumann–Morgenstern utility theory in decision analysis.

CHAPTER 9

Selection and interpretation of diagnostic tests

Do that test only if the results could change what you do for the patient.

(Anonymous)

This clinical precept is familiar to students of medicine. It is a challenge to the student to be thoughtful about ordering tests and diagnostic procedures. The purpose of this chapter is to provide a logical, patient-centered approach to selecting and interpreting diagnostic tests. By selection, we mean the decision to order a test. Interpretation is more difficult to define. Some would say it means "to explain what the test results mean." That definition is a good start toward the one we proposed in Chapter 4: "now that I know the post-test probability of disease, what shall I do?"

These two ideas, selection and interpretation, are linked to a third idea, trying to predict the effect of test results on patient care, something to do before ordering a test but also after you know the results.

This chapter has nine parts. An illustrative test ordering problem, the selection of tests for suspected brain tumor, appears at several points in the chapter.

Medical Decision Making, Second Edition. Harold C. Sox, Michael C. Higgins and Douglas K. Owens.

9.1   Taking action when the consequences are uncertain: principles and definitions

9.1.1   Three principles of decision making

The following principles lead directly to a method for deciding when a diagnostic test will alter the patient's treatment:

1. *Knowing the patient's true state is often unnecessary*: Clinicians' terminology often seems to imply that they cannot start treatment without being sure of the patient's true state, particularly when they use the term "make a diagnosis" to indicate that they believe that a disease is definitely present. They also use the term "ruling out a diagnosis" to indicate that they believe that disease is definitely absent, which would correspond to a probability of disease equal to 0. If action depended on "making a diagnosis" or "ruling out disease," clinicians would be compelled to ascertain each patient's true state before starting treatment. In fact, they often do not know the patient's true state when they start treatment.

   Every practicing clinician understands the distinction between *knowing* that a disease is present and *acting* as if it were present. When the probability of a disease is 0.95, there is a small chance that it is not present yet clinicians often start treatment as if they were certain of the true state of the patient. In practice, the terms "making a diagnosis" and "ruling out disease" mean the following:
   - making a diagnosis: knowing that more information would not change a decision to act as if the patient had the suspected disease;
   - ruling out a disease: knowing that more information would not change the decision to act as if the patient did not have the suspected disease.

2. *Treatment error is always a possibility when the diagnosis is uncertain*: Figure 9.1 is a reminder of the implications of probability in medicine. Each point on a probability scale corresponds to a population in which some patients are diseased (solid circles) and some are not diseased (open circles).

   If a clinician elects to treat a patient when the probability of disease is greater than 0 and less than 1.0, some patients will receive treatment for

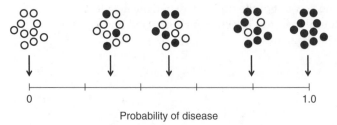

Probability of disease

Figure 9.1 The correspondence of probability and hypothetical populations of patients. The solid circles represent diseased persons.

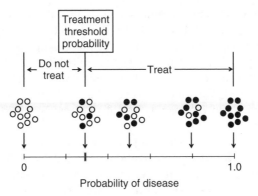

Figure 9.2 Treatment population when the diagnosis is not certain.

a disease that they do not have. Figure 9.2 illustrates this for a situation in which the treatment threshold probability is 0.25.

According to Figure 9.2, some patients would receive treatment even though they do not have disease. If the treatment was risky and the disease was not very serious, the damage they incur could outweigh the benefit to the diseased patients.

3. *The need for diagnostic certainty depends on the penalty for being wrong*: How sure must a clinician be before starting treatment? The need for diagnostic certainty depends on the penalty for being wrong about the patient's true state. Several examples will illustrate this point.

Example 1: Suppose that you are an internist seeing a patient with sudden onset of stabbing pain in the right anterior chest a week after total knee replacement. The physical examination is normal, with no swelling above or below the knee on the side of the surgery. Despite the physical examination, you strongly suspect a pulmonary embolism (PE), but your pre-test probability is 0.75 (pre-test odds 3:1), so you are not sure. You obtain a contrast CT scan of the chest. To your surprise, it does not show any evidence of PE. Should you send the patient home without starting treatment, start anticoagulation (the correct treatment for venous thrombosis and PE) or obtain a pulmonary arteriogram?

This question restates the classic dilemma that clinicians face when managing a high-stakes condition like PE. Failure to treat when the patient has a blood clot in the leg (a common occurrence after surgery on the leg) could result in a second, perhaps fatal PE. Treating with anticoagulants when the patient does not have a blood clot occasionally results in serious bleeding that can be fatal.

You start by removing your smart phone from your pocket. You have downloaded a program developed for a study of computer-assisted management of suspected PE. You enter the pre-test odds of PE (3:1).

The computer program reminds you of the likelihood ratio negative (LR−) of a contrast CT scan (0.10). It calculates the post-test odds of PE (post-test odds = pre-test odds × likelihood ratio) as 3:1 × 0.10 = 0.3:1, which is equivalent to a 0.23 post-test probability of PE. You think to yourself, "I'm surprised the post-test probability of PE is so high after a negative contrast CT scan. However, that probability of PE is too high for me to withhold anticoagulation. Shall I treat now or do a pulmonary arteriogram?"

Your smart phone-based computer program can help you to answer this question. Based on information provided by its creators, it says "either strategy is reasonable. A pulmonary arteriogram nearly always detects a PE, and false-positive results are rare. If it is negative, the post-test probability of PE is so low that you should not treat. If it's positive, you are certain of the diagnosis. The probability that the arteriogram will be positive is 0.23." You decide to obtain the arteriogram, and it shows a pulmonary embolus.

Comment: The only part of this story that may be unclear to the reader is the judgment about when to treat a PE. The treatment threshold probability is surprisingly low (~0.10) due to the favorable balance of harms and benefits of anticoagulation for known PE. So, the patient's post-test probability of PE (0.23) is well above the threshold for starting treatment. However, the pulmonary arteriogram could change the management of this patient if it is negative (remember that its sensitivity is close to 1.0). So, testing is reasonable in this situation, but so is treating (especially if the arteriogram is not available).

Example 2: A pediatrician is examining an adolescent with a sore throat. The patient has low-grade fever, a confluent tonsillar exudate, and very tender anterior cervical lymph nodes. The pediatrician estimates the probability of streptococcal pharyngitis to be 0.50 and gives the patient an injection of benzathine penicillin without obtaining a test for beta-hemolytic streptococcal infection

Comment: The pediatrician is willing to treat even though the probability of treating someone who does not have a strep infection is 0.50 because she believes that the consequences of this error are minor and she would not trust a negative throat culture in this patient. The pediatrician bases the decision to treat without a culture on the safety of treatment with penicillin. A small penalty for error allows a larger margin for error.

9.1.2   The meaning of the treatment-threshold probability

The preceding examples illustrated one point in common: the relationship between the willingness to treat and the probability of disease. These examples

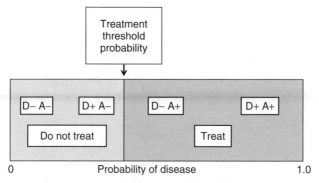

Figure 9.3 The treatment-threshold probability defines four groups of patients. $D+$ denotes disease present. $D-$ denotes disease absent. $A+$ denotes action taken (such as treatment given). $A-$ denotes action withheld.

illustrated implicitly the concept of a *disease probability threshold*. This concept is the key to understanding when a person should start treatment for a disease when still uncertain about the diagnosis. It addresses directly the question "when am I sure enough to act as if I am certain?"

Definition of treatment-threshold probability: The probability of disease at which one should be indifferent between giving treatment and withholding treatment.

The treatment threshold divides patients into those who receive treatment and those who do not. Referring to Figure 9.2, recall that both groups comprise patients who have the target condition and patients who do not have it. Figure 9.3 illustrates these four groups of patients.

As shown in Figure 9.3, patients whose true state ($D+$ or $D-$) is unknown can be in one of four states following a decision to take action ($A+$) or to withhold action ($A-$). We call these states "disease-treatment states." These terms will be used frequently in this chapter:

- *Diseased and treated*: Potentially a nice state to be in, depending on the seriousness of the disease and the effectiveness of treatment. Denoted by $D+A+$.
- *Diseased and not treated*: Usually the worst state to be in, unless the disease is something minor like an upper respiratory infection, and the treatment is unpleasant. Denoted by $D+A-$.
- *Not diseased and treated*: Often an acceptable state to be in, less so if the treatment has unpleasant or serious side effects. Denoted by $D-A+$.
- *Not diseased and not treated*: The best state to be in. Denoted by $D-A-$.

9.2 The treatment-threshold probability

In the first part of this chapter, we learned that the treatment threshold reflects the tradeoffs between the harms and benefits of the treatment options. The

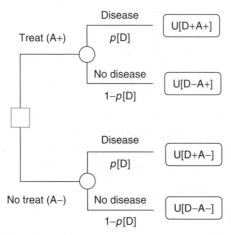

Figure 9.4 The decision between treatment and no treatment. U[D+A+] denotes the patient's utility for the state of being diseased and being treated.

goal of this section is to derive a mathematical expression for this relationship. The derivation of this relationship is straightforward.

Consider the following situation. The clinician has completed the history and physical examination, has done all the recommended diagnostic tests, and must now choose whether to treat or to withhold treatment. The situation may be represented by a simple decision tree (Figure 9.4).

To decide between these alternatives, we must calculate the expected utility of each alternative. As expected utility decision makers, we will then choose the treatment alternative with the highest expected utility. The expected utility (EU) is obtained by averaging out at the chance nodes. This process is expressed in the following equations:

$$EU[A-] = p \times U[D + A-] + (1 - p) \times U[D - A-] \qquad (9.1)$$

$$EU[A+] = p \times U[D + A+] + (1 - p) \times U[D - A+] \qquad (9.2)$$

These two equations may be represented graphically by plotting the expected utility of the $A+$ and $A-$ alternatives against p, the probability of disease (Figure 9.5).

To maximize the patient's welfare, the clinician should choose the alternative that has the highest expected utility. Figure 9.5 shows that the preferred option depends on the probability of disease. When the probability of disease is low, the "no treatment" option has the highest expected utility and should be preferred. When the probability of disease is high, the "treat" option has the highest expected utility and should be preferred. At one probability of disease, the expected utilities of the two options are equal: the point where the two curves intersect. At this point (denoted by C), the clinician should be indifferent between treating and withholding treatment. This point is the treatment threshold probability (denoted by p^*).

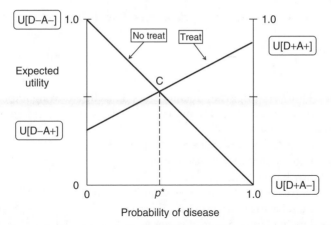

Figure 9.5 Expected utility of the treat (A+) and no treatment (A−) options, as derived from Equations 9.1 and 9. 2. The line that runs from the upper left corner to the lower right corner represents Equation 9.1, the expected utility of no treatment (A−) as a function of the probability of disease (p). The line running from lower left to upper right represents Equation 9.2, the expected utility of treatment (A+) as a function of the probability of disease.

To decide which action to take, the clinician need only estimate the probability of disease and compare it to the treatment-threshold probability. This approach to decision making is remarkably simple in principle, since one must only learn how to estimate the treatment-threshold probability.

To calculate the threshold-treatment probability, proceed as follows. The expected utility of the two decision alternatives (A+ and A−) are equal at the treatment-threshold probability. Therefore, set Equation 9.1 equal to Equation 9.2 and solve for p^*, the treatment-threshold probability:

$$\frac{p^*}{1-p^*} = \frac{U[D-A-] - U[D-A+]}{U[D+A+] - U[D+A-]} \tag{9.3}$$

This expression may be solved for p^*, the treatment-threshold probability, by rearranging terms and substituting the following definitions:

$$H = U[D-A-] - U[D-A+]$$

H is the net harm of treating patients who do not have the target condition as if they did have it. They cannot benefit from treatment. Therefore, any effects of treatment are a "harm" of treatment.

The second definition is

$$B = U[D+A+] - U[D+A-]$$

B is the net benefit of treating diseased patients, and is therefore the difference in utility between treating and not treating a diseased person.

Solving Equation 9. 3 for p^* by substituting H and B, we get

$$p^* = \frac{H}{H + B} \qquad\qquad (9.4)$$

Equation 9.4 is a very important relationship. It has three strong implications:
1. The harms and benefits of treatment affect the threshold-treatment probability in revealing ways.
    A low treatment-threshold probability is due to:
     • high benefit to diseased patients;
     • low harms to non-diseased patients.
    A high treatment-threshold probability is due to:
     • high harms to non-diseased patients;
     • low benefit to diseased patients.

2. *The treatment-threshold probability is usually lower than 0.50* because the benefits of most treatments exceed their harms. As an extreme example, consider the example of deciding when to give penicillin for suspected pneumococcal pneumonia. Penicillin is a safe drug for those who do not have a penicillin allergy, and it is very beneficial for patients with pneumococcal pneumonia. With minimal harms and a large benefit, you would expect a low treatment-threshold probability. Conclusion: if you have any reason to suspect pneumococcal pneumonia, you should start penicillin.

3. *p^* depends only on the patient's utilities for the disease-treatment states.* It does not depend on the probability that these states will occur. Since p^* depends on the utilities for the disease-treatment states, it will reflect the outcomes of those states their probabilities relative to one another, and the patient's utilities for those outcomes.

    For an example of calculating p^*, imagine treating a patient with penicillin for suspected pneumococcal pneumonia-. First, calculate the harms, remembering that $H = U[D - A-] - U[D - A+]$:

    $U[D-A-]$ is how a person would feel about not having pneumonia and not getting treated for it. On a scale of 0 to 1.0, where 0 is the worst possible outcome (immediate death) and 1.0 is a person's current health, the person would probably say that $U[D-A-]$ is 1.0.

    $U[D-A+]$ is how a person would feel about not having pneumonia but being treated for it anyway. This disease-treatment state occurs when the clinician starts treatment before knowing the patient's true state, as shown in Figure 9.6. In this example, a patient treated with penicillin has three outcome states: no allergic reaction, a non-fatal reaction (a rash, wheezing, non-fatal anaphylactic shock), and fatal anaphylactic shock. Imagine that the probabilities of these three states are 0.99, 0.0099, and 0.0001, respectively, and the patient's utilities for these states are 1.0, 0.90, and 0. Because these outcomes of an

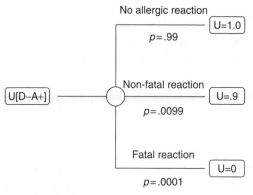

No allergic reaction

U=1.0

p=.99

U[D–A+]

Non-fatal reaction

U=.9

p=.0099

Fatal reaction

U=0

p=.0001

Figure 9.6 A tree representing the $D-A+$ state.

allergic reaction occur by chance, we can use a tree to calculate the expected utility of the $D-A+$ state (Figure 9.6).

The expected utility of the $D-A+$ state is the sum over the three outcome states of the products of the probability of each state times the patient's utility for that state (= (0.99×1.0) + $(0.0099 \times 0.90) + (0.0001 \times 0))\ 0.9989$).

Remembering that $H = U[D - A-] - U[D - A+]$, $H = 1.0 - 0.9989 = 0.0011$.

Now, calculate the benefits, remembering that $B = U[D + A+] - U[D + A-]$.

$U[D+A+]$: To calculate this utility, assume that the only long-term outcome states of pneumonia are recovery or death. The patient's utilities for these outcomes states are 1.0 and 0. The recovery rate with treatment of pneumococcal pneumonia is 0.99. $U[D+A+]$ is 0.99 times U(recovery), which equals 1.0, plus 0.01 times U(death), which equals 0. $U[D+A+]$ is therefore 0.99.

$U[D+A-]$: In this disease-treatment state, the patient has pneumonia and recovers spontaneously. A hypothetical recovery rate without treatment is 0.50, so $U[D+A-]$ is 0.50 times the utility for recovery $(U = 1.0) = 1.0$.

Thus, $B = 0.99 - 0.50 = 0.49$.

Therefore, the treatment threshold is

$$p^* = \frac{H}{H + B} = \frac{0.0011}{0.0011 + 0.49} = 0.0022$$

The threshold treatment probability is a valuable tool for decision makers. Clinicians typically decide which action to take (treat or do not treat) by subjectively weighing the harms and benefits of treatment against the clinical characteristics of the patient. The treatment-threshold probability transforms this intuitive, improvised process into a precise, consistent method to aid decision making. As shown in Figure 9.5, when the threshold-treatment probability and the probability of disease are known, the clinician can identify the action that will maximize the patient's expected utility.

However, understanding this model of decision making is the easy part. Implementing it is hard work. The task of determining the treatment-threshold probability requires a decision model and the patient's utilities for the outcomes that the patient may experience.

The meaning of "treatment"

We have referred to "treatment" as if it were a therapy to be given when the probability of disease exceeded the threshold probability. Another, broader view is that the clinician commits to a course of action. The course of action could be starting a treatment or it could be doing a definitive test to decide whether to start treatment. Thus, "treatment" in the broadest sense is an algorithm that prescribes each action. Reflecting this definition of "treatment," we have used the symbols $A+$ (for "take definitive action") and $A-$ ("withhold definitive action"). Thus, the disease-treatment state $D+A+$ means "the patient has the target condition and definitive action was taken."

9.3 The decision to obtain a diagnostic test

9.3.1 The criteria for diagnostic testing

These are as follows:

1. *When the pre-test probability exceeds the treatment threshold:* Is treatment always indicated when the probability of disease is above the treatment threshold? Not necessarily. Treating when the probability of disease is above the treatment-threshold probability exposes non-diseased patients to potential harm without prospect of benefit (Figure 9.1). We can avoid this outcome if a negative test result reduced the probability of disease to a point below the treatment-threshold probability, so that the action with the highest expected utility would be "do not treat" (see Figure 9.7).

   • Criterion 1: Do a test only if a test result could lower the probability of disease enough to cross a treatment threshold.

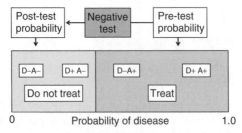

Figure 9.7 A negative test result lowers the probability of disease past the threshold probability.

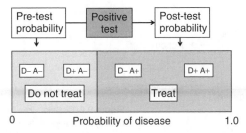

Figure 9.8 A positive test result raises the probability of disease past the threshold probability.

Whether a test result could meet this criterion depends on its test performance (sensitivity, specificity, likelihood ratio-negative), the pre-test probability, and the treatment threshold probability.

2. *When the pre-test probability of disease is lower than the treatment threshold:* Should treatment always be withheld when the probability of disease is lower than the threshold-treatment probability? Not necessarily. Looking at Figure 9.1, you see that some patients with a low probability actually do have the target condition. They are likely to experience harm unless they receive treatment. Avoiding these harms altogether is not realistic since it would require a zero probability of the target condition in order to justify withholding treatment. However, if a test could raise the probability of disease past the treatment threshold, treatment would maximize the treated patient's expected utility (Figure 9.8). Of course, it might not be reasonable to do the test if the probability of a positive result was very low, as occurs when the pre-test odds are very low or the test result has a low sensitivity ($p+|D$).

   • Criterion 2: Do a test only if a test result could raise the probability of disease enough to cross a treatment threshold (Figure 9.8).

The two criteria are equivalent. They restate in technical language the teaching precept that you should test only if the result could change your management of the patient.

Test if the result could move the probability of disease past a treatment threshold.

Thus, one role of testing is to reduce the chance that treatment will be given or withheld when additional information could improve a decision. In this chapter, this basic principle will be transformed into a method for deciding which patients will benefit from a diagnostic test.

9.3.2   A method for deciding to perform a diagnostic test

We learned how the clinician can make a treatment decision in the special circumstance of having already obtained as much information as can possibly

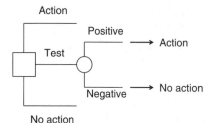

Action

Test

Positive → Action

Negative → No action

No action

Figure 9.9 Decision tree for choosing between testing and taking action.

be obtained (Section 9.2). We now use similar reasoning to derive a method for deciding whether to obtain more information before making a treatment decision. The decision problem is represented by the tree shown in Figure 9.9.

To decide between these alternatives, we must calculate the expected utility of each alternative and choose the treatment alternative with the highest expected utility. Since the patient's true state and the outcome of the test are unknown, the decision alternatives are represented by the trees depicted in Figure 9.10.

The probabilities at the chance nodes that depict the outcome of the test are written in conditional probability notation. For example, if the patient

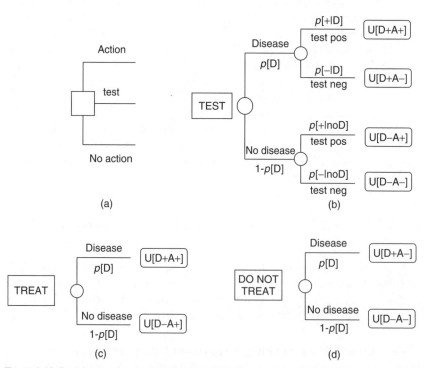

Figure 9.10 Decision tree for choosing between testing and taking action. In this figure, "action" is equivalent to "TREAT."

is diseased and the test is positive, the probability of the test being positive is the conditional probability, $P[+|D+]$ ("probability of a positive test given that disease is present"). Using this notation, we may calculate the expected utility of the test option by averaging out at the chance nodes in the tree for the TEST option in Figure 9.9:

$$EU[\text{Test}] = P[D] \times P[+|D] \times U[D+A+] + P[D] \times P[-|D] \times U[D+A-]$$
$$+ (1 - P[D]) \times P[+|\text{no } D] \times U[D-A+] \times (1 - P[D]) \times P[-|\text{no } D]$$
$$\times U[D-A-]$$

Recall the following definitions from Chapter 4:

$P[+|D]$ = true-positive rate of test (TPR or sensitivity)
$P[-|D]$ = false-negative rate of test (FNR)
$P[+|\text{no } D]$ = false-positive rate of test (FPR)
$P[-|\text{no } D]$ = true-negative rate of test (TNR or specificity)

Substituting these equalities into the equation for $EU[\text{Test}]$, we obtain Equation 9.5, which is the expected utility of the test option. Equation 9.5 includes a term for the utility of the test, $U(T)$, to take account of any effects of experiencing the test (e.g., some patients experience claustrophobia when placed in the narrow confines of the magnetic resonance imaging scanner):

$$EU[\text{Test}] = P[D] \times \text{TPR} \times U[D+A+] + P[D] \times (1 - \text{TPR}) \times U[D+A-]$$
$$+ (1 - P[D]) \times \text{FPR} \times U[D-A+] + (1 - P[D]) \times (1 - \text{FPR})$$
$$\times U[D-A-] + U(T) \tag{9.5}$$

The equations for the expected utility of the treat $(A+)$ and no treat $(A-)$ options are obtained by averaging out at the chance nodes in the trees for these options (Figure 9.10). The same equations were used in Section 9.2 to derive the expression for the treatment-threshold probability:

$$EU[A-] = P[D] \times U[D+A-] + (1 - P[D]) \times U[D-A-] \tag{9.6}$$

$$EU[A+] = P[D] \times U[D+A+] + (1 - P[D]) \times U[D-A+] \tag{9.7}$$

Abbreviations:

$U[\ ]$: the utility of a disease-treatment state.

$U[T]$ is the net utility of the test. $U[T]$ is determined by the patient's and clinician's attitudes toward such factors as the cost of the test, its morbidity and mortality, and reassurance provided by the test for psychological or medical–legal reasons.

$U[T]$ has a negative sign if the net effect of experiencing the test is undesirable. Thus, the test would reduce the expected utility of the test option in Equation 9.5.

$U[T]$ has a positive sign if the net effect of experiencing the test is desirable (the reassurance it provides outweighs the unpleasant aspects of the test). Thus, the test would increase the expected utility of the test option in Equation 9.5.

The name "net utility of the test" could lead to confusion of $U[T]$ with EU[Test], the expected utility of testing. Equation 9.5 shows that $U[T]$, the net utility of experiencing the test, is a component of EU[Test], along with the consequences of true-positive and false-positive test results.

We represent Equations 9.5–9.7 graphically by plotting the expected utility of the decision alternatives (test, treat, or no treat) against $p[D]$, the probability of disease. The slope and vertical axis intercepts of each of the lines are determined by the utility of the disease-treatment states, and, in the case of the testing option, by the true-positive rate and false-positive rate of the test. The utility of the test, $U(T)$, does not change the slope of the line corresponding to the test option, but it does alter the point at which the line intercepts the vertical axes.

To maximize the patient's welfare, the clinician should choose the alternative that has the highest expected utility. Figure 9.11 shows that the preferred option depends on the probability of disease:

Low probability of disease: Below a certain probability, no treatment is always preferred because an abnormal test result could not increase the probability of disease enough to cross the treatment threshold (p^*) and change management.

High probability of disease: Above a certain probability, treatment is always preferred because a negative test result could not reduce the probability of disease enough to cross the treatment threshold and change management.

Intermediate probability of disease: The testing option is preferred because a test result could alter the probability of disease enough to cross the treatment threshold and alter management.

9.3.3 The threshold probabilities for testing

The patient should prefer the alternative with the highest expected utility at the patient's pre-test probability of disease. The three solid lines in Figure 9.11 represent the expected utilities of the no treat, test, and treat options at each probability of disease. As shown in Figure 9.11, the probability scale is divided into three zones by two probabilities. These two probabilities are defined by the points where the lines intersect; at the leftmost of these intersections, the patient should be indifferent between no treatment ($A-$) and testing.

Definition of no treatment–test threshold: The probability at which one should be indifferent between no treatment and testing. We denote the no treatment–test threshold probability by $p1$ (Figure 9.12).

Below this threshold probability, the post-test probability after a positive test result is below the treatment threshold, and the test result would not affect management. In effect, if $p1$ is the pre-test probability, the post-test probability after a positive test is the treatment threshold, p^* (Figure 9.12).

Definition of test–treatment threshold: The probability at which one should be indifferent between testing and treatment. We denote the test–treatment threshold probability by $p2$ (Figure 9.13).

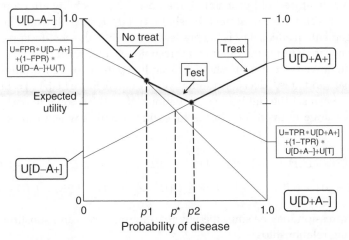

Figure 9.11 Relationship between the pre-test probability of disease and the expected utility of the test, treat, and no treatment options. The expressions for the expected utilities of these decision alternatives when $P[D] = 0$ and $P[D] = 1.0$ appear along the vertical axes. The labels within the graph denote the action with the highest expected utility at each probability of disease.

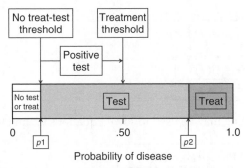

Figure 9.12 The no treatment–test threshold probability.

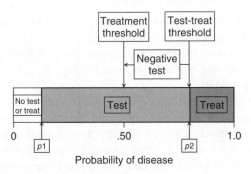

Figure 9.13 The test–treatment threshold probability.

Above this threshold probability, the post-test probability after a negative test result is above the treatment threshold, and the test result would not affect management. In effect, if $p2$ is the pre-test probability, the post-test probability after a negative test is the treatment threshold, p^* (Figure 9.13).

At the lower of these threshold probabilities, the expected utilities of the "no treat" and "test" decision alternatives are equal. Since $EU[A-] = EU[\text{Test}]$ at $p1$, we can set the right side of Equations 9.5 and 9.6 equal to one another and rearrange terms to obtain the following equation which can be solved for $p1$:

$$p1 \times \{\text{TPR} \times U[D + A+] + (1 - \text{TPR}) \times U[D + A-] - U[D + A-]\} + U(T)$$

$$= [1 - p1] \times \{U[D - A-] - \text{FPR} \times U[D - A+] - (1 - \text{FPR}) \times U[D - A-]\}$$

This expression may be simplified by rearranging terms and substituting the following relationships:

$H = U[D - A-] - U[D - A+]$ the cost of treating well patients

$B = U[D + A+] - U[D + A-]$ the benefit of treating diseased patients

$p1 \times (\text{TPR} \times B) + U(T) = (1 - p1) \times (\text{FPR} \times H)$
   Solving this expression for $p1$,

$$p1 = \frac{\text{FPR} \times H - U(T)}{\text{FPR} \times H + \text{TPR} \times B} \tag{9.8}$$

The same reasoning may be used to solve Equations 9.5 and 9.7 for $p2$:

$$p2 = \frac{(1 - \text{FPR}) \times H + U(T)}{(1 - \text{FPR}) \times H + (1 - \text{TPR}) \times B} \tag{9.9}$$

Equations 9.8 and 9.9 divide the probability scale into three sections corresponding to the no treat, test, and treat options (Figure 9.11). The clinician can use Figure 9.11 and the patient's pre-test probability of disease to decide what action will maximize the patient's expected utility. To achieve this goal is to accomplish a great deal.

Equations 9.8 and 9.9 and the pre-test probability of disease are sufficient to choose the decision alternative with the highest expected utility. These equations do not include a term for p^*, the treatment-threshold probability. Therefore, we are not required to determine p^* to solve the decision problem. Nevertheless, we shall focus in this chapter on how to determine the treatment-threshold probability. The clinician can use it (p^*) to judge if the solution to the decision problem makes clinical sense. This external check for clinical realism may prevent uncritical acceptance of the results of the analysis.

$p*$, the treatment-threshold probability, is related to H and B, the costs and benefits of treatment (see Equation 9.4). From this relationship, $p1$ and $p2$ may be obtained in terms of $p*$:

$$p^* = \frac{H}{H+B} \qquad (9.4)$$

Equation 9.4 may be solved for B in terms of H and $p*$. Substituting this expression for B in Equations 9.8 and 9.9, we obtain the following relationships between $p*$ and $p1$ and $p2$:

$$p1 = \frac{\text{FPR} \times p^* - \left[\frac{U(T)}{H}\right] \times p^*}{\text{FPR} \times p^* + (1 - p^*) \times \text{TPR}} \qquad (9.10)$$

$$p2 = \frac{(1 - \text{FPR}) \times p^* + \left[\frac{U(T)}{H}\right] \times p^*}{(1 - \text{FPR}) \times p^* + (1 - p^*) \times (1 - \text{TPR})} \qquad (9.11)$$

In many clinical situations, the utility of undergoing the test, $U(T)$, is small compared to the utility of experiencing the disease-treatment states. In these cases, the term for $U(T)$ may be set to zero. When $U(T)$ is zero, 9.10 and 9.11 can be derived using Bayes' Theorem where $p*$ is the post-test probability and $p1 < p*$ and $p2 > p*$ are the prior probabilities respectively. Solving these equations for $p1$ and $p2$ will get 9.10 and 9.11. These relationships underscore the point that $p*$ is the post-test probability when $p1$ and $p2$ are the prior probabilities.

9.4 Choosing between diagnostic tests

This advanced topic can be omitted on a first reading without loss of continuity.

The reasoning used to decide whether a test should be performed may be extended to the choice between tests. Consider the case of choosing between two tests, T_1 and T_2 (we will discuss the possibility of doing various combinations of the two tests subsequently). The decision maker now has four options:

Strategy	Test decision	Treatment decision
1	Do not test	Do not treat
2	Do not test	Treat
3	Do T_1	Treat only if T_1 is positive
4	Do T_2	Treat only if T_2 is positive

The strategy with the highest expected utility should be the preferred alternative. To calculate the expected utilities of these strategies, apply the reasoning used in the case of one test. (Subscripts are used to denote which of the two tests is intended, and p represents the probability of disease.) This approach results in the same decision tree as shown in Figure 9.9 except for one more subtree corresponding to the additional test. This tree would yield four equations (the additional one corresponding to the EU of T_2), where FPR_2 and TPR_2 denote the false-positive rate and true-positive rate for T_2:

$$EU[A+] = p \times U[D + A+] + (1 - p) \times U[D - A+] \tag{9.12}$$

$$EU[A-] = p \times U[D + A-] + (1 - p) \times U[D - A-] \tag{9.13}$$

$$\begin{aligned} EU[T_1] = {} & p \times TPR_1 \times U[D + A+] + p \times (1 - TPR_1) \times U[D + A-] \\ & + (1 - p) \times FPR_1 \times U[D - A+] \\ & + (1 - p) \times (1 - FPR_1) \times U[D - A-] + U(T_1) \end{aligned} \tag{9.14}$$

$$\begin{aligned} EU[T_2] = {} & p \times TPR_2 \times U[D + A+] + p \times (1 - TPR_2) \times U[D + A-] \\ & + (1 - p) \times FPR_2 \times U[D - A+] \\ & + (1 - p) \times (1 - FPR_2) \times U[D - A-] + U(T_2) \end{aligned} \tag{9.15}$$

Using these equations, the expected utility of each decision alternative may be plotted against the probability of disease (Figure 9.14). The slope of each of the lines and their vertical axis intercepts are determined by the utility of the disease–treatment states, and, in the case of the testing options, by the true-positive rates and false-positive rates of the two tests and their respective $U(T)$s.

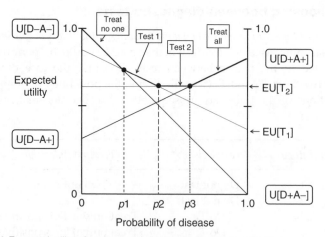

Figure 9.14 Expected utility of two test options and the treatment options.

The alternative with the highest expected utility at each pre-test probability of disease is the preferred alternative. The choice between the two tests depends on the pre-test probability of disease:

1. The lowest of the three threshold probabilities, $p1$, may be calculated by setting $EU(A-)$ equal to $EU(T_1)$ and $EU(T_2)$, solving each equation for p, and choosing the test corresponding to the lowest value of p to be Test 1 and assigning the lowest value of p to $p1$.
2. The highest of the three thresholds, $p3$, may be calculated by setting $EU(A+)$ equal to the expected utility of the remaining test, solving the resulting equation for p, and assigning that value of p to be $p3$.
3. The intermediate threshold, $p2$, is obtained by setting $EU(T_1)$ equal to $EU(T_2)$ and solving for p.

The appropriate action depends on the pre-test probability of disease as shown in the following table:

Pre-test P[D]	Test decision	Treatment decision
$P[D] < p1$	Do not test	Do not treat
$p1 < P[D] < p2$	Do T_1	Treat only if T_1 is positive
$p2 < P[D] < p3$	Do T_2	Treat only if T_2 is positive
$P[D] > p3$	Do not test	Treat

In Figure 9.14, note that if the line corresponding to $EU(T_2)$ is a little lower, $EU(T_1)$ will always exceed $EU(T_2)$. In that case, one should not choose T_2 at any probability of disease. T_1 will dominate.

9.5 Choosing the best combination of diagnostic tests

This advanced topic can be omitted on a first reading without loss of continuity.

9.5.1 Principles for choosing a combination of diagnostic tests

When two or more tests are available, the clinician may want to decide between doing both tests, one test, or neither test. This topic is discussed at length in an article by Doubilet (1983). In principle, the choice between combinations of tests is an extension of the approach already used.

Consider the situation in which there are two tests available, and the clinician can choose to do either test, both tests, neither test, or a second test conditional upon the results of the first test. In principle, the clinician may treat or withhold treatment with each combination of test results. However, for some combinations of test results some of the treatment decisions are illogical are unreasonable as management strategies and can be eliminated. Ten mutually exclusive strategies are listed in the table. The clinician's task is to choose the strategy that has the highest expected utility for a patient whose prior probability of the target condition is p.

Strategy	First stage	Second stage	Action
1	T_1	No tests	Treat only if $T_1 +$
2	T_1	T_2 if $T_1 +$	Treat only if $T_1 +$ and $T_2 +$
3	T_1	T_2 if $T_1 -$	Treat if $T_2 +$
4	T_2	No tests	Treat only if $T_2 +$
5	T_2	T_1 if $T_2 +$	Treat only if $T_2 +$ and $T_1 +$
6	T_2	T_1 if $T_2 -$	Treat if $T_1 +$
7	T_1 and T_2	No tests	Treat if $T_1 +$ and $T_2 +$
8	T_1 and T_2	No tests	Treat if $T_1 +$ or $T_2 +$
9	No tests	No tests	Treat no one
10	No tests	No tests	Treat everyone

Each action depicted in the table is a gamble, since the clinician does not know the true state of the patient at the time of deciding to treat or not. To solve this problem, start with a decision tree that represents the choice between all 10 strategies. This tree has 10 subtrees, each depicting the consequences of one of the strategies. Using the subtree for each strategy, form an equation for calculating the expected utility of the corresponding subtree; the equations will be similar to those shown for the choice between two tests but more complex. To calculate the expected utility of each strategy as a function of the probability of disease, substitute all possible values of $p[D]$ into the corresponding equation. In a graph of these findings, the slope of the line corresponding to each equation is a function of the utility of the disease-treatment states for each strategy and the performance characteristics and the disutility of the test combination. The intersections of the lines represent the threshold probabilities at which one strategy becomes preferred to another. This relationship is depicted in simplified form in Figure 9.15.

The strategy that is in the patient's best interests is the strategy with the highest expected utility at the patient's pre-test probability of disease.

One problem with modeling strategies for using several diagnostic tests in combination is being sure that the tests are conditionally independent, which is seldom known for a combination of tests. Chapter 5 contains a discussion of this problem.

9.5.2 Using a computer to choose the best decision option

The reader may wonder if this elegant conceptual model is a practical decision-making aid. Developing decision models of complex problems, finding the data required by the parameters of the models, and solving the resulting equations to obtain the threshold probabilities can be the work of many months. If all this work was expended to solve one patient's decision problem, the effort would not be sustainable. However, computer programs to represent and solve the decision models make these models available to anyone.

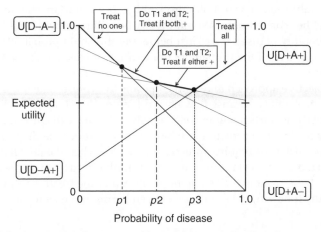

Figure 9.15 Expected utility of various combinations of tests and test results.

The data required by the threshold model are obtained from several sources. Methods for estimating the pre-test probability are discussed in Chapter 3. Obtaining reliable information from the medical literature on the true-positive rate and false-positive rate of a diagnostic test is discussed in Chapter 5. The remaining hurdle is measuring the net harms and benefits of treatment and setting the threshold-treatment probability. This problem is the heart of the matter. We discuss it in the next section.

9.6 Setting the treatment-threshold probability

To choose between treatment and testing strategies, the clinician must either estimate p^*, the treatment-threshold probability, directly or calculate it from the net benefits (B) and harms (H) of treatment. We next discuss four approaches to setting the treatment threshold probability.

1. Subjective estimation of p^*
2. Subjective estimation of the ratio of treatment harms to benefits (H/B)
3. Use life expectancy to estimate the ratio of harms to benefits (H/B)
4. Use the patient's utilities for the disease-treatment states to estimate treatment harms and benefits.

9.6.1 Estimate p^* subjectively

The clinician must first think about the danger of taking the wrong course of action: either providing treatment when disease is absent or withholding treatment when disease is present. Then, the clinician must ask:

At what probability of the disease would I be indifferent between treating and withholding treatment?

Having established a threshold probability, the clinician should test the strength of her convictions: "Would I really be willing to withhold treatment if the probability of disease was just below my threshold probability? Would I be willing to treat if the probability of disease were just above the threshold probability?"

The subjective approach may lead clinicians to overestimate the treatment-threshold probability because they have difficulty abandoning the traditional teaching that one starts treatment only when certain of the diagnosis. Clinicians do think about starting treatment when uncertain about the diagnosis when urgent circumstances require immediate action or when the penalty for error is small. Two barriers stand in the way of thinking this way for less urgent problems. First, most clinicians do not realize that the treatment threshold is given by the following relationship between harms and benefits of treatment:

$$p^* = \frac{H}{H + B} \tag{9.4}$$

This equation means that p^* will usually be less than 0.50. Second, because clinicians often do not know the sensitivity or specificity of the tests that they order they cannot estimate the effect of false-positive and false-negative results on the probability of the target condition.

9.6.2 Subjectively estimate the ratio of harms to benefits (*H*/*B*)

The clinician must compare in a subjective, global way the net harms of treating the well (H) to the net benefits of treating the sick (B). From this comparison, the clinician will derive the ratio of treatment harms for the well (H) to treatment benefit for the sick (B). The following relationship, which is derived from Equation 9.4, is used to calculate the threshold treatment probability:

$$p^* = \frac{\dfrac{H}{B}}{1 + \dfrac{H}{B}} \tag{9.12}$$

Example 1: A neurologist considers the effect of treatment for a brain tumor for a patient with a headache and progressive hemiplegia.
- *Benefits*: The prognosis is very bad without treatment, but even with treatment the patient may not be cured or may be permanent impaired due to brain damage during surgery.
- *Harms*: Performing a craniotomy only to find that the patient does not have a brain tumor can cause permanent disability as well as pain and expense.

The neurologist may conclude that the ratio of harm to benefit is about 1:2, which corresponds to a treatment-threshold probability of 0.33.

Example 2: The pediatrician whose patient has a sore throat considers the treatment threshold for streptococcal pharyngitis.

- *Benefits*: The benefit of treatment with penicillin is modest: penicillin will prevent rheumatic fever, which has become a rare disease, and will speed resolution of symptoms by a day or so.
- *Harms*: The risk of treating the well is a serious allergic reaction to penicillin, which can occur even after asking about a history of penicillin allergy.

In contrast to suspected brain tumor, the harms and benefits of treating the patient with sore throat are small. However, Equation 9.12 shows that the treatment threshold is determined by the ratio of harm to benefit, not the magnitude of harms and benefit. The pediatrician decides that the benefits of treatment slightly outweigh the harms (H/B is $1/3$). The corresponding treatment threshold is 0.25. The pediatrician must test this conclusion by asking if she would withhold treatment if the probability of streptococcal pharyngitis were 0.20.

The relationship between p^* and H/B is instructive (Figure 9.16). As the ratio of H to B rises, p^* changes rapidly when the harms-to-benefit ratio is less than 1.0, which should usually be the case, and more slowly with higher ratios.

9.6.3 Use life expectancy to calculate p^*

The relationship between p^* and the net harms (H) and net benefits (B) of treatment is given by Equation 9.4:

$$p^* = \frac{H}{H + B} \tag{9.4}$$

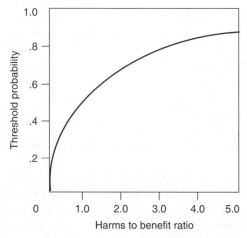

Figure 9.16 Relationship between treatment-threshold probability and the ratio of net costs to net benefits.

In this relationship, B and H are differences in utility:

$$B = U[D + A+] - U[D + A-]$$
$$H = U[D - A-] - U[D - A+]$$

Using a measure of preference, utility, to characterize the benefits and costs of treatment means that the decision alternative with the highest expected utility *should* be preferred. We lose this advantage when we use life expectancy to calculate H and B. Life expectancy is not a measure of preference unless one assumes that life in all outcome states is equally preferred. However, since some patients cannot participate in utility assessment, the clinician may have to use length of life in an outcome state to measure the benefits and costs of treatment.

Example: In our running example of a patient with a suspected brain tumor, the neurologist may use life expectancy to estimate p^* because the patient's illness has impaired his intellectual capacity, and he has no immediate family. She estimates that craniotomy for tumor has a 3% rate of perioperative mortality, 10% of all untreated patients with a brain tumor survive five years, and 63% of treated patients survive five years. The patient's normal life expectancy is 21 years. Using the declining exponential approximation of life expectancy (DEALE) (Section 7.3 of Chapter 7), she estimates the following life expectancies:

Disease-treatment state	Life expectancy
A+D+	11.0 years
A−D+	2.2 years
A−D−	21.0 years
A+D−	20.0 years

$$H = 21.0 - 20.0 = 1.0 \text{ years}$$
$$B = 11.0 - 2.20 = 8.8 \text{ years}$$

$$p^* = \frac{H}{H + B} = \frac{1,0}{1.0 + 8.8} = 0.099$$

Using life expectancy to estimate the treatment-threshold probability requires two assumptions:
- all outcome states are equally preferred by the patient;
- each year of life in each outcome state is equally preferred.

Neither of these assumptions is realistic. Therefore, the clinician should make every effort to use utility as the measure of the costs and benefits of treatment. If the patient cannot cooperate, a relative, a friend, or even the clinician can act as the patient's agent in responding to the utility assessment questions.

9.6.4 Use the patient's utilities for the disease-treatment states to estimate treatment harms and benefits

The best way to determine p^* is to assess the patient's utilities for the disease-treatment states $B = U[D+A+] - U[D+A-]$ and $H = U[D-A-] - U[D-A+]$ and solve Equation 9.4 for p^*:

$$p^* = \frac{H}{H+B}$$

Since H and B are differences in utility, making assumptions about the patient's preferences for quality of life or length of life is unnecessary. Furthermore, to assess utility, the clinician and the patient must talk candidly about the consequences of the decision alternatives, which sets the stage for informed consent and shared responsibility for decision making.

Consider each of the disease-treatment states in the example of suspected brain tumor in a 55-year-old man:

- $D-A-$: The patient does not have brain tumor, and receives no treatment for brain tumor, nor is subject to the risk of dying from surgery. This 55-year-old man's life expectancy is 21 years.
- $D-A+$: The patient does not have a brain tumor, but surgery is performed because the evidence strongly suggested that brain tumor was present. If the patient survives surgery, he has a normal life expectancy.
- $D+A-$: The patient has a brain tumor, but surgery is not performed because the evidence was not strong enough to justify surgery. The outcome is death with an average survival of 2 years.
- $D+A+$: The patient has a brain tumor, and surgery is performed. If the patient survives surgery, there is a 48% chance of cure and a normal life expectancy of 21 years. If the tumor is not curable, life expectancy is estimated to be 2 years.

In two of these disease-treatment states ($D+A+$ and $D-A+$), the final outcome is uncertain: death may occur in the perioperative period, after a gradual decline of several years (in the case of $D+A+$), or after several decades of normal life. We can take one of two approaches to assessing the patient's utility for these complex states.

Method 1: Write a description of the expected course in each disease-treatment state and find the patient's indifference probability for the following generic standard reference gamble (Figure 9.17):

The problem with Method 1 is that evaluating complex disease-treatment states is difficult for patients. In the scenario for the $D+A+$ disease-treatment state, the outcome of surgery for a suspected brain tumor and whether cure will be achieved are uncertain. In addition, the patient may live a normal life or may live two years with progressive brain tumor. Sorting out all of these variables is a hard cognitive task, especially since the patient must also cope with the probabilities of these outcomes.

Method 2: The preferred approach is to represent uncertainty in the disease-treatment states by trees comprising chance nodes. The structure of the tree

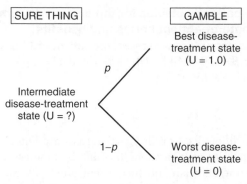

Figure 9.17 Directly assessing the utility for a disease-treatment state.

reflects the medical facts. The probabilities at the chance nodes are obtained from the clinician's experience or the medical literature. A representation of the outcome of the $D+A+$ disease-treatment state is shown in Figure 9.18. The patient will experience one of three possible outcomes:
- perioperative death from surgery;
- death from incurable brain tumor (life expectancy of two years);
- normal life expectancy, albeit with residual left-sided weakness that surgery did not cure.

This approach greatly simplifies the problem of assessing the patient's utility. The outcomes, their interrelationships, and their probabilities are explicit. The utility of each of these outcomes is quite easily assessed with the direct assessment shown in Figure 9.19.

After assessing the utilities for each outcome, the clinician places them in the trees representing the disease-treatment states and calculates the expected utility of the disease-treatment state.

By disaggregating a complex disease-treatment state into its component outcomes, the utility assessment scenarios can describe a single health state

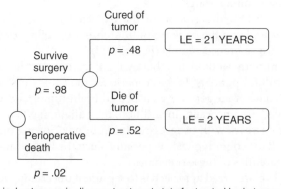

Figure 9.18 Clinical outcomes in disease-treatment state for treated brain tumor.

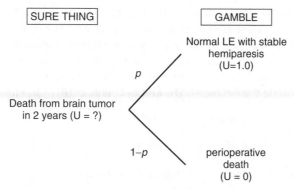

Figure 9.19 Standard reference gamble for directly assessing the utility of one of the outcomes of the disease-treatment state for treated brain tumor.

rather than a sequence of health states. Utility assessment for a single health state should be relatively easy for the patient. Of course, disaggregation creates more outcome states, which means more utility assessments to perform. Nonetheless, Method 2 is usually better.

To assess the treatment-threshold probability, follow a sequence of five steps:

Step 1: Identify the outcomes for each disease-treatment state. If a disease-treatment state has more than one outcome, do the following:
1. Create a tree to represent the chance events that lead to the outcomes.
2. Assign a probability to each chance event.

Step 2: Assess the utility of each outcome state identified in Step 1:
1. List each outcome state.
2. Rank the outcome states in order of preference.
3. Assign a utility of 1.0 to the most preferred outcome and a utility of 0 to the least preferred outcome.
4. Create a standard reference gamble for each intermediate outcome.
5. Create a scenario for outcome state.
6. For each standard reference gamble, directly assess the conditions for indifference between the gamble and the sure thing. Usually, this step means determining the patient's indifference probability.
7. Solve for the unknown utility in each standard reference gamble.

Step 3: Using the trees from Step 1 and the utilities from Step 2, calculate the expected utility of each disease-treatment state

$$U[D + A+] \qquad U[D + A-]$$

$$U[D - A-] \qquad U[D - A+]$$

(a) If the disease-treatment state has only one outcome, use the utility of that outcome state, as measured in Step 2.

(b) If the disease-treatment state has several outcomes, substitute their utilities (measured in Step 2) into the tree (from Step 1) that represents the disease-treatment state. Calculate the expected utility of the disease-treatment state by calculating the expected utility at each chance node, working from right to left in the tree.

Step 4: Calculate the net harms (H) and net benefits (B) of treatment:

$$B = U[D + A+] - U[D + A-]$$
$$H = U[D - A-] - U[D - A+]$$

Step 5: Calculate the treatment threshold probability

$$p^* = \frac{H}{H + B}$$

Example: Application to the patient with a suspected brain tumor

To illustrate Method 2 for estimating the treatment threshold, we return to our running example of the neurologist's patient with progressive hemiparesis (weakness of one side of the body) and headache.

Step 1 Identify the outcomes for each disease-treatment state

D−A−: You do not have a tumor, and surgery will not be necessary. The hemiparesis will stabilize and you will live out your remaining life span of 21 years. The only outcome of this disease-treatment state is:

- stable hemiparesis and normal length of life.

D+A−: An operation is not performed. As time goes on your weakness and headache worsen, and it becomes apparent that you have an incurable brain tumor. After about two years of worsening headaches and weakness, you slip into a coma and die. The only outcome of this disease-treatment state is:

- progressive hemiparesis and death in two years.

D−A+: Brain surgery is performed, and there is a 9% chance of leaving the hospital alive. The operation will show that you do not have a brain tumor. Therefore, if you survive the operation, you will have your normal life span of 21 years. Your hemiparesis will stabilize after surgery. This disease-treatment state has two outcomes:

- perioperative death;
- stable hemiparesis and normal length of life.

This disease-treatment state has more than one outcome, and it should be represented by the tree depicted in Figure 9.20.

D+A+: Brain surgery is required, but there is a 97% chance of leaving the hospital alive. If surgery does not cure the tumor, life expectancy is 2 years, and the hemiparesis will gradually worsen. If surgery does cure the tumor, life expectancy is 21 years, and the hemiparesis will stabilize or improve.

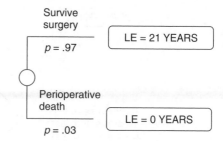

Figure 9.20 Model of the outcome of performing a craniotomy in a patient who does not have a brain tumor (health state $D-A+$).

This disease-treatment state has three outcomes:
- perioperative death;
- no cure of brain tumor: progressive hemiparesis and death in two years;
- cure of brain tumor with stable hemiparesis and normal length of life.

We used this disease-treatment state earlier as the example of Method 2. Figure 9.21 depicts the tree.

Step 2 Assess the utility of each outcome state identified in Step 1
- List and rank the outcomes and assign a utility of 1.0 to the most preferred outcome and 0 to the least preferred outcome.

Life expectancy	Clinical state	Operation	Utility
21 years	Stable hemiparesis	No	1.0
21 years	Stable hemiparesis	Yes	?
2 years	Progressive hemiparesis	No	?
2 years	Progressive hemiparesis	Yes	?
0 years	Perioperative death	–	0

- Create a standard reference gamble for each intermediate state.

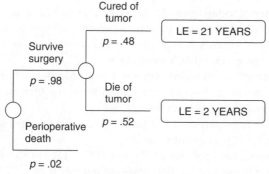

Figure 9.21 Model of the outcome of performing a craniotomy in a patient who has a brain tumor (health state $D+A+$).

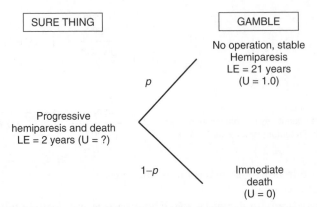

Figure 9.22 Standard reference gamble for assessing the utility of progressive hemiparesis and death from brain tumor.

We will illustrate the utility assessment process for one of the intermediate outcome states: no operation and progressive hemiparesis with death in two years from brain tumor. The standard reference gamble is shown in Figure 9.22.

Now follow the five steps to assessing a utility using a standard reference gamble.

Step 1: Create a scenario for the standard reference gamble:

The patient imagines that he has been told that he has a life expectancy of two years during which he will experience progressive hemiparesis to the point of being confined to bed. This outcome may be avoided by taking a chance on a painless but risky procedure, which will result either in a normal life expectancy with stable hemiparesis or immediate death.

Step 2: Determine the probability of success in the gamble between the best and worst outcomes that would leave the patient indifferent between the gamble and the sure thing:

In this case, the clinician should determine the patient's indifference probability for the standard gamble shown in Figure 9.22. The patient decides that he would be willing to gamble on the risky procedure when the probability of success was as low as 0.25 in order to avoid progressive disability and certain death in two years.

- Solve for the unknown utility in terms of known utilities.

At the indifference probability (π), the utility of the intermediate outcome is equal to the expected utility of the gamble

U(progressive hemiparesis, LE 2 years) $= \pi \times U$(stable hemiparesis, LE 21 years) $+ (1 - \pi) \times U$(perioperative death)

- U(progressive hemiparesis, LE 2 yrs) $= 0.25 \times 1.0 + 0.75 \times 0 = 0.25$
- His utility for the intermediate state is therefore 0.25.

The rest of the intermediate states' utilities are shown in the following table:

Life expectancy	Clinical state	Operation	Utility
21 years	Stable hemiparesis*	No	1.0
21 years	Stable hemiparesis	Yes	0.98
2 years	Progressive hemiparesis	No	0.25
2 years	Progressive hemiparesis	Yes	0.23
0 years	Perioperative death	–	0

*Comment: Stable hemiparesis is not perfect health, but it is the best that this patient can expect, so we assign it a utility of 1.0. If recovery of normal motor function were possible, we would model the problem differently and assign a utility of 1.0 to the state of normal motor function.

Step 3: Calculate the expected utility of each disease-treatment state:

$$U[D + A+] \quad U[D + A-]$$
$$U[D - A-] \quad U[D - A+]$$

Two of the disease-treatment states have only one outcome. The utility of these outcomes may be taken directly from the table. There is only one outcome to the $D-A-$ state, and its utility is 1.0. There is only one outcome to the $D+A-$ state, and its utility is 0.25, as described above.

The other two outcome states, $D+A+$ and $D-A+$, have several outcome states. The expected utilities of these states are obtained by averaging out the trees for these two states after first substituting the utilities from the table at the appropriate places in the trees (Figures 9.23a and b).

Disease-treatment state (D−)	Utility	Disease-treatment state (D+)	Utility
$U[D-A-]$	1.0	$U[D+A+]$	0.57
$U[D-A+]$	0.95	$U[D+A-]$	0.25

Step 4: Calculate the net harms (H) and net benefit (B) of treatment:

$$H = U[D - A-] - U[D - A+] = 1.0 - 0.95 = 0.05$$
$$B = U[D + A+] - U[D + A-] = 0.57 - 0.25 = 0.32$$

Step 5: Calculate the treatment threshold probability:

$$p^* = \frac{H}{H + B} = \frac{0.05}{0.32 + 0.05} = 0.135$$

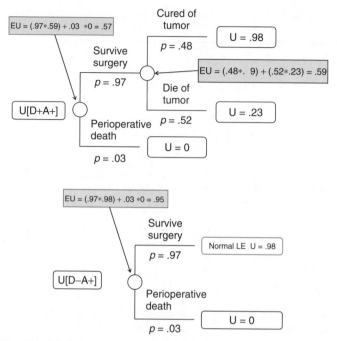

Figure 9.23a and b Calculating the expected utility of the disease-treatment states.

Comment: Thus, according to this analysis of a very difficult dilemma, the neurologist should recommend treatment if the clinical probability of brain tumor is 0.135 or more. Below that probability, watchful waiting is in order to see if the condition is stable or progresses in the next month. The latter would raise the probability of brain tumor.

The reader might wonder if the neurologist should ask the neurosurgeon to perform a craniotomy on her patient. The treatment threshold probability is 0.135, and the probability of tumor is approximately 0.25, according to the history and physical examination. Surgery appears to be in the patient's best interests. Although neurosurgeons do not like to perform craniotomy when the chance of finding a tumor is only 25%, craniotomy would be indicated if no other information could be obtained, given the patient's preferences for the outcomes he faces. In fact, diagnostic tests could be performed. If these tests were negative, the probability of tumor might be below the treatment threshold, and performing a craniotomy would not be in the patient's best interests.

Direct assessment of the patient's utilities requires the most effort of any of the methods for estimating the treatment-threshold probability. When the decision involves substantial risk and cost, an understanding of the patient's preferences is very important. The clinician can then approach a difficult decision with confidence that choosing the decision alternative with

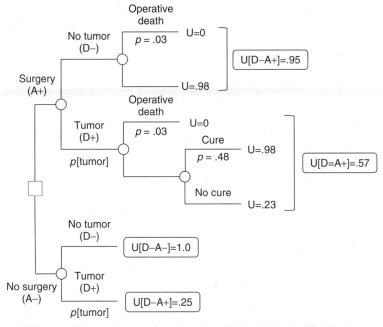

Figure 9.24 An alternative way to calculate the treatment-threshold probability by using a decision tree, which in this case is for choosing between surgery and no surgery for suspected brain tumor. To calculate the treatment-threshold probability, set the expected value of surgery equal to the expected value of no surgery and solve for the probability of brain tumor.

the highest expected utility will maximize the patient's chance of having a favorable outcome of the illness.

Rather than calculate the harms and benefits of treatment (H and B), an equivalent way to determine the treatment-threshold probability is to use the decision tree shown in Figure 9.24. The only unknown in the tree is P[tumor], so setting the expected utility of surgery equal to the expect utility of no surgery and solving for p^* will give the probability of tumor at which the two actions have the same expected utility, which is the definition of the treatment-threshold probability.

9.7   Taking account of the utility of experiencing a test

This chapter is based on the fundamental principle that tests should be obtained only when the results could alter patient management. Other factors may influence the decision to perform a diagnostic test:

- *The cost of the test*: Health insurance is widely available, and patients usually do not have to pay for the entire cost of a diagnostic test. Most insurance plans have a co-payment arrangement whereby the patient pays a fraction of the expense of services. Cost will be a factor if the patient must pay for all or part of the test. Regardless of who pays, the ethics of professionalism in medicine now recognize that the physician has an obligation to take costs into account, not only to one of her patients, but, in the setting of limited societal resources for health care, also to society as a whole.

- *The patient's need for reassurance*: A test may be warranted only because the patient seems especially likely to benefit from the reassurance that the test result may provide. If the patient seems especially worried or asks that a test be done, the first step is to give additional verbal reassurances. If reassurance and explanation of the limited value of the test both fail to alleviate the patient's concern, the test may be ordered. However, the clinician has no ethical obligation to order a test against her better judgment about what is best for the patient. Some would go further and argue that ordering a useless test wastes societal resources.
- *"Defensive medicine"*: This book approaches decision making from the patient's perspective. However, clinicians sometimes take into account their own interests when ordering a test. Concern about indiscriminant malpractice claims sometimes leads clinicians to order diagnostic tests when they believe that the chance of a clinically significant abnormality is below what can be justified on clinical grounds. The best defense against a successful malpractice suit is a careful clinical evaluation, including diagnostic tests when medically indicated, discussion with the patient, the family, and colleagues, and clear documentation of findings, assessment, and consultation.
- *Unpleasant effects of the test*: Many tests cause non-fatal adverse effects, including bleeding, discomfort during the procedure, or psychological stress.

We use Equation 9.5, repeated here, to calculate the expected utility of doing a test:

$$EU[\text{Test}] = P[D] \times \text{TPR} \times U[D + A+] + P[D] \times (1 - \text{TPR}) \times U[D + A-]$$
$$+ (1 - P[D]) \times \text{FPR} \times U[D - A+] + (1 - P[D]) \times (1 - \text{FPR})$$
$$\times U[D - A-] + U(T)$$

This equation includes a term for the utility of the test, $U(T)$, to take account of any effects of experiencing the test. $U(T)$ has a negative sign if the net effect of experiencing the test is undesirable. Therefore, an unpleasant test reduces the expected utility of the test (as calculated with Equation 9.5) by an equal amount ($U(T)$) at each probability of disease. The effect is to shift the line representing Equation 9.5 downward without changing its slope (Figure 9.25). As seen in Figure 9.25, a patient's attitude toward a disagreeable test narrows the range of disease probability within which the test is indicated.

Examining Equations 9.8 and 9.9 leads to the same conclusion. An unpleasant test (for which $U(T)$ has a negative sign) increases $p1$ and decreases $p2$,

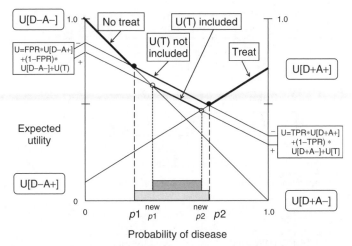

Probability of disease

Figure 9.25 Effect of considering the net effects of experiencing the test. The heavy line represents the action with the highest expected utility. Taking into account the utility of unpleasant test lowers the expected utility of testing so that the line representing testing intersects the lines representing no treat and treat at a lower point on each line (the + and − signs adjacent to both ends of the two "test" lines indicate which line includes U(T) and which does not). The lower point of intersection narrows the range of probabilities at which testing is the preferred option from the light-shaded band to the narrower dark-shaded band of probabilities.

narrowing the range of probabilities within which testing is the preferred option:

$$p1 = \frac{\text{FPR} \times -U(T)}{\text{FPR} \times H + \text{TPR} \times B} \tag{9.8}$$

$$p2 = \frac{(1 - \text{FPR}) \times H + U(T)}{(1 - \text{FPR}) \times H + (1 - \text{TPR}) \times B} \tag{9.9}$$

Figure 9.26 summarizes the effect of an unpleasant test on the probabilities at which testing is preferred. The result makes common sense. The criterion for doing an unpleasant test should be more stringent.

Assessing the utility of undergoing a test

The scenario for assessing the patient's utility of a test ($U(T)$) must describe the pleasant and unpleasant aspects of the test. The patient must then consider the generic standard gamble shown in Figure 9.27.

For the experience of undergoing a MRI of the head prior to having surgery for suspected brain tumor, the standard reference gamble would have the appearance shown in Figure 9.28.

The description of the MRI would include the risk of death (nil) and complications (very low) and unpleasant feelings (mostly claustrophobia from having to lie in a long, narrow, close-fitting cylinder within a large noisy machine for 15–20 minutes).

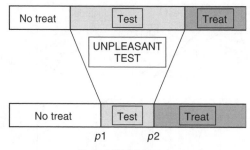

Figure 9.26 Effect of an unpleasant test on the range of probabilities within which testing is the preferred option.

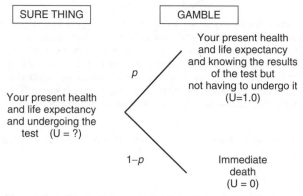

Figure 9.27 Generic standard reference gamble for determining $U(T)$, the patient's utility for undergoing a test.

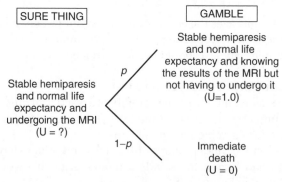

Figure 9.28 Standard reference gamble for determining the utility $U(T)$ of a MRI of the head.

To assess the patient's utility, the clinician asks him to imagine that the information to be provided by the procedure could be obtained without doing an arteriogram. What risk of death would be acceptable to avoid the arteriogram? The patient had a MRI of his spine a few years earlier and had to concentrate very hard to avert feelings of panic from being in a very confined space. Given this experience and the clinical situation, the patient may decide that he would take up to a 0.2% chance of death to avoid this procedure and still have the information it would provide. Since the patient's indifference probability is 0.002, his utility for undergoing the test would be 0.998. The difference between his utility for undergoing the test and knowing the results (0.998) and his utility for knowing the results without undergoing the test (1.0) is −0.002, the utility of the test. Since the experience of having the test is undesirable, $U(T)$ has a negative sign.

Most tests are virtually risk-free and do not produce much discomfort. Patients would not risk death to avoid these tests. Thus, their disutility is negligible and can be disregarded. Such would doubtless be the case for a CT scan of the head.

9.8 A clinical case: test selection for suspected brain tumor

To illustrate the selection and interpretation of diagnostic tests, we will use threshold probabilities to select tests for the neurologist's patient with headache and progressive hemiparesis (weakness of one side of the body). This patient's pre-test probability of brain tumor is 0.25. As described in Section 9.6 of this chapter, the treatment-threshold probability, as determined by the patient's utilities for the disease-treatment states, is 0.135. Although the pre-test probability exceeds the treatment threshold, the diagnosis is in doubt, and the treatment for the leading diagnosis is a major surgical procedure. Other possible diagnoses include brain abscess, cerebral aneurysm, brain metastasis, demyelinating disease (multiple sclerosis), and brain cyst. Intuitively, a test seems indicated.

The logical first choice for a diagnostic test in this situation is a MRI scan of the head. This test has superseded the head CT scan for suspected brain tumor.

The performance of the MRI scan in brain tumor is difficult to determine with certainty. For this illustrative example, the author elicited this information from a neurosurgeon who specializes in brain tumor treatment:
- MRI scan sensitivity (TPR) = 0.98
- MRI false-positive rate (FPR) (1 − specificity) = 0.03

Other data for this analysis are from the example in Sections 9.6 and 9.7:
- $H = U(D-A-) - U(D-A+) = 1.0 - 0.95 = 0.05$
- $B = U(D+A+) - U(D+A-) = 0.57 - 0.25 = 0.32$
- The treatment threshold (obtained in Section 9.6) = 0.135
- The pre-test probability $(p) = 0.25$
- $U(T)$ for the MRI scan is −0.002 (see Section 9.7).

Since the pre-test probability exceeds the treatment threshold, the only test result that could change management is a negative result. In other words, treatment is indicated unless the probability of brain tumor after a negative CT scan is below the treatment threshold ($p^* = 0.135$). If the pre-test probability is higher than $p2$, the probability of tumor after a negative CT scan will be above p^*. The first priority, therefore, is to calculate $p2$:

$$p2 = \frac{(1 - \text{FPR}) \times p^* + \left[\frac{U(T)}{H}\right] \times p^*}{(1 - \text{FPR}) \times p^* + (1 - p^*) \times (1 - \text{TPR})}$$

$$p2 = \frac{(1 - 0.03) \times 0.135 + \left[\frac{-0.002}{0.03}\right] \times 0.135}{(1 - 0.03) \times 0.135 + (1 - 0.135) \times (1 - 0.98)}$$

$$= \frac{0.131 - 0.009}{0.131 + 0.0173} = 0.82$$

$$p1 = \frac{\text{FPR} \times p^* - \left[\frac{U(T)}{H}\right] \times p^*}{\text{FPR} \times p^* + (1 - p^*) \times \text{TPR}}$$

$$p1 = \frac{0.03 \times .0135 - \left[\frac{-0.002}{0.03}\right] \times 0.135}{0.03 \times 0.135 + (1 - 0.135) \times 0.98} = \frac{0.0041 + 0.009}{0.0041 + 0.85} = 0.015$$

The testing zone defined by $p1$ and $p2$ is very wide, which befits the MRI scan with its very high sensitivity and low false-positive rate. The pre-test estimate of disease probability in this patient is 0.25, which lies between $p1$ and $p2$ in the testing-preferred zone. Therefore, the MRI scan should be performed (Figure 9.29).

The interpretation of the MRI scan was "mass lesion in the frontal lobe, compatible with neoplasm." The next task is to calculate the post-test probability of brain tumor corresponding to this result and consult with the neurosurgeon about her willingness to operate on the patient without further confirmation of the diagnosis.

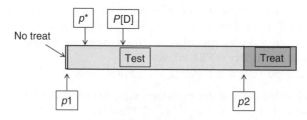

Probability of brain tumor

Figure 9.29 Analysis of the decision to perform a CT scan of the brain in a suspected brain tumor. $p1$ is 0.015, $p2$ is 0.82. Because $P[D]$ is in the test zone between $p1$ and $p2$, the neurologist should do the MRI scan.

Pre-test probability of brain tumor $= 0.25$
TPR of MRI scan $= 0.98$
FPR of MRI scan $= 0.03$
Using Bayes theorem,

$$P[\text{tumor if MRI+}] = \frac{P[\text{tumor}] \times \text{TPR}}{(P[\text{tumor}] \times \text{TPR}) + (1 - P[\text{tumor}]) \times \text{FPR}}$$

$P[\text{tumor if MRI+}] = 0.92$

The neurosurgeon says, "I would prefer not to operate with this degree of uncertainty if it is possible to avoid it. The MRI is the best test we have. Perhaps we should follow the patient closely for the next few weeks and see if his neurological deficit progresses a little. That would convince me that we are dealing with an expanding mass lesion, and I'd feel much better about operating."

With no imaging test options, the neurosurgeon is using the test of time to characterize the lesion physiologically. If it grows, it needs surgery. Sometimes, the test of time is best.

9.9   Sensitivity analysis

Testing the stability of a decision analysis is essential. In one-way sensitivity analysis, the clinician substitutes the lowest plausible value for a variable and recalculates the expected utility of the decision options. The process is repeated for the highest plausible value. If the preferred decision option remains the same, the variable is not critical to the decision. If it does change, the variable is a driver of the decision. This process may be repeated for all of the variables in the model. Sensitivity analysis is particularly important for testing the trustworthiness of the model when the analysis leads to unexpected conclusions.

Sensitivity analysis for the threshold model involves the following variables:
- the true-positive rate and false-positive rate of the test;
- the pre-test probability of disease;
- the threshold treatment probability;
- $U(T)$, the utility of the test.

Two-way sensitivity analysis for the pre-test probability and treatment-threshold probability

A two-way sensitivity analysis is shown in Figure 9.30, which depicts the MRI scan for suspected brain tumor. In a two-way sensitivity analysis for a decision analysis, the model calculates the expected value for the decision options for every combination of two variables. In Figure 9.30, the two variables are the pre-test probability and the treatment threshold probability. Figure 9.30 shows the range of values for the two variables at which the no test-no treat, the TEST, and the treat-no test options each have the highest expected value.

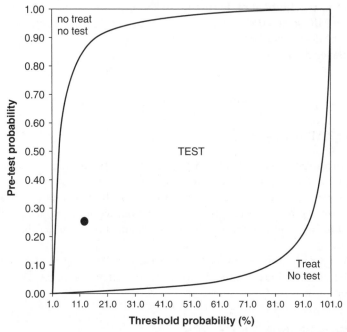

Figure 9.30 Two-way sensitivity analysis for MRI scan in suspected brain tumor: effect of uncertainty in the pre-test probability and treatment-threshold probability. The assumed sensitivity and specificity are 0.98 and 0.97 respectively. The solid circle represents the pre-test probability and treatment-threshold probability for the patient in the example. The concave downward curve represents $p2$, and the concave upward curve represents $p1$.

Each point on the upper curve is a value for $p2$, which was calculated using Equation 9.11 with the treatment-threshold probability on the horizontal axis. Each point on the lower curve is a value for $p1$, which was calculated using Equation 9.10 with the treatment-threshold probability on the horizontal axis. The space enclosed within the axes is divided up into three zones. Each point within the space corresponds to one combination of pre-test probability and treatment-threshold probability:

- When the pre-test probability (vertical axis) exceeds $p2$ for any value of p^*, the patient should receive treatment without prior testing. Thus, treatment is indicated for combinations of the pre-test probability and the treatment-threshold probability that lie in the upper left zone.
- When the pre-test probability is lower than $p1$ for any value of p^*, the patient should not receive treatment. Thus, treatment is not indicated for combinations of the pre-test probability and the treatment-threshold probability that lie in the lower right zone.
- For intermediate values of the pre-test probability, the test should be performed. Thus, testing is indicated for combinations of the pre-test probability and the treatment-threshold probability that lie in the middle

zone. The large area of the test zone is consistent with the high sensitivity and specificity of the MRI scan for brain tumor.

For the case of the patient whose pre-test probability of brain tumor is 0.25 and whose threshold-treatment probability is 0.135 (indicated by a solid circle), the clinician can be confident in recommending a MRI scan, since the solid circle representing the patient is far from the boundaries of the test zone. Figure 9.30 shows that a MRI scan would be indicated over a wide range of pre-test probabilities and treatment-threshold probabilities.

Sensitivity analysis for the true-positive rate and false-positive rate of the test

Using Equations 9.10 and 9.11, we can extend the sensitivity analysis to take into account uncertainty in the true-positive rate and false-positive rate of the MRI scan (Figure 9.31). The upper curve (concave downward) that is closest to the 45 degree line represents $p2$ with a 0.87 test true-positive rate and a 0.13 false-positive rate. The lower curve (concave upward) that is closest to the 45 degree line represents $p1$ with the same combination of test performance measures. Even if these extreme values are assumed for the true-positive rate and false-positive rate of the MRI scan, testing is still indicated for a wide range around the patient's values for the pre-test probability and the threshold-treatment probability.

Sensitivity analysis for the utility of the test

The disutility of the test, $U(T)$, can affect the decision to test. As seen in Figure 9.22, a patient's attitude toward a disagreeable test narrows the range of disease probability for which the test is indicated.

The relationship between $U(T)$ and the range of probability of brain tumor in which a MRI scan is preferred is shown in the following table, which was calculated using Equations 9.10 and 9.11, substituting several values for $U(T)$:

$U[T]$	$p1$	$p2$	Range of $P[D]$ in which testing is preferred
0	0.003	0.74	0.003 to 0.74
−0.005	0.018	0.61	0.018 to 0.61
−0.01	0.033	0.49	0.033 to 0.49
−0.02	0.063	0.23	0.063 to 0.23
−0.03	0.094	−0.02	Never

This table shows that if a test is very unpleasant, the range of disease probability in which testing is preferred narrows appreciably. When $p2$ is negative, the expected utility of the treat option equals the expected utility of

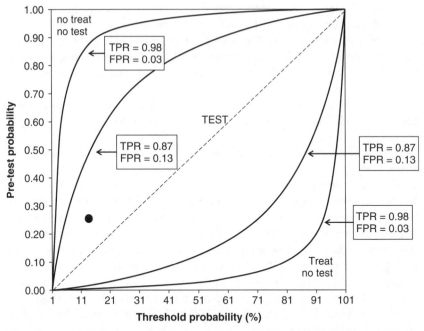

Figure 9.31 Effect of uncertainty in test true-positive rate and false-positive rate on the decision to perform a MRI scan for suspected brain tumor. The solid circle represents the pre-test probability and treatment-threshold probability for the patient. The concave downward curves represent $p2$, and the concave upward curves represent $p1$.

the test option at a point to the left of the zero point on the horizontal axis, which means that the treat option is always preferred to the test option.

Summary

1. If a diagnostic test result cannot change the management of the patient, do not do the test.
2. To determine whether a test can change the management of the patient, the following are required:
   - the pre-test probability of disease;
   - the true-positive rate of the test ($P[+|D]$, TPR, sensitivity);
   - the false-positive rate of the test ($P[+|no\ D]$, FPR, 1 − specificity);
   - the treatment threshold probability (p^*).
3. The treatment threshold (p^*) is a measure of the balance between the benefits of treatment to patients with the target condition and the harms of treatment to other patients. We discuss several ways to obtain the threshold-treatment probability:

- a subjective estimate of p^* using the relationship

$$p^* = \frac{H}{H+B}$$

- estimating the ratio of harms of the treatment to its benefits (H/B) and calculating the treatment threshold as

$$p^* = \frac{\dfrac{H}{B}}{1 + \dfrac{H}{B}}$$

- measuring the patient's utility for the four disease-treatment states and calculating the threshold-treatment probability as

$$p^* = \frac{H}{H+B}$$

where $H = U[D-A-] - U[D-A+]$ and $B = U[D+A+] - U[D+A-]$.

4. Definitions:
   - No treatment-test threshold $(p1)$: The probability at which one should be indifferent between testing and not treating. Equivalently, it is the probability of disease below which the post-test probability of disease cannot exceed the treatment threshold.
   - Test-treatment threshold $(p2)$: The probability at which one should be indifferent between testing and treating. Equivalently, it is the probability of disease above which the post-test probability of disease cannot exceed the treatment threshold.
5. The equations for calculating the testing thresholds are

$$p1 = \frac{\text{FPR} \times p^* - \left[\frac{U(T)}{H}\right] \times p^*}{\text{FPR} \times p^* + (1 - p^*) \times \text{TPR}}$$

$$p2 = \frac{(1 - \text{FPR}) \times p^* + \left[\frac{U(T)}{H}\right] \times p^*}{(1 - \text{FPR}) \times p^* + (1 - p^*) \times (1 - \text{TPR})}$$

$U(T)$ is the utility of undergoing the test. It has a negative sign if the net effect of the test is unpleasant. For many tests, it is so small that it can be ignored, but for unpleasant tests it can be large enough to have a significant effect on the range of probabilities in which testing is the preferred option.

6. Application of threshold model to patient care:
   Step 1: Estimate the pre-test probability of disease (p), using the methods described in Chapter 3 (Figure 9.32).

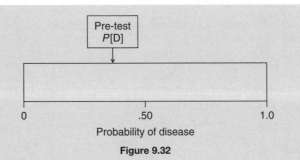

Figure 9.32

Step 2: Estimate the treatment threshold (p^*), using one of the four methods described in an earlier section of this chapter. Estimate the disutility of the test if appropriate (Figure 9.33).

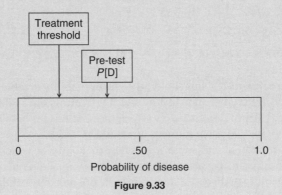

Figure 9.33

Step 3: Calculate the no treatment–test threshold ($p1$) and the test-treatment threshold ($p2$), using p^* and the true-positive rate (TPR) and false-positive rate (FPR) of the test (Figure 9.34).

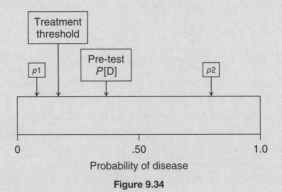

Figure 9.34

Step 4: Interpretation (Figure 9.35):
• *Do not test* if the pre-test probability is less than $p1$ or greater than $p2$.

The test result, positive or negative, will not change the estimate of disease probability enough to cross the treatment threshold and therefore change management.

- *Test* If the pre-test probability lies between $p1$ and $p2$.

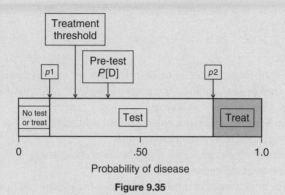

Figure 9.35

Step 5: Perform sensitivity analysis to check the stability of your conclusions.

Bibliography

Doubilet, P. (1983) A mathematical approach to interpretation and selection of diagnostic tests. *Medical Decision Making*, **3**, 177–96.

This article describes very clearly how the decision threshold concept for test ordering can be extended to tests that have multiple discrete results or continuous results. This article is the logical next step for the reader who understood this chapter and wants to learn more.

Greenes, R.A., Cain, K.C., Begg, C.B. and colleagues (1984) Patient-oriented performance measures of diagnostic tests: I, II and III. *Medical Decision Making*, **4**, 7–46.

Three articles which extend the ideas in this chapter, particularly in indicating the likelihood that a test will alter management and in showing the relationship between prior estimated probability of disease and the treatment threshold.

Hershey, J.C., Cebul, R.D., and Williams, S.V. (1986) Clinical guidelines for using two dichotomous tests. *Medical Decision Making*, **6**, 68–78.

An extended discussion of the principles discussed in Section 9.5: choosing the best combination of several diagnostic tests.

Pauker, S.G. and Kassirer, J.P. (1975) Therapeutic decision making: a cost-benefit analysis. *New England Journal of Medicine*, **293**, 229–34.

A threshold approach to therapeutic decision making.

Pauker, S.G. and Kassirer, J.P. (1980) The threshold approach to clinical decision making. *New England Journal of Medicine*, **302**, 1109–17.

An extension of the threshold approach to test ordering decisions. This chapter is based on the ideas in this article.

CHAPTER 10

Cost-effectiveness analysis and cost–benefit analysis

The purpose of this chapter is to help the reader understand how clinicians and policy makers can include the costs of medical care into decision making for patients. The chapter has four parts:

10.1 The clinician's conflicting roles: patient advocate, member of society, and entrepreneur

10.1.1 The clinician as advocate for the patient

One of the clinician's roles in society is to be an advocate for the patient. Individual patients expect clinicians to do what is best for them, even when the needs of society conflict with the patient's needs. Thus, a woman with leukemia expects her clinician to write a letter protesting the refusal of the government health insurance program to pay the costs of an experimental treatment. At times, the needs of society conflict with the patient's needs. Thus, the government might reject the appeal saying spending the money on programs to reduce premature birth is more important to the public than spending it on an unproven, costly treatment for the woman. Thus, both the patient and those who pay for health care have an interest in how a clinician practices medicine.

The problem is far more complex than the interaction between three parties: the clinician, the patient, and society. Society is an aggregation of individuals, and individuals' values may depend on whether they benefit from a patient care decision or whether it costs them money. The taxpayer who votes for a senator who promises to cut the cost of government health programs

Medical Decision Making, Second Edition. Harold C. Sox, Michael C. Higgins and Douglas K. Owens.
© 2013 John Wiley & Sons, Ltd. Published 2013 by John Wiley & Sons, Ltd.

may become a beneficiary of those programs. The man who switches health insurance companies to save a few dollars in premium costs will eventually become ill and insist upon an expensive test that has little chance of altering the course of his care.

So far, the focus of this book has been the individual patient. The reader has learned how to identify the decision alternative that maximizes the patient's expected utility. One view of the clinician's role in society holds that the clinician should always choose the action that maximizes the patient's expected utility, even though it consumes resources that are no longer available for the care of others. Thus, if the patient is worried about a rare but serious disease, the clinician should order a costly test that will reduce the patient's uncertainty from 1 in 1000 (0.001) to 1 in 10 000 (0.0001). According to this view, it is unethical to do slightly less than what would maximize your patient's utility in order to benefit someone else.

The experienced clinician will recognize that this ethical position is unrealistic in practice, however vehemently he may endorse it in casual conversation. Imagine yourself in the following common situation:

The coronary care unit is full, and the head nurse has just called you about a patient in the emergency room with an acute myocardial infarction. She reminds you that one of your patients has been in the coronary care unit for two days with a small myocardial infarction. He is doing well and has a much better outlook than the other patients in the coronary care unit. The person in the emergency room will benefit much more from that coronary care unit bed than your patient, so the head nurse asks you to move your patient.

Although unlikely, your patient might have a complication of his myocardial infarction after he has been transferred to a less intensively staffed part of the hospital, where a complication that might be handled successfully in the coronary care unit could prove fatal. If your sole motivation is to maximize your patient's expected utility, you should keep him in the coronary care unit a few more days. However, recognizing that others have a right of access to a limited resource, you agree to transfer your patient. You have made a decision that maximizes the expected utility of the acute myocardial infarction patients in the hospital.

This example demonstrates that clinicians often make decisions that expose their patients to a slightly increased risk of harm in order to assure the best use of a shared resource.

The changing relationship between the payer, the clinician, and the patient

In the first half of the twentieth century, most patients bore the cost of illness from their savings. The clinician had to forgo expensive diagnostic tests or find alternatives to costly drugs. The patient and the clinician were partners in trying to assure good care at low cost because people had a tangible, personal interest in minimizing the costs of their health care to a minimum.

With the advent of access to health insurance for most people, health care costs became a shared concern because more costly care for some patients meant more costly insurance premiums for everyone. With health insurance, other people share in an individual patient's expenses. Thus, the cost of medical care has become a concern of groups of people rather than the individual patient. In this new, relatively depersonalized environment, the clinician has been able to act as the patient's advocate without much experiencing much resistance.

The cost of an individual's care is again becoming an issue in the United States. To get insurance, the patient must usually agree to pay part of the cost of many services (co-payment), and often the patient pays all of the costs up to an amount (the deductible) above which the insurance pays most of the costs. Here, the clinician and the patient may work together to minimize costs to the patient. Many people are in health plans in which the health plan receives a lump sum to care for all the patient's health care needs, an arrangement that provides a strong incentive for clinicians to avoid unnecessary expense, which is desirable. However, the clinician's role as patient advocate may conflict with self-interest when the health plan pays a bonus to physicians who successfully control costs. In either situation, understanding the relationships between the costs of medical services and their benefits may help the clinician and the patient to make good decisions together. The subject of this chapter is how to characterize the efficiency of health care services by measuring their costs and their effectiveness.

10.1.2 Principles for allocating scarce resources

There are several principles that might be used to allocate a scarce resource:

- **Maximize health outcomes at any cost**: The clinician has a professional duty to maximize her patient's well-being. Expending additional resources may increase the chance of survival or functional recovery however slightly.
- **Minimize cost**: If taken to an extreme, this approach would often result in poor health outcomes.
- **Maximize outcomes without exceeding the available resources**: Expend resources on health care as long as the additional cost for each additional unit of benefit is less than would be derived from using the money in another way (such as recreation).

The principal goal of this chapter is to describe two ways to characterize decision alternatives by taking into account their costs. The two methods, **cost-effectiveness analysis** and **cost–benefit analysis**, are often used to help make decisions for allocating resources. These resources may be owned jointly (by the clients of an insurance company) or individually (by a person who must make a co-payment for a service covered partially by health insurance).

10.2 Cost-effectiveness analysis: a method for comparing management strategies

Cost-effectiveness analysis is a method for comparing decision alternatives by their relative costs and effectiveness.

Definition of cost-effectiveness analysis: "A method designed to assess the comparative impacts of expenditures on different health interventions" (Gold *et al.*, 1996).

Equivalently, cost-effectiveness analysis compares management strategies by a measure such as cost per unit of output, where output is an outcome such as additional years of life, utility, or additional cases of newly detected disease.

Note that both of these definitions contain the word "comparative." *Cost-effectiveness analysis always compares strategies.* The method may compare two services by their **incremental cost-effectiveness**, the difference in cost divided by the difference in outcomes. The standard of comparison may be another treatment or it may be usual care.

When comparing two treatments, Treatment *A* and Treatment B, the incremental cost-effectiveness of Treatment A relative to B is

$$\text{incremental C-E} = \frac{\text{costs with A} - \text{costs with B}}{\text{life expectancy with A} - \text{life expectancy with B}}$$

where C-E is cost-effectiveness

10.2.1 Using cost-effectiveness analysis to set institutional policy

Cost-effectiveness analysis may be used to set a policy that others will follow. Consider the problem of the administrator of a group practice who must decide between three strategies for coping with a disease. A consultant has just presented the administrator with the following table:

Strategy	Cost	Life expectancy
A	$9400	19.60
B	$10 000	19.64
C	$10 000	19.28

The administrator notes right away that choosing between these strategies will require a compromise: Strategy A is the least expensive, and Strategy B leads to the longest average survival. In deciding whether the additional effectiveness of Strategy B is worth the extra cost, the administrator calculates the incremental cost-effectiveness of Strategy B. Strategy B costs $600 more per patient than Strategy A and prolongs life two weeks (0.04 years) longer than Strategy A. The administrator shakes his head in frustration. He realizes that he understands the problem much better than before hiring the consultant, but he still does not know which strategy to recommend.

Cost-effectiveness analysis has provided this administrator with additional insight: he knows now that he does not have a clear choice. To understand his dilemma, let us go back to the beginning and find out how the analysis was performed.

The administrator of a hospital-based group practice must decide whether to accede to the wishes of the chief of urology who has asked the hospital to purchase an instrument that dissolves kidney stones by ultrasonic waves. The urologist proposes that all patients who do not pass their kidney stone within 48 hours should undergo the ultrasound treatment. He argues that the machine will reduce the number of patients who will have to undergo surgery for kidney stones. Avoiding surgery will be especially important for patients whose risk of death from surgery is increased because of their poor medical condition.

The administrator asks the consultant to investigate this request. After investigation, the consultant comes up with the following facts:

Fatality rate with surgery:
  low-risk patients: 2%
  high-risk patients: 10%
Success rate of treatment:
  ultrasonic therapy: 80% for all patients
  surgery: 100% for all patients who survive surgery
Prevalence of patients at high risk from surgery: 20%
Cost to the practice of treatments:
  ultrasonic treatment: $2000 (includes the purchase price of the ultrasound equipment amortized over its lifetime)
  surgery: $10 000

After hearing these facts, the administrator is convinced that the ultrasound machine may be beneficial to some patients, but he is worried about the cost of purchasing the machine. Perhaps he could send patients who are too sick for surgery to a nearby hospital that has recently purchased an ultrasound machine. He suggests that the consultant look into a resource-sharing arrangement whereby low-risk patients would have surgery and high-risk patients would be sent to the nearby hospital.

The consultant negotiates the following arrangement. The neighboring hospital will charge $4000 for an ultrasonic treatment. If the ultrasonic treatment fails, the patient will undergo surgery at the neighboring hospital, which will charge the practice $15 000 to perform the surgery.

The administrator asks the consultant to analyze the choice between:
- surgery for all patients (the current mode of treatment);
- ultrasonic treatment for all patients (with surgery for those whose kidney stones resist ultrasonic treatment);
- surgery for low-risk patients (ultrasonic treatments at the neighboring hospital for high surgical risk patients).

The administrator asks the consultant to analyze the problem in terms of costs and length of life for the average kidney stone patient, who is 55 years old and has a 20-year life expectancy.

The consultant uses the following sequence to perform the analysis.

I. Define the problem to be solved and the precise objectives

The problem: Which of three strategies for treating patients who have kidney stones that do not pass spontaneously should the administrator recommend for adoption by the practice?

The objectives: Predict the consequences of the three strategies by analyzing the expected costs and expected survival for 55-year-old patients. If possible, identify a dominant solution which will maximize survival and minimize costs. If there is no dominant solution, use incremental cost-effectiveness analysis to characterize the decision alternatives.

II. Define the consequences of each decision alternative
The consultant represents the problem by a decision tree in which the probabilities and outcomes are those identified in the first phase of her investigation. For convenience, the trees for each decision alternative are displayed separately (Figures 10.1, 10.2, and 10.3).
The analyst identifies two types of outcomes: survival and costs.

Survival:
- Immediate death due to surgery: life expectancy 0 years.
- Survive surgery and live to one's normal life expectancy of 20 years.

Treatment costs per patient:
- **Option 1**: Purchase ultrasound equipment
  - successful ultrasound treatment: $2000
  - ultrasound fails, surgery required: $2000 + $10 000.
- **Option 2**: Surgery for all patients: $10 000.

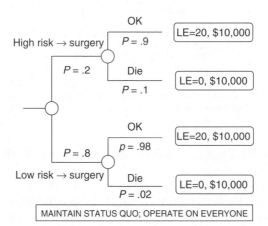

Figure 10.1 Outcomes of operating within the practice on all patients with kidney stones.

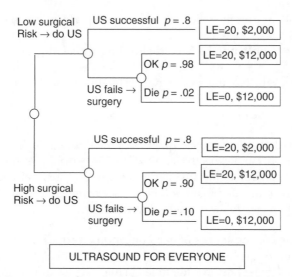

Figure 10.2 Outcomes of a strategy of selective use of surgery and ultrasonic treatment (US) within the group practice for kidney stones that do not pass spontaneously.

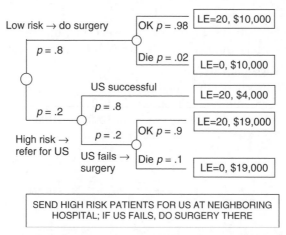

Figure 10.3 Outcome of doing surgery within the practice on low-risk patients with kidney stones that do not pass spontaneously and sending high-risk patients to another hospital for ultrasound treatment (US) (and surgery if it is unsuccessful).

- **Option 3**: Send high surgical risk patients to neighboring hospital for ultrasound:
    - low-risk patients (surgery at practice): $10 000
    - high-risk patients with successful ultrasound: $4000
    - high-risk patients who require surgery after unsuccessful ultrasound: $4000 + $15 000.

III. Average out and fold back the decision tree
The results are shown in the following table:

Strategies	Expected cost	Life expectancy of patients
Option 1: Buy ultrasound for practice	$4000	19.86 years
Option 2: Send high-risk patients to neighboring hospital for ultrasound	$9400	19.60 years
Option 3: Operate on everyone	$10 000	19.28 years

What does this analysis mean? To interpret it, examine each of the columns of the table in turn.

Expected cost: The expected cost of each of the three decision alternatives was obtained by averaging out and folding back, using cost as the measure of outcome.

	Operate on everyone	Buy ultrasound for your practice	High-risk patients are sent to nearby hospital
Expected cost	$10 000	$4000	$9400

Interpretation: Purchasing the ultrasound machine is the least costly alternative, presumably because most patients can be treated with ultrasound and do not require a $10 000 surgical operation. Referral of all patients to the near-by hospital is expensive because of its high charges for ultrasound and surgery if needed.

Life expectancy: The life expectancy of the patients is obtained by averaging out and folding back the decision trees, using life expectancy as the measure of outcome.

	Operate on everyone	Buy ultrasound for your practice	High-risk patients are sent to nearby hospital
Life expectancy	19.28 years	19.86 years	19.60 years

Interpretation: Purchasing the ultrasound machine leads to the longest expected length of life, presumably because fewer than 10% of the patients are subjected to the risk of death from surgery. In contrast, many more patients undergo surgery if one chooses the other two decision alternatives.

Purchasing the ultrasound machine for the practice leads to the lowest costs for the practice and the longest life expectancy for the patient. Since purchasing the ultrasound machine is preferred on the basis of costs and survival, it is said to *dominate* the other choices. The hospital administrator is relieve to learn that he does not need to analyze the tradeoff between cost and survival.

As the administrator is about to place the order, he learns about a worldwide shortage of materials for a crucial part in the new version of the ultrasound machine. The company has shut down its production line and has no idea when this model will become available again. The alternative is to buy an older, more expensive model, which is less effective in dissolving the kidney stones. The probability of success is only 0.50 with the older machine. The cost to the practice of each procedure will be $5000 with the older machine. However, the neighboring hospital, which has the new ultrasound machine, can still offer the procedure for $4000. Your consultant repeats the analysis after substituting the revised cost of an ultrasound treatment to the practice. She presents the following table:

Strategies	Average cost	Life expectancy of patients (years)
Option 2: Buy ultrasound for practice	$10 000	19.64
Option 1: Send high-risk patients to neighboring hospital for ultrasound	$9400	19.60
Option 3: Operate on everyone	$10 000	19.28

The situation is now quite different. The least expensive alternative is different than the alternative that produces the longest life expectancy for patients. None of the options dominates. The administrator could choose on the basis of either cost or survival, but he chooses to use incremental *cost per year of survival*, which is a measure of cost-effectiveness. First, he must decide which two of the alternatives to choose between.

Option 3 is as costly as Option 2 and more costly than Option 1. Option 3 also leads to a lower life expectancy than either Option 1 or 2, so it is inferior to both, and the choice is between Option 1 and Option 2. Option 2 is more costly than Option 1 but less effective, so choosing between them is difficult.

The administrator notes that patients' life expectancy will be slightly better if the practice buys its own ultrasound machine. How much will he have to pay to avoid the potential loss of life from doing surgery on all low-risk patients and sending high-risk patients to the neighboring hospital? How will that cost per years of life gained compare to other decisions that the practice has made recently? The average cost per procedure of buying the ultrasound machine is only $600 more than if high-risk patients are sent to the other hospital. The incremental cost-effectiveness of buying the ultrasound machine is calculated as follows:

$$\text{incremental C-E} = \frac{\text{cost (Option 1)} - \text{cost (Option 2)}}{\text{life expectancy with 1} - \text{life expectancy with 2}}$$

$$\text{incremental C-E} = \frac{\$10\,000 - \$9400}{19.64 \text{ years} - 19.69 \text{ years}} = \frac{\$600}{0.04} = \$15\,000/\text{YLS}$$

In this example, YLS is "year of life saved," the difference in life expectancy between Option 1 and Option 2.

The improvement in life expectancy that can be obtained by buying the ultrasound machine will cost an additional $15 000 per additional year of life gained. To decide if the expenditure is warranted, the administrator should measure the incremental cost-effectiveness of interventions in other diseases treated in the practice. Perhaps another investment will yield a greater prolongation of life at less cost than buying ultrasonic treatment of kidney stones. In the event, $15 000 per year of life saved compares very favorably to the cost-effectiveness of services that everyone seems to agree are an efficient use of resources. In fact, the rather arbitrary dividing line between what is and what is not cost-effective is between $50 000 and $100 000 per year of life saved, so this expenditure is certainly defensible in a presentation to the hospital board of trustees.

Cost-effectiveness analyses often express the gain to the patient as quality-adjusted life years (QALYs) gained rather than life years saved. As described in Section 8.9 in Chapter 8, QALYs are life years in a health state multiplied by a measure of the quality of life in the health state, such as utility. Since a cost-effectiveness analysis of an intervention applies to a population that uses the intervention, the analysis would use the average utility in the target population. The dividing line between what is and what is not cost-effective is actually expressed as cost per QALY. In this example, the two outcomes states are normal health ($U = 1.0$) or death ($U = 0$), so life years saved and QALYs gained are the same.

10.2.2 Flat-of-the-curve medicine

Often, one must choose from among several ways to use a service. For example, in screening for cancer of the cervix, one can obtain a Papanicolau smear at any frequency, from every three months to every ten years or more. To help analyze this problem, some investigators plot the cost of adopting each policy against its effectiveness (Figure 10.4). This topic is discussed by Garber and Phelps (1997).

This analysis shows the small increment in effectiveness in relation to the high cost of more intensive screening for this hypothetical cancer. Practicing medicine with policies that provide a relatively small incremental benefit for the added cost is sometimes called "flat-of-the-curve medicine." How should

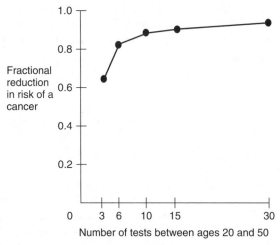

Figure 10.4 Incremental costs and incremental effectiveness of several methods for screening for a hypothetical cancer.

one use the information in Figure 10.4 to choose a policy for cancer screening? In principle, one should adopt the most intensive screening program that has a higher incremental cost-effectiveness than alternative uses for the resources. Cost-effectiveness analysis is a method for comparing decision alternatives, but to decide whether any alternative is cost-effective, a decision maker must have a criterion for cost-effectiveness. Athough $50,000 per QALY is often used, it has neither a theoretical basis nor a valid empirical rationale. The consensus of expert opinion rejects a general criterion for cost-effectiveness (Gold *et al.*, 1996). Cost–benefit analysis, our next subject, provides an alternative approach for deciding if a program is worth undertaking.

10.3 Cost–benefit analysis: a method for measuring the net benefit of medical services

Definition of cost–benefit analysis: A comparison in which the costs and benefits of a service or services are both expressed in same units.

To use cost–benefit analysis to compare different programs or policies, the analyst may calculate net benefits by subtracting costs from benefits $(B - C)$. Analysts also use the ratio of benefits to costs to compare policies, although net benefit provides a more easily explained rationale for making a decision.

10.3.1 The distinction between cost–benefit analysis and cost-effectiveness analysis

Many people have difficulty distinguishing between cost–benefit analysis and cost-effectiveness analysis. The distinction is quite subtle but is very important.

Cost-effectiveness analysis is helpful for comparing alternatives but is otherwise a limited measure for decision making. It can guide the choice between alternatives (pick the one with the most favorable cost-effectiveness ratio). However, to decide if any alternative is worth doing one must choose an arbitrary threshold of cost-effectiveness. For example, you should have no difficulty choosing between services whose cost-effectiveness ratios are $200 000 per life year saved and $300 000 per life year. To decide whether either of the services is worth its cost, you must first establish a cost-effectiveness threshold (e.g., $50 000 per life year gained). A cost-effectiveness threshold is arbitrary because the unit of measure of costs (currency) is different than the unit for measuring effectiveness. Therefore, the units of cost-effectiveness do not have a natural, common-sense meaning that can serve as a framework for setting a threshold.

This limitation becomes clearer when we contrast cost-effectiveness with **cost–benefit analysis**, in which the measure of benefit and cost is monetary. Because the two measures have the same units (currency), the difference between them has the common-sense, real-world meaning of profit or loss, which is a natural criterion for deciding if a service is worth doing.

Cost–benefit analysis is a method for deciding between alternatives but also a method for deciding whether a service is worth doing. Another advantage: choosing between policies with different outcomes is possible if the outcomes can be transformed into the same monetary measure, such as dollars.

10.3.2 Placing a monetary value on human life

Although cost–benefit analysis is potentially very powerful, it has one major drawback. Cost is usually expressed in units of currency (dollars, pounds, or yen). The outputs of a service must also be in units of currency. The analyst faces a very difficult problem: how does one place a monetary value on health outcomes? The output of many policies is additional years of healthy life. Therefore, to apply cost–benefit analysis to medical problems, one must ask, "How does one place a monetary value on an additional year of life?" The methods for converting benefits to monetary terms are not entirely satisfactory:

How were past decisions valued? The size of an investment by society in a program designed to save lives and the number of lives actually saved is one measure of the value that society places on a life. However, these societal investments occur in a context that is unique to each occurrence. Generalizing from one such situation to another is risky.

The human capital method: This approach values a policy by its effect on the patient's lifetime earnings. A life saved at age 55 years means 10 more years of gainful employment. The monetary value of that period in the workforce can be calculated with methods to be described in this chapter.

The human capital approach is widely used, although it has a number of deficiencies. By valuing everything by anticipated income, the human capital approach implies that the life of a person with a lifetime income of $100 000 is worth twice as much as a person with a lifetime income of $50 000. This notion may have validity in economic terms, but it feels somehow unfair. The human capital approach also assumes that people are unwilling to pay more than their remaining lifetime earnings to avoid death. People with savings or a home might be willing to spend heavily from these reserves to avoid death. The next measure of the value of life is the amount that people are willing to pay to avoid death or disability.

Willingness to pay: The willingness-to-pay method helps people to express a value for life by saying how much they would be willing to pay for a program that would decrease the probability of death by a stated amount.

The subject might be told:

> Suppose that the probability that you will die from a stroke is 0.01 during your remaining lifetime. What is the most that you would be willing to pay over your lifetime for a program that would reduce this risk by 50%?

The subject might reply: "$2000."

Interpretation: A lifetime probability of 0.01 is equivalent to a risk of 10 stroke deaths per 1000 individuals. A reduction by 50% would eliminate 5 deaths per 1000 individuals. This person is willing to pay $2000 to reduce the probability of death by 0.005 (5 lives saved per 1000 persons).

By asking such questions of a community sample, one can derive an estimate of the value that the populace places on saving a life. However, what one is willing to pay is likely to depend on the exact circumstances. The premise of the willingness-to-pay approach is that a person who is willing to pay $2000 to reduce the probability of death by 0.005 would be willing to pay $400 000 ($2000 divided by 0.005) to avert the loss of their life. Many would question that premise.

Obtaining a consistent value for a human life with the willingness-to-pay approach is difficult for other reasons. People's willingness to pay increases with the risk of death. Does this mean that the value that is placed on life depends on the risk of losing it? Wealthy people are generally willing to pay more for a program to reduce the risk of death than poor people. People are more willing to pay when they personally benefit from a program than when they are asked to pay for a program that will benefit others.

Clinicians may not accept the results of cost–benefit analysis because it is so difficult to develop a consensus opinion on the monetary value of a year of human life. Most clinicians who are interested in analyzing tradeoffs between clinical strategies use cost-effectiveness analysis. Perhaps policy makers should be paying more attention to the principal advantage of cost–benefit analysis: because the costs and benefits of a program are both measured in units of currency, they can express the tradeoff between them with a tangible measure that the public can understand (profit or loss in units of currency).

10.3.3 Should clinicians take an interest in cost–benefit analysis?

The problems with applying cost–benefit analysis seem remote from daily practice. The individual clinician is not concerned with allocating effort between programs to improve the health of the community. The clinician's primary responsibility is to look after the interests of the patient. However, the choices open to the clinician may be affected by resource allocation decisions that are based on cost–benefit analysis. Policy makers must deal with such methods when they try to decide whether to allocate scarce federal resources to screening programs to detect disease in young people or programs to treat chronic disease in old people. If clinicians want policy makers to listen to them, they should understand the methods that policy makers depend on and help them to apply these methods to the world of medical practice.

10.4 Measuring the costs of medical care

Cost-effectiveness analysis depends on accurate inputs. The most important concept is that the cost of an intervention includes *both* the cost of the intervention itself *and* the downstream costs (or savings) that occur because of the intervention. For example, a cost-effectiveness analysis of the use of implantable cardioverter defibrillators includes not only the cost of the defibrillator itself, but also the cost of all of the care that occurs because the defibrillator was implanted, including follow-up visits and treatment of complications. Likewise, a cost-effectiveness analysis of anticoagulation therapy to prevent stroke would include the cost savings for each stroke prevented.

The costs due to an intervention include changes in the use of the following (Gold *et al.*, 1996, Chapter 6):

- health care resources;
- non-health-care resources (e.g., transportation);
- informal caregiver time;
- the patient's time (e.g., the time required to undergo a treatment).

Of these, the use of health care resources is typically the most important component of costs. However, for some interventions, other categories of costs also may be important. The analyst should assess the relative importance of the different types of costs on a case-by-case basis. Drummond *et al.* (2005), and Gold *et al.* (1996), provide comprehensive coverage of cost estimation. Chapters 6 and 7 of the Gold *et al.* book are the source of this chapter's framework for considering costs and discounting.

10.4.1 The direct costs of care

The direct costs of care include the value of the resources used to provide an intervention. The analyst should define resources broadly and include goods (e.g., drugs, devices), services (e.g., labor costs), and other resources (see Gold *et al.*, 1996, p. 179). The direct costs include the cost of the intervention and the costs of its adverse effects and later consequences (either good or bad). Thus, the direct costs include the direct health care costs, direct non-health-care costs, and the opportunity costs of time spent by informal caregivers in giving care and by the patient in receiving care. To take one of these, the direct health care costs include hospital costs, outpatient costs, the costs of tests, drugs, and health care personnel. As an example of the direct health care costs, the analyst should consider the following:

Hospital costs:

Hotel costs associated with hospitalization:
administration
plant operation and maintenance
depreciation of capital equipment.
Other routine costs of hospitalization:
food
nursing care
supplies
medical records.
Ancillary costs:
operating rooms
anesthesia
radiology
clinical laboratories
drugs.
Clinicians' professional fees.

Outpatient care:

Clinicians' professional fees (including the costs of running an office practice)
Diagnostic tests
Drugs and supplies
Transportation to the clinician's office.

Charges are generally an unreliable indicator of the cost of a service. Providers set charges for use in negotiations with payers and usually do not reveal the cost of producing a service. Depending on the services that a patient requires, total charges and total costs may be similar or widely divergent.

As a practical approach to estimating the true costs of a service, many analysts use as a surrogate the reimbursement from payers (which typically differs from charges). For example, in the United States, the reimbursement that Medicare pays represents the cost of care to the government. A common approach to estimating the cost of hospitalization for older patients is to use the reimbursement from Medicare based on Diagnosis Related Groups (DRG). This approach avoids the difficulty of having to account separately for the different categories of hospital costs. However, analysts should be aware that reimbursement is not always a good indicator of the true costs of care.

10.4.2 Productivity costs

Productivity costs, sometime referred to as indirect costs, include the costs from lost work due to illness or death. These costs to productivity occur because patients are unable to use their time gainfully when they are receiving medical services. Productivity costs include wages that patients would have received but did not because illness prevented them from working.

Guidelines for the conduct of cost-effectiveness analyses in the United States (see Gold *et al.*, 1996, pp. 181–3) suggest that assessment of the quality of life should take into account the patient's feelings about lost productivity. Therefore, the analyst should not include productivity costs separately in the numerator of a cost-effectiveness analysis because including them would, in effect, count them twice. However, if the quality of life assessments do not include the implications of decreased productivity, the analyst may choose to include productivity costs in the analysis.

The calculation of productivity costs usually assumes that the patient is an average wage earner. Thus, analysts use average age- and gender-specific values for wages. While this approach to valuing time is tractable, it is objectionable because wages – but not necessarily the value of time – vary by age and gender, which leads to systematically undervaluing the time of the young and women. Further details about this approach are available in Gold *et al.* (1996), and Drummond *et al.* (2005).

10.4.3 Discounting future costs

Some of the costs of an intervention may occur in the future. Most of us would rather pay $100 in 10 years' time than pay it today. As long as the interest rate on investments exceeds the rate of inflation, we should invest the $100 and earn interest for 10 years rather than paying the $100 today. Thus, the value of a future cost depends on when it is incurred. The best way to avoid confusion is to estimate all future costs as if they had been incurred in the present. **Discounting** is the process for calculating the **present value** of money that will be spent in the future. The **discount rate** is the annual rate at which money is discounted. Theoretical arguments about how to choose the discount rate notwithstanding, most analysts follow the current guidelines in the United States, which suggest a rate of 3% and rates from 0% to 7% in sensitivity analyses (see Gold *et al.*, 1996, Chapter 7). The discount rate may need revision as economic conditions change.

The present value of a future expense is given by the formula

$$P = \frac{S}{(1+r)^N}$$

where P = present value, S = future value of expense, r = discount rate and N = number of years until an expense is incurred

Assuming a discount rate of 7%, the present value of a $1000 cost that is incurred 10 years from now is

$$P = \frac{1000}{(1+0.07)^{10}} = \frac{1000}{1.96} = \$508$$

Summary

1. The clinician has an ethical obligation to be the patient's advocate. However, when resources are limited, the clinician will often have to take into account the needs of other patients or society as a whole. The Charter for Professionalism (2001) is a consensus document that emphasizes this dual obligation.
2. When resources are limited, clinicians and policy makers must identify inefficient management strategies and improve them. The methods for characterizing efficiency are called "cost-effectiveness analysis" and "cost–benefit analysis."
3. Cost-effectiveness analysis is a method for comparing clinical strategies. The basis for comparison is the relationship between the costs of the compared management strategies and their clinical effectiveness. Lacking a criterion for cost-effectiveness, it is not possible to say if a service or policy is cost-effective.
4. Cost–benefit analysis measures the net benefits and costs in the same units (usually currency) and can therefore be used to decide if a management strategy or public health policy will be of net benefit to society.

Problems

1. Suppose that one of your patients is trying to decide between an intrauterine device (IUD) and an oral contraceptive. One of her concerns is cost which she will have to cover herself during the five years that she plans to practice birth control. The initial cost for an IUD is $40. An examination, costing $20, will be necessary at the end of each of the five years the device is in place. The cost of oral contraceptives and the necessary annual examinations is $30 for each year of use plus another $20 at the end of the last year of use. The schedule for these costs is as follows:

	IUD	Oral contraceptive
Initial cost	$50	$30
Cost at year 1	$20	$30
Cost at year 2	$20	$30
Cost at year 3	$20	$30
Cost at year 4	$20	$30
Cost at year 5	$20	$20

Taking into account an annual discount rate of 0.08, which form of birth control is cheaper? Ignore any costs that may be due to complications or unplanned pregnancies.

Bibliography

Drummond, M.F., Sculpher, M.J., Torrance, G.W., O'Brien, B.J., and Stoddart, G.L. (2005) *Methods for the economic evaluation of health care programmes*, 3rd ed., Oxford University Press, Oxford.

This is an excellent comprehensive textbook that covers a broad range of economic evaluations.

Eddy, D.M. (1980) *Screening for Cancer: Theory, analysis, and design*, Prentice Hall, Englewood Cliffs, NJ.

This book describes an influential mathematical model of cancer screening. The author's rigorous mathematical approach will be difficult for most readers, but the book is strongly recommended for the adventurous reader.

Eddy, D.M. (1983) A mathematical model for timing repeated tests. *Medical Decision Making*, **3**, 45–62.

The issues that influence policy for screening for disease are clearly outlined in this description of a mathematical method for deciding when to perform periodic screening tests.

Garber, A.M. and Phelps, C.E. (1997) Economic foundations of cost-effectiveness analysis. *Journal of Health Economics*, **16**(1), 1–31.

The theoretical foundation, including ideas about choosing a cost-effectiveness threshold.

Gold, M., Siegel, J.E., Russell, L.B., and Weinstein, M.C. (1996) *Cost-effectiveness in health and medicine*, Oxford University Press, New York.

This book is still the bible for cost-effectiveness analysis.

Owens, D.K., Qaseem, A., Chou, R., and Shekelle, P., for the Clinical Guidelines Committee of the American College of Clinicians (2011) High-value, cost-conscious health care: concepts for clinicians to evaluate benefits, harms, and costs of medical interventions. *Annals of Internal Medicine*, **154**, 174–80.

A tutorial that covers the concepts of cost-effectiveness analysis for clinicians.

Russell, L.B., Gold, M.R., Siegel, J.E., Daniels, N., and Weinstein, M.C. (1996) The role of cost-effectiveness analysis in health and medicine. *Journal of the American Medical Association*, **276**(14), 1172–7.

This article discusses the potential role of cost-effectiveness in medicine.

Weinstein, M.C. and Stason, W.B. (1977) Foundations of cost-effectiveness analysis for health and medical practices. *New England Journal of Medicine*, **296**, 716–21.

An excellent introduction to cost-effectiveness and cost–benefit analysis. The reference list contains many classic articles on measuring the monetary value of a human life.

Weinstein, M.C., Fineberg, H.V., and colleagues (1980) *Clinical Decision Analysis*. W.B. Saunders, Philadelphia, pp. 228–65.

This book chapter explains how to measure the different types of health care costs.

Weinstein, M.C., Siegel, J.E., Gold, M.R., Kamlet, M.S., and Russell, L.B. (1996) Recommendations of the Panel on Cost-Effectiveness in Health and Medicine. *Journal of the American Medical Association*, **276**(15), 1253–8.

This article summarizes the recommendations of the expert panel whose report appears in the book by Gold *et al.* (1996).

CHAPTER 11

Medical decision analysis in practice: advanced methods

The purpose of this chapter is to show the reader how the concepts covered in the book are used in real-world analyses. These real-world analyses are much more complex than the examples used in previous chapters, but the underlying concepts are the same. The models we discuss here have been published in medical journals, and each required over a year of full-time effort to develop. The chapter has four parts:

11.1   An overview of advanced modeling techniques

Many of the real-world problems that people analyze are quite complex. In this book, we showed how to use decision trees to represent a decision problem. Analysts typically use a decision tree to represent problems in which all the events occur either immediately or within a short time frame (as shown in Chapter 6). If events may occur at different points in time, decision trees may become very large and difficult to understand. In general, for clinical problems in which events occur over long time horizons (e.g., cancer), events occur repeatedly, or one group interacts with another, the decision tree representation usually is not sufficient. We will discuss briefly several advanced modeling methods that can represent such events faithfully. The publications at the end of the chapter provide more detailed explanations of these methods.

Medical Decision Making, Second Edition. Harold C. Sox, Michael C. Higgins and Douglas K. Owens.
© 2013 John Wiley & Sons, Ltd. Published 2013 by John Wiley & Sons, Ltd.

11.1.1 When are advanced modeling approaches needed?

The decision about when to use more advanced methods depends on the decision problem. Modeling approaches other than decision trees are usually needed when the clinical problem:

- requires representing the natural history of a chronic disease (e.g., cancer);
- has events that occur over long time horizons (e.g., heart disease);
- has events that can occur multiple times (e.g., opportunistic infections in people living with HIV);
- requires representing transmission of an infectious disease (e.g., HIV, tuberculosis, influenza);
- involves interactions among groups (e.g., patients and clinicians in a model that addressed how to treat patients more efficiently);
- involves resource constraints (e.g., a limited number of hospital beds in a model that addressed how to triage patients in an influenza pandemic).

Each of these situations would be difficult to represent in a decision tree. For complex problems with long time horizons, the decision tree would become too large. For problems that require modeling interactions over time among groups, the decision tree is not suitable because it cannot depict such interactions.

11.1.2 Types of modeling approaches

A variety of modeling frameworks are suitable for representing complex medical decision problems. All of the approaches described here use computer-based mathematical simulations. The analysts can implement these models in software developed specifically for the modeling approach, in more general programming software, and for some of the approaches, in spreadsheet software.

The most common type of model used in medicine currently is the state-transition model (see Siebert *et al.*, 2012). This general term describes several modeling approaches that we will define and explain briefly. Interested readers should read the publications at the end of the chapter for more detail and guidance on how to develop these models.

State-transition models characterize the health states of a disease (e.g., HIV) or of an epidemic (e.g., the at-risk population) as a sequence of transitions from one state of nature (or health state) to another. For example, a health state-transition model of the natural history of HIV infection in a given individual might define health states in terms of CD4 lymphocyte counts or HIV-RNA levels. Analysts can use state-transition models to estimate the changes in length and quality of life and costs for a cohort of persons who undergo a particular intervention, either preventive or therapeutic. They allow for a running tally of all clinical events, the length of time spent in each health state, and the costs and quality of life associated with each health state. These, in turn, make it possible to compute overall performance measures such as average life expectancy, quality-adjusted life expectancy, cost, and cost-effectiveness.

There are several types of state-transition models. **Markov models**, introduced in Chapter 7, are a special class of state-transition models. They are relatively easy to specify and are used widely. As explained in Chapter 7, the Markov assumption specifies that the probability of transition to another state depends only on the current health state. Because past history is often important in clinical problems, the Markov health states must be specified with care to avoid violations of the Markov assumption. For example, the probability of recurrence of breast cancer may depend on how many years have elapsed since treatment. To represent this clinical history in a Markov model therefore often requires expanding the number of health states. A breast cancer model might need to include a state for each year after initial treatment (e.g., year 1, year 2, ..., year 20). Markov models are very useful, but if the relevant clinical history is very complex, the models may require so many health states that they become difficult to develop, debug, and understand.

In such situations, another approach is to use a generalized health state-transition model, often called an "individual-level state-transition model," or **microsimulation model**. These models provide a means of flexibly modeling events over time when the clinical history is complex. In this framework, the model comprises specific individuals that have particular attributes (such as age and gender) and can have a complex history (such as a history of a disease, associated treatment, and complications). As time progresses in the model, the history of each person can develop as events occur (e.g., a stroke) according to specified probabilities. This approach allows for complex histories, but the analyst must model the history of each of many individuals (usually thousands or more), so this approach is often more computationally intensive than are Markov models. For an example, see the paper by Bendavid and colleagues (2008) at the end of the chapter.

For problems in which the population-wide effects of an infectious disease are important, **dynamic transmission models** are a useful approach (see the paper by Pitman and colleagues, 2012). These models divide the population into compartments (e.g., the infected population and the uninfected–susceptible population), and the transitions between the compartments occur as specified by systems of equations. These equations account for the fact that the number of people in one compartment influences the rate of transition to other compartments. For example, up to a point, as the number of people in the infected population increases, transmission becomes more likely. Then at some point, transmission slows because there are fewer uninfected people to become infected. See the article by Long and colleagues (2010) for an example.

Other types of models

We also note two additional modeling approaches that do not fall into the category of state-transition models. **Discrete-event simulation models** can be used for a variety of applications (see the by Karnon and colleagues, 2012). In these models, *entities* (e.g., a patient) have *attributes* (e.g., demographic information and clinical history), are subject to *events* (e.g., a stroke), can interact with other entities (e.g., patients, physicians), and use *resources* (e.g., money or a hospital bed). These models allow for complex interactions over time. Discrete-event simulation models are particularly useful when interactions between agents are important, or when there are resource constraints. **Network models** are used less often than are other types of models, but can be useful when detailed disease transmission patterns are especially important. For example, an analysis of how influenza spreads in a population might use a network model that captures detailed relationships between people, such as family members, co-workers, and classmates.

11.1.3 Choosing among modeling approaches

The choice of a modeling approach depends on the purposes of the analysis, the problem under consideration, and the expertise of the analyst. For some problems, several different approaches may be applicable. In the example we will turn to next, we used a Markov model to evaluate the cost-effectiveness of screening for HIV. This problem can also be analyzed with microsimulation models, dynamic transmission models, or discrete event simulation models.

The choice between a Markov model and a microsimulation model depends in large part on the complexity of the history and the number of health states required to represent the problem. If the natural history of the disease, or the clinical history, is very complex, a microsimulation model may be preferable, although Markov models and other approaches may be useful as well. In the example of HIV screening in the next section, the screening and treatment Markov model had several hundred health states. Although the model was still manageable, a microsimulation approach would have also been a good option. Analysts often find that the complexity of the model and health condition is not fully apparent until the project is far along. Consultation with an experienced decision modeler is advisable before starting a project.

If a major focus of the analysis is to determine the population-wide effects of an intervention for an infectious disease, a dynamic transmission model is often preferred, although microsimulation models are also an option. A network model is especially useful for a detailed analysis of disease transmission patterns.

The goal in choosing a modeling framework is to use an approach that can capture the necessary complexity to represent a problem faithfully, while preserving its essential features in a form that an expert colleague can understand well enough to offer useful criticism. The word "transparency" is often used to describe this characteristic of a model. Transparency is important for both the modeling team and the end user of the analysis. Highly complex models are more difficult to develop and debug. They are also more difficult for readers to understand, and to the extent that critical readers cannot understand the model, they will be more skeptical of the results. Unfortunately, despite the desire for simplicity, most challenging medical problems require relatively sophisticated models. At this level, peer review – an essential element of science – becomes very difficult.

In the next section, we turn to an extended example of a Markov-model-based analysis of the health and economic outcomes of HIV screening.

11.2 Use of medical decision-making concepts to analyze a policy problem: the cost-effectiveness of screening for HIV

In the second and third parts of this chapter, we illustrate analyses of real-world problems using the concepts covered in the book. The first example is an analysis of a policy question: Is routine screening for HIV cost effective? We will discuss several aspects of the analysis, and interested readers may want to read the journal article by Sanders *et al.* (2005).

11.2.1 The policy question

The problem we will assess is whether routine, voluntary HIV screening is cost effective. This question is important because, at the time of the analysis, national guidelines for screening recommended risk-based screening in many settings. The guidelines recommended that clinicians screen people who had behaviors that put them at increased risk for HIV infection (such as having multiple sexual partners or injection drug use). Although this approach seemed as if it should be efficient because only people at increased risk would be screened, it had not been successful. Many high-risk patients were not screened and were therefore diagnosed with HIV very late in the course of disease when they could not receive the maximum benefit from antiretroviral therapy. An alternative strategy would be to screen all patients, regardless of risk. But such a strategy could have high total costs, and it was not known whether routine screening of all patients would be cost effective relative to practice at the time.

11.2.2 Steps of the analysis

The main steps in such an analysis are listed in Table 11.1. The first step is to define the problem, objectives, and perspective. Then the analyst should identify the alternatives, choose a modeling framework, and structure the problem. Structuring the problem includes defining chance events and the sequence of decisions and chance events. Depending on the condition under study, it may also include defining and modeling the natural history of the disease. The next step is to define the probabilities of chance events, which requires reviewing the available evidence on the natural history of disease, the accuracy of diagnostic tests, and the benefits and harms of interventions or treatments. If the analysis is a cost-effectiveness or cost–benefit analysis, the analyst will need to estimate costs, and discount costs and benefits appropriately (see Chapter 10). Then the analyst can calculate the expected

Table 11.1 Steps in performing an analysis.

---

1. Define the problem, objectives, and perspective
2. Identify alternatives
3. Choose the modeling framework
4. Structure the problem, define chance events, represent the time sequence
5. Determine the probability of chance events
6. Value the outcomes
7. Estimate costs
8. Discount costs and health outcomes appropriately
9. Calculate the expected value (utility) and costs of each alternative
10. Calculate cost-effectiveness, eliminate dominated alternatives
11. Analyze uncertainties
12. Address ethical issues
13. Discuss results

Based on data from: Office of Technology Assessment, *The Implications of Cost-Effectiveness Analysis of Medical Technology*, US Congress, 1980.

value (utility) and costs of the alternatives, calculate cost effectiveness, analyze uncertainties, address ethical issue, and discuss the results.

We will illustrate some of these steps in the next sections.

11.2.3   Define the problem, objectives, and perspective

The problem is whether routine HIV screening is cost effective. The objective of the analysis is to estimate the health benefits, costs, and cost-effectiveness of HIV screening. We will evaluate this problem from the societal perspective, which considers all benefits and all costs, regardless of who benefits or who pays.

11.2.4   Identify alternatives and choose the modeling framework

The alternatives we will compare are routine voluntary screening of all patients presenting for medical care, and a strategy in which only patients who presented with symptoms or signs that suggested HIV would be tested. To choose the modeling framework, we first consider the natural history of HIV. Without treatment, HIV infection causes progressive destruction of the immune system and susceptibility to infections that healthy people do not get. These infections, called opportunistic infections, occur over time as the immune system becomes weaker. As of 2013, HIV requires lifelong treatment. Therefore, to understand the long-term benefits and costs of a screening program, we need a modeling framework that enables us to model medical events and costs that occur over the entire lifetime of the cohort that will be screened (or not screened). Because of the long time horizon, a decision tree is not practical, as it require hundreds or thousands of chance nodes to represent the uncertain events that could occur over many years. The options include Markov models, microsimulation models, and dynamic transmission models.

For this analysis, we chose a Markov model because we believed it would be more transparent and more easily debugged. In the end, because of the complicated history associated with antiretroviral treatment, the model contained a large number of health states, so a microsimulation model would also have been a good alternative approach for representing the complex treatment history. Another analysis was published at the same time based on a microsimulation model (see the article by Paltiel and colleagues (2005) noted at the end of the chapter). Our analysis did account for HIV transmission to partners, but did not model population-wide effects of HIV transmission. A dynamic transmission model would be an alternative for a more complete analysis of transmission, but we wanted to model treatment regimens in substantial detail. A detailed treatment model would be more challenging in a dynamic transmission model because of the large number of compartments the model would require.

11.2.5 Structure the problem, define chance events, represent the time sequence

An analysis of screening must represent both the events related to screening and the events related to treatment that follows screening. We must model treatment because the benefit of screening comes from treatment, presumably earlier treatment than would be prescribed in the absence of screening. An analysis of the cost-effectiveness of screening therefore includes the costs of screening and the costs, benefits, and harms of treatment over the lifetime of the patient.

Modeling the time course of disease

To understand how treatment affects length and quality of life with HIV, we must model the events that occur during HIV disease. As HIV disease progresses, a certain kind of white blood cell, called a CD4 lymphocyte, declines in number, which reflects progressive immune system destruction. HIV replicates rapidly and clinicians can measure ribonucleic acid (RNA) from the virus in the blood, which is called the viral load. If HIV antiretroviral therapy is successful, viral replication is stopped and the viral load drops and becomes undetectable in the blood. With successful antiretroviral therapy, CD4 counts generally increase or remain stable, but if viral replication begins again and remains unchecked, CD4 counts drop. Opportunistic infections and death occur when the CD4 count gets low. Although we will not explore these details further, the actual model that we used to analyze screening and treatment contained health states that represented screening status, CD4 count, viral load, and antiretroviral treatment regimens. As noted, this complexity resulted in a Markov model with several hundred health states. The technical appendix for the published paper by Sanders *et al.* (2005) contains further details about the model.

To illustrate the concept of modeling the course of HIV disease, Figure 11.1 shows a simplified schematic of a Markov model of disease and treatment

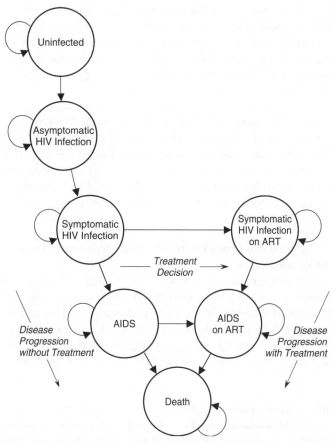

Figure 11.1 Schematic diagram of a Markov model of HIV disease. The circles indicate health states and arrows indicate allowed transitions between health states. Arrows that point downward indicate transitions due to disease progression. Arrows that point from left to right indicate transitions that occur because of the initiation of treatment. ART = antiretroviral therapy.

health states. In the figure, we have grouped stages of HIV disease into asymptomatic (high CD4 counts), symptomatic (medium CD4 counts), and AIDS (low CD4 counts). In this type of figure, circles represent health states and arrows represent the allowed transitions among health states. An arrow that loops back to the same health state indicates that a person could stay in the same health state during the next cycle. The schematic shows the transitions associated with the natural history of untreated HIV, and the transitions to health states associated with antiretroviral treatment.

Modeling screening

Our model of HIV screening must reflect both the outcomes of testing and the effect of treatment on the course of HIV disease. A possible structure is

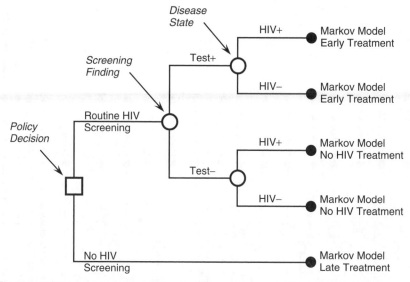

Figure 11.2 Decision tree representation of a HIV screening model. The square indicates a decision and circles indicate chance events. At the end of each branch in the decision tree, a Markov model is attached, similar to the Markov model in Figure 11.1.

shown in Figure 11.2. The model reflects the outcomes of testing in a decision tree, followed by Markov models that reflect early treatment in the Screening strategy and later treatment in the No Screening strategy.

This structure, with modifications to make it more realistic, could represent a one-time screening program in which all patients are screened at the initiation of the program. However, a more realistic scenario is that screening would occur over time rather than all at once. In addition, another important question is whether screening should be repeated. Guidelines at the time our analysis was performed called for periodic screening of high-risk individuals; the model in Figure 11.2 could not address repeat screening.

To address repeat screening, say every year or every five years, we could use the structure shown in Figure 11.3. In this figure, the Markov model is represented in a tree format rather than as circles and arrows as in Figure 11.1. Figures 11.1 and 11.3 show two alternative methods for representing the Markov model schematically, but the underlying model itself is the same. Health states shown as circles in Figure 11.1 (Uninfected, Asymptomatic HIV Infection, Symptomatic HIV Infection, and AIDS) are shown in Figure 11.3 as branches in a tree, with "Markov" in the circle to indicate that it is a Markov node. In this format, we denote the possible transitions from a health state as branches in the tree, rather than as arrows. For example, the branches from the uninfected health state are labeled Become Infected and Stay Uninfected. These correspond to the arrows from the uninfected health state in Figure 11.1.

In Figure 11.3, we represent whether or not someone is screened as a chance node at the end of each branch in the Markov model, rather than as a decision

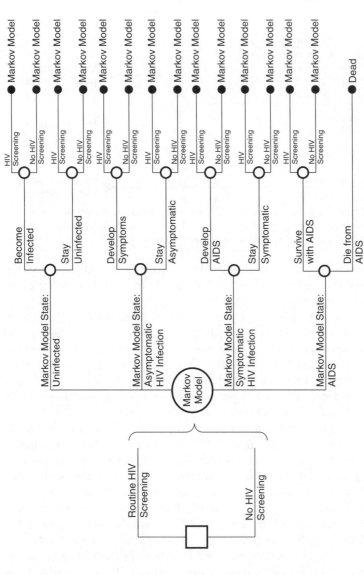

Figure 11.3 Tree representation of a Markov model of HIV screening. In the diagram, the Markov model depicted in Figure 11.1 is shown as a tree structure. After the decision to screen or not, the Markov model has the health states Uninfected, Asymptomatic HIV Infection, Symptomatic HIV Infection, and AIDS. The branches of the tree after these states indicate the allowed transitions to other health states in the Markov model. The last chance node in each branch indicates that screening could occur during that cycle of the Markov model. At the end of each branch, Markov Model indicates that the next cycle of the Markov model then begins. (From Sanders *et al*. Cost effectiveness of screening for HIV in the era of highly active antiretroviral therapy. *New England Journal of Medicine* 2005; 352:570–585 Copyright © 2005, Massachusetts Medical Society. Modified with permission from Massachusetts Medical Society.)

node in the decision tree. Although whether someone is screened is actually a decision, the standard Markov model has chance nodes only, not decision nodes. To work around this constraint, we use the chance node to represent screening. We can model periodic screening by setting the probability of screening to 1 in the years that screening occurs and 0 in the other years, or we can model ongoing screening by having a probability of screening each year.

People identified as having HIV, either through screening or case finding, can begin antiretroviral treatment if they are eligible. Figure 11.1 shows treatment-associated health states. We model the benefit of treatment as a reduction in the probability of transitioning to more advanced states of HIV disease or to death.

Our next step is to determine the probability of chance events in the model.

11.2.6 Determine the probability of chance events

When the analyst believes the structure of the model adequately represents the clinical problem, the next step is to specify the probability of chance events (see the paper by Briggs and colleagues, 2012). To do so, the analyst will review the relevant medical literature. This process is labor intensive. The model we used for evaluating the cost-effectiveness of HIV screening had over 80 parameters, many of which were chance events.

Although the analyst may not be able to perform a comprehensive review of the literature for all model parameters, he should do so for all important parameters. For example, the probability of transitioning to more advanced HIV disease for patients who are on treatment depends on the effectiveness of antiretroviral therapy. To estimate the relevant probabilities, we reviewed the available literature on the effectiveness of antiretroviral therapy. This task alone required substantial effort. Other important parameters included the sensitivity and specificity of the tests used to screen, the probability of death by stage of HIV infection, the probability of HIV transmission to sexual partners, and the probability of treatment failure.

Given that a complex model may have many parameters and a comprehensive review of the literature is time intensive, how can an analyst approach this task efficiently? For important parameters, we recommend that the analyst search for high-quality systematic reviews, and then update those reviews selectively as necessary. The analyst may also search for clinical prediction rules that help estimate probabilities for specific clinical settings or risk factors (see Chapter 3). We also recommend using the model early in the process to help determine which parameters are crucial to the analysis. To do this, the analyst can perform a preliminary review of the literature and consult experts to get rough estimates of the model parameters. The analyst can then use sensitivity analysis to determine which parameters are most important. The sensitivity analyses can direct the effort of the subsequent literature review. The analyst can use this process iteratively to use resources efficiently in the literature review. The analyst should also aim to estimate a probability distribution for important parameters, rather than a single point estimate of the probability, because such distributions are necessary to perform probabilistic sensitivity analysis (see Section 3.8).

When the analyst is convinced that he has the best estimates possible for the important model parameters, he can move to the next step, valuing the outcomes.

11.2.7 Value the outcomes

The analyst can now turn to valuing the outcomes. He could use any of the metrics we have discussed in previous chapters, including life expectancy or quality-adjusted life years (QALYs). We chose to use QALYs as our primary metric because HIV and antiretroviral therapy affect both length and quality of life. If we used life expectancy only, we would not capture the effect of screening and treatment, for better or worse, on quality of life. Estimation of how screening changes quality of life is challenging, however, so we also used life expectancy as an outcome.

Quality of life is important in the HIV screening analysis because untreated HIV reduces quality of life, screening may reduce or increase quality of life, and treatment, at least for patients with advanced disease, increases quality of life. The effect of screening itself on quality of life is complex. You could imagine that a person with asymptomatic HIV infection might feel that their quality of life had been diminished by discovering through screening that they had HIV. Alternatively, a person with symptoms from HIV might find quality of life to be improved by effective therapy. Studies in the literature suggest that both of these scenarios do occur.

To estimate QALYs, we had to specify the quality of life associated with each health state in the Markov model. Using the health states in Figure 11.1 as an example, we note that we must estimate the quality of life for people who are uninfected, and for people both on and off treatment with asymptomatic HIV, symptomatic HIV, and AIDS. To do this, we reviewed the literature to find quality of life estimates for these health states. Many studies have measured the quality of life with HIV based with standard gambles, time tradeoffs, and with other quality of life assessment instruments such as the health utilities index and the EQ-5D. See the study by Joyce *et al.* (2009) for an example of a study that used all of these quality of life assessment instruments.

11.2.8 Estimate costs and discount outcomes

To estimate the costs associated with an intervention, the analyst must determine the cost of the intervention itself and the costs of any subsequent care that occurred because a person decided to undergo the intervention (see Chapter 10). We include these subsequent costs because they result from use of the intervention; these downstream costs would not have occurred had the intervention not been performed.

For our HIV screening example, this principle means that we must estimate the cost of screening and of all care that follows screening. The screening costs include the cost of the initial and confirmatory tests and the cost of associated counseling. The analyst should also include the costs of follow-up tests or treatment that result from a false-positive test result, and, if there are any, the costs from a false-negative test result. The treatment costs include the costs of tests, office visits, procedures, drugs, and hospitalizations.

For an analysis that uses a Markov model or other state-transition model, the analyst must assign costs for each health state. We used the literature to estimate the cost of the health states depicted in Figure 11.1. The cost of care increases as HIV disease progresses, therefore the annual cost for a patient with asymptomatic HIV infection is less than the annual cost for a patient with more advanced disease.

As explained in Chapter 10, the analyst should discount costs. By using appropriate formulas, the analyst can specify the Markov model so that the model discounts future costs appropriately. The further a cost occurs in the future, the more it will be discounted. If the analysis has a long time horizon, the effect of discounting may be substantial. For example, HIV treatment costs that occur 15 to 20 years in the future will have less influence on cost-effectiveness than do treatment costs that occur in the first 5 years.

11.2.9 Calculate the expected utility, costs, and cost-effectiveness

Once the analyst has specified the probability of chance events, estimated costs, and valued the outcomes, he can analyze the model to calculate expected utility, costs, and cost-effectiveness. In a Markov model, this analysis occurs differently than in the decision trees that we evaluated in earlier chapters. While a decision tree is evaluated by averaging and rolling back the tree from right to left (see Chapter 6), a Markov model is evaluated as a mathematical simulation that begins at a specified time and goes forward in time until predetermined stopping criteria are met.

For our HIV screening example, we can think of the model as performing two mathematical simulations: one for the Screening strategy and one for the No Screening strategy. Let us consider the Screening strategy first. The software for the model begins the analysis at time 0 and, as time moves forward, the model keeps track of how long an individual spends in each health state. For example, a person might spend a year in the uninfected state before becoming infected, and then progress through each of the health states associated with HIV disease. The person would be diagnosed as having HIV (depending on when screening occurs), and then be treated. At each new cycle of the Markov model, people either stay in the same health state or transition to other health states according to the specified transition probabilities. Based on these transition probabilities, the model determines the duration of time a person is in each health state. The model also accounts for the quality of life and costs in the health states. To calculate life expectancy, QALYs, and total costs, the model sums these amounts (with appropriate discounting) over all the health states. The model also performs the same simulation for the No Screening strategy.

The results of the analysis for HIV screening are given in Table 11.2. The table shows the lifetime costs and benefits of each strategy, based on a prevalence of undiagnosed HIV infection of 1%. We note that No Screening is the least expensive strategy, and the least effective. The one-time screening strategy costs $194 additional dollars over the lifetime of the person screened and increases life expectancy by 5.48 days and quality-adjusted life expectancy by 4.70 days relative to the No Screening strategy. We emphasize that a cost-effectiveness analysis estimates the incremental benefit and incremental costs of one strategy relative to another. Screening every five years results in slightly higher costs ($206 per person screened) and slightly larger increases in life expectancy (1.52 days) and QALYs (1.31 days) than does one-time screening.

The increases in life expectancy and QALYs are approximately five days per person screened. You may wonder if such a benefit is important. To understand this result, we first note that the analysis assumes that the prevalence of undiagnosed HIV infection is 1%. This prevalence means that of 100 people who are screened, 99 do not have HIV infection and receive no benefit from screening, while 1 person does have HIV and will receive a benefit of approximately 1.5 additional years of life (see the published study by Sanders *et al.* (2005) for more detail). The fairly large benefit to the one person is averaged across all 100 people screened, which results in *per person* benefit of about five quality-adjusted days. Of course, a specific individual either receives no benefit or a relatively large benefit, but our results represent the average per person benefit for each person screened. Although the per person benefit is modest, the total benefit from the screening program may be very substantial. For example, a program that screened 1 million people would result in almost 13 000 additional quality-adjusted life *years* in the screened population.

We can also calculate the incremental cost-effectiveness ratio of screening compared to case finding from the results in Table 11.2. One-time screening costs $15 078 per QALY gained. This result means that if we implement a screening program, we would expect to spend about $15 000 dollars for each additional QALY gained from screening. In the United States, that would be considered good value. Screening every five years relative to one-time screening costs $57 138 per QALY gained. In our example, repeated screening is less efficient use of resources than is one-time screening.

11.2.10 Evaluate uncertainty

In Chapter 6, we discussed how to do sensitivity analyses and why they are important. We now discuss sensitivity analysis in the context of the HIV screening example.

The most important sensitivity analysis of the HIV screening analysis assessed how the cost-effectiveness of screening changed with the prevalence of undiagnosed HIV infection. The reason this analysis was important is that it answered a key clinical question. The Centers for Disease Control and Prevention (CDC) HIV screening guideline recommended routine screening

Table 11.2 Health outcomes, costs, and cost-effectiveness of HIV screening.

Strategy	Lifetime cost ($)	Incremental cost ($)	Life expectancy (years)	Incremental life expectancy (days)	Incremental cost effectiveness ($/LY)	Quality-adjusted life expectancy (years)	Incremental quality-adjusted life expectancy (days)	Incremental cost-effectiveness ($/QALY)
No screening	52 623		21.015			18.576		
One-time screening	52 816	194	21.030	5.48	12 919	18.589	4.70	15 078
Screening every 5 years	53 022	206*	21.034	1.52*	49 509*	18.592	1.31*	57 138*

*Relative to one-time screening.

LY = life year, QALY = quality-adjusted life year. Based on a prevalence of 1% of undiagnosed HIV infection, and includes the benefit from reduction in transmission. Health and economic outcomes were discounted at 3%, including benefits and costs of transmission to partners.

Based on data from Sanders *et al.* (2005).

only if the prevalence of HIV was above 1%. If screening were cost effective at a lower prevalence than 1%, routine screening might be warranted in more clinical settings.

The results of the sensitivity analysis indicated that screening was cost effective even at a much lower prevalence than 1%. At a prevalence of 0.5%, one-time screening cost about $19 000 per QALY gained. Even at a prevalence of 0.05%, 20 times lower than the CDC guideline threshold for routine screening, the cost-effectiveness of screening was approximately $50 000 per QALY gained, which most observers would agree is good value in the United States.

The critical insight from the sensitivity analysis was that routine screening was cost effective even at a much lower HIV prevalence than was recommended in guidelines at the time. We discuss the implications of this finding in the next section.

11.2.11   Address ethical issues, discuss results

The analyst should always consider whether important ethical issues are germane to the analysis. Ethical questions may include whether a policy is fair to all individuals, whether a policy might benefit one group at the expense of the other, whether the analysis fairly captures benefits and harms, and whether the policy may have unintended consequences. Ethical considerations shaped several aspects of HIV screening policy, including recommendations that screening should be voluntary, that people should be informed before testing is initiated, and that people diagnosed with HIV should be protected from stigmatization.

The final step in an analysis is to discuss the importance and implications of the results and the limitations of the analysis. The content of this discussion depends on the nature of the problem, the context for the analysis, the intended audience, and goals of the analysis. The purpose of the discussion is to help the reader to understand the insight that the analysis provides and to appreciate limitations of the data or analytic approach.

For our HIV screening example, the finding that screening is cost effective at low prevalence had important implications. The analysis we have described, and an independent analysis by Paltiel and colleagues (2005) had similar results. In part based on these studies, the CDC recommended routine screening in all health care settings in which the prevalence of HIV was above 0.1%, a threshold that was 10 times lower than the previously recommended prevalence of 1% for routine screening. Because there were few, if any, health care settings with a documented prevalence less than 0.1%, the new guideline was essentially a recommendation to switch from risk-based screening to routine voluntary screening in health care settings. This new recommendation represented a major change in screening policy.

We will now turn to an example in which we evaluated a testing strategy for a complicated diagnostic problem.

11.3 Use of medical decision-making concepts to analyze a clinical diagnostic problem: strategies to diagnose tumors in the lung

We now turn to an example that evaluates a challenging diagnostic and treatment problem (this example is based on the article by Gould *et al.*, 2003; the reader can refer to this article and its appendix for details of the analysis, assumptions, inputs, and results). The question is how best to evaluate and manage an abnormality on a chest x-ray known as a solitary pulmonary nodule. A solitary pulmonary nodule is a circumscribed lesion on a chest x-ray and may be caused by lung cancer or by other disease processes, such as infectious or inflammatory diseases. The clinician has many possible diagnostic tests to choose from. This problem has high stakes for the patient, as prompt diagnosis of cancer is important because treatment may be life-saving. Alternatively, an erroneous diagnosis of cancer could result in unnecessary surgery or other treatments.

11.3.1 Define the problem, objectives, and perspective

The problem we will address is the cost effectiveness of alternative management strategies for patients with a solitary pulmonary nodule on chest x-ray. The management strategies include both the diagnostic evaluation and the treatment.

11.3.2 Identify alternatives and choose the modeling framework

The diagnostic tests we will consider are computed tomography (CT), which localizes the nodule within the lung, and positron emission tomography (PET). PET scans measure the metabolic rate of tissues; because malignant tumors have increased metabolic rate, PET scans can also distinguish cancer from benign lesions. The strategies to manage pulmonary nodules include surgical resection, transthoracic needle biopsy, and watchful waiting. Surgical resection is the definitive treatment if the nodule is malignant and the cancer has not spread to other locations. However, the surgery has risks, and clinicians would not want to recommend lung surgery to a patient who did not have lung cancer. Transthoracic needle biopsy is a technique for sampling the tissue from the nodule to see if it is cancer. The watchful waiting strategy involves repeating the imaging test (CT or PET) periodically to see if the nodule is getting bigger. If the nodule stays the same size, it is unlikely to be cancer.

We will use a hybrid modeling strategy: a decision tree to represent the multiple possible initial strategies, followed by a Markov model that represents the natural history of lung cancer and the effect of treatment. We could have also chosen a microsimulation modeling framework.

11.3.3 Structure the problem, define chance events, represent the time sequence

We start by defining the initial decision a clinician must make, as shown in Figure 11.4. As shown by the decision node labeled with an A, the options

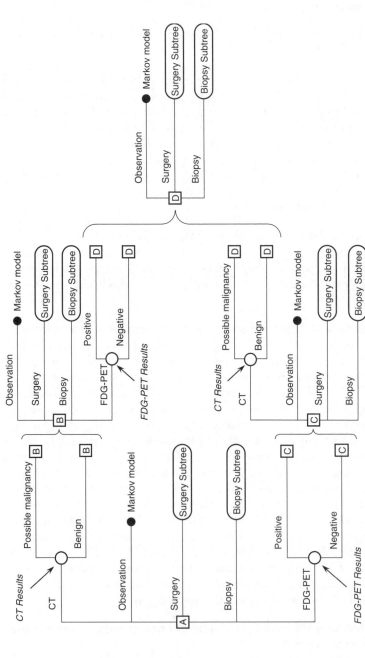

Figure 11.4 Decision tree representation of the evaluation of a solitary pulmonary nodule. The decision node labeled A indicates the initial alternatives the clinician can choose. Decision node labeled B indicates the management choices after an initial CT scan. The decision node labeled C indicates the management choices after an initial PET scan. The decision node labeled D indicates management choices after both PET and CT. See Figure 11.5 for the structure of the Biopsy Subtree and the Surgery Subtree. CT = computed tomography; FDG-PET = 18-flourodeoxyglucose positron emission scanning. (Modified from Gould MK *et al.* Cost effectiveness of alternative management strategies for patients with solitary pulmonary nodules. *Annals of Internal Medicine* 2003; **138**, 724–735, with permission from the American College of Physicians.)

the clinician could choose are imaging with CT or PET, observation (watchful waiting), immediate surgery, or transthoracic biopsy. The decision tree in Figure 11.4 shows the events that could occur after each of these choices. If the clinician chooses to perform a CT scan, the scan could be negative (i.e., indicate that the nodule is benign) or positive, which indicates that the nodule is possibly malignant. A CT scan cannot prove that a nodule is malignant, so we will use the phrase "possibly malignant" to denote a positive CT. The clinician must then decide what to do about the results of the CT scan; the decision node labeled B shows the options. The clinician could choose observation, surgery, biopsy, or further imaging with PET scan. If the clinician chooses further imaging with PET scan, then she must decide what to do, as shown by decision node D, about the results of the PET scan. Figure 11.5 shows the subtrees for biopsy and surgery, which indicate the events that can occur if the clinician chooses those options.

Note that the time sequence of the decisions is represented by their place within the decision tree. Going from left to right in Figure 11.4, decision A occurs first, and decisions B, C, and D occur subsequently or not at all, depending on the clinician's choice for decision A. We can see from the tree that decision D occurs only if the clinician chooses to obtain both CT and PET.

The decision tree captures the complexity of the choices facing the clinician. We can evaluate 40 clinically plausible strategies, based on different choices at decisions A, B, C, and D.

11.3.4 Determine the probability of the chance events

As in our previous example, to determine the probability of chance events, the analyst should search the literature carefully, seeking out the best available evidence, which is usually found in systematic reviews, and clinical prediction rules for estimating the probabilities in the model. For this analysis, we had to determine the prior probability that a solitary pulmonary nodule is malignant given the patient's history and the features of the nodule on the chest x-ray. Other important information is the sensitivity and specificity of the diagnostic tests, and the probability of the outcomes of surgery and biopsy, including complications. We combined the results of studies of the sensitivity and specificity of CT and PET so that we could obtain the most valid estimates of test performance. We also developed a model of the natural history of lung cancer, which included estimates of the rate of growth of malignant tumors, the probability of death from cancer at different stages, and the probability of recurrence of cancer for various stages of cancer and treatments. The estimates of these and all other input parameters are available in the appendix of the article by Gould *et al.* (2003).

11.3.5 Value the outcomes

Because lung cancer affects both length and quality of life, we chose to measure the outcomes for management of lung nodules in QALYs. To do so, we estimated the mortality with lung cancer, the effectiveness of treatment,

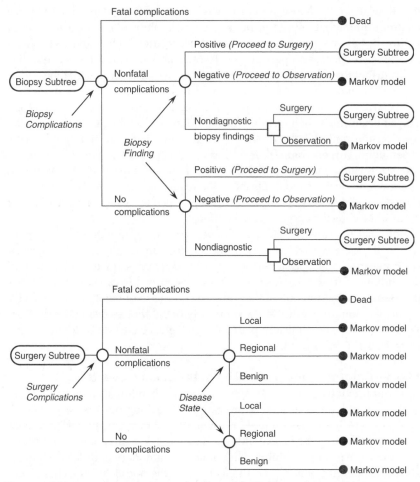

Figure 11.5 Biopsy and surgery subtrees for Figure 11.4. The biopsy and surgery subtrees indicate the chance events and outcomes that occur after a decision to perform a biopsy or surgery. (Modified from Gould MK *et al*. Cost effectiveness of alternative management strategies for patients with solitary pulmonary nodules. *Annals of Internal Medicine* 2003; **138**, 724–735, with permission from the American College of Physicians.)

and the quality of life with lung cancer, with lung cancer treatment (e.g., with a partial or complete resection of the lung), and with complications of treatment. We also estimated decrements in quality of life caused by diagnostic biopsy and surgery. Invasive procedures will reduce quality of life for a while, even if no complications occur. Modeling these changes is straightforward.

11.3.6 Estimate costs and discount outcomes

To evaluate the cost-effectiveness of management strategies for pulmonary nodules, we estimated the costs of the tests and treatment alternatives. These include the cost of CT, PET, biopsy, surgery, costs of complications, the cost of cancer treatment, including the cost of follow-up care, and long-term costs associated with cancer and other conditions that cause pulmonary nodules. We also estimated the costs of health care unrelated to cancer that patients would receive over their lifetime. We included these costs because a treatment that changes length of life will change the cost of non-cancer care over a lifetime.

11.3.7 Calculate expected utility, costs, and cost-effectiveness

The analysis resulted in estimates of the costs, life expectancy, QALYs, and cost-effectiveness of each of the 40 clinical strategies, at different pre-test probabilities. Here, we will focus on the main clinical insights from the analysis. First, CT scan was the initial best choice unless the pre-test probability of cancer was greater than 0.9. When the pre-test probability of cancer was greater than 0.9, surgery was the preferred option. Second, the choice of subsequent management strategy after CT scan depends strongly on the pre-test probability of cancer. That is, the strategies that were most effective and cost-effective varied depending on the pretest probability of disease. This finding reinforces the lessons of previous chapters about the importance of pre-test probability on the interpretation of diagnostic tests (see the article by Swensen and colleagues (1977) for a clinical prediction rule to estimate the probability that a pulmonary nodule is malignant). Third, PET, a very expensive test, could still be cost effective, if clinicians used it selectively.

Figure 11.6 shows the next preferred test after CT based on the pre-test probability of disease. The top panel in the table shows the next test after a positive (possibly malignant) CT result, and the bottom panel shows the next test after a negative (benign) CT result. At low pre-test probabilities (0.05 to 0.1), after a positive CT, the post-test probability is sufficiently high (0.10 to 0.20) that biopsy is preferred (top panel). At pre-test probabilities between 0.10 and 0.55, PET is preferred as the next test after a positive CT. At higher pre-test probabilities, surgery is preferred without further testing. In contrast, if at low pre-test probabilities (0.05 to 0.10), CT is negative, then the post-test probability of cancer is less than 0.01, and watchful waiting is preferred, as shown in the bottom panel of Figure 11.6.

The results of the analysis are summarized in a clinical algorithm in Figure 11.7. The algorithm stratifies patients by pre-test probability as low (0.1 to 0.5), intermediate (0.51 to 0.76), and high (0.77 to 0.9), and shows the preferred sequence of tests and treatment. For example, for a patient with a low pre-test probability, a possibly malignant result on CT is followed by PET. If the PET is positive, surgery is the best option. If the PET is negative, needle biopsy is the best option to ensure the PET result is not a false negative. An algorithm is a good way to show the results of a complex analysis.

11.3.8 Evaluate uncertainty

The sensitivity analyses showed that the pre-test probability of cancer, the sensitivity of CT, the diagnostic yield of biopsy, and the utility of watchful

	Recommended Test Sequence – Possible Malignant CT Results			
Next test after CT:	Biopsy	FDG-PET	Surgery	Surgery (No CT)
Pre-test Probability (%)	5 10	15 20 25 30 35 40 45 50	55 60 65 70 75 80 85	90 95 100
Post-test Probability (%)	10 20	28 35 42 48 54 59 64 69	73 76 80 84 87 90 93	95 98 100

	Recommended Test Sequence – Benign CT Results			
Next test after CT:	Watchful Waiting	Biopsy	FDG-PET	Surgery (No CT)
Pre-test Probability (%)	5 10 15 20	25 30 35 40 45 50 55 60 65 70 75	80 85	90 95 100
Post-test Probability (%)	<1 <1 1 2	2 3 3 4 5 6 7 8 10 13 16	20 26	36 54 100

Figure 11.6 Recommended test sequences and post-test probability after an initial CT scan for evaluation of a solitary pulmonary nodule. The top panel shows the preferred next test after a CT scan result that indicated a possibly malignant nodule. The pre-test probability indicates the probability of cancer before the CT is performed. The post-test probability indicates the probability of cancer after the CT result. For example, if the pre-test probability of cancer is 25%, the post-test probability after a positive CT is 42% and the preferred next action is PET scan. The bottom panel shows the preferred tests and post-test probability if the CT suggests the nodule is benign. CT = computed tomography; FDG-PET = 18-flourodeoxyglucose positron emission scanning. (Modified from Gould MK *et al.* Cost effectiveness of alternative management strategies for patients with solitary pulmonary nodules. *Annals of Internal Medicine* 2003; **138**, 724–735, with permission from the American College of Physicians.)

waiting could affect the preferred option at different stages of the management of the patient with a solitary pulmonary nodule.

Sensitivity analysis on one and two variables can provide key insights into the effects of uncertainty on decision making. However, for most analyses, the true value of many model parameters is uncertain. To address this problem, the analyst can perform probabilistic sensitivity analysis. **Probabilistic sensitivity analysis** evaluates the impact of uncertainty about many or all model parameters simultaneously. To do such an analysis, the analyst must estimate probability distributions for each important model parameter. In the analysis, the software randomly selects a value for each parameter from its distribution, and evaluates the model based on the chosen set of parameters to estimate costs, benefits, and cost-effectiveness. This process is then repeated 1000 to 10 000 times, each time with a new set of values for the model parameters, with each value chosen randomly from the probability distribution of the parameter. The result of the probabilistic sensitivity analysis is an estimate of costs, benefits, and cost-effectiveness (relative to the appropriate next best

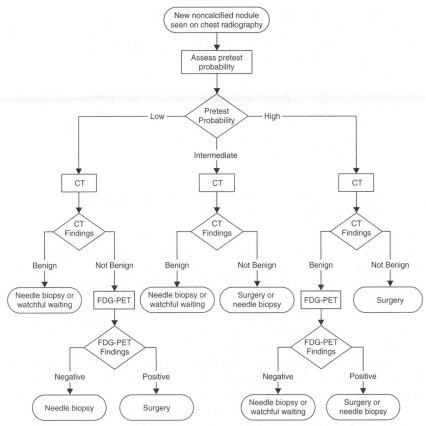

Figure 11.7 Algorithm for the evaluation of solitary pulmonary nodule, stratified by pre-test probability. The algorithm indicates the preferred strategy for evaluation of a solitary pulmonary nodule for low, intermediate, and high pre-test probabilities of cancer. CT = computed tomography; FDG-PET = 18-flourodeoxyglucose positron emission scanning. (Modified from Gould MK *et al*. Cost effectiveness of alternative management strategies for patients with solitary pulmonary nodules. *Annals of Internal Medicine* 2003; **138**, 724–735, with permission from the American College of Physicians.)

strategy) for each decision option for each of the 1000 to 10 000 runs of the model. With these results, the analyst can calculate the probability that the cost-effectiveness of a strategy is below a chosen threshold (say, $100 000 per QALY gained), accounting for the uncertainty in all model parameters chosen by the analyst. For example, if the cost-effectiveness of a decision option was less than $100 000 per QALY gained in 600 of 1000 model runs, then the probability of that strategy being cost effective (for that threshold) would be 60%.

In our pulmonary nodule example, probabilistic sensitivity analysis indicated that for patients with low and high pre-test probability of cancer, strategies that included PET were cost effective (at a threshold of $100 000 per QALY) in 77% and 99% of simulations, respectively.

11.3.9 Address ethical issues, discuss results

The important lesson from this example is that decision models can help us understand complex diagnostic and treatment problems. How to evaluate and treat a pulmonary nodule is complicated because the clinician can choose from several diagnostic tests, which can be done in different sequences, and from several treatment options. The analysis helped us choose the most effective and cost-effective strategies from among 40 clinically plausible options. The example also shows how the concepts of sensitivity, specificity, and pre-test and post-test probability are essential to understanding complicated real-world medical decision problems.

11.4 Use of complex models for individual-patient decision making

Our example of the evaluation of a solitary pulmonary nodule illustrates how complex some medical decisions can be. The examples we have discussed show analyses that help inform clinical decisions, such as whether to screen for HIV or how to evaluate possible lung cancer. Although our lung cancer example showed the importance of the pre-test probability of cancer in choosing a management strategy, we did not discuss other characteristics of the patient that might be very important for individual patient decisions. For example, what if the patient had other illnesses that would make surgery more risky? And should older patients – who are at greater risk of death from other cause – be treated the same as younger patients? How should patients' utilities be incorporated into a decision? The sophisticated models we have discussed in this chapter took several years and cost well over $100 000 to develop. Given the effort and expense needed to develop such models, you might well ask how clinicians and patients could use these models for individual decisions. We now address this topic.

How to use decision models for patient-specific decision making is an active area of research. Computer-based programs that aim to help clinicians or patients make clinical decisions are called **decision support systems**. Among the many types of decision support systems, we will focus on a specific example: a prototype system that uses the decision model we just discussed to help clinicians evaluate solitary pulmonary nodules. Systems such as the one we will discuss seem promising, but whether they will prove useful in day-to-day clinical practice is a research question that has not yet been addressed.

11.4.1 The Alchemist decision support system

The Alchemist decision support system uses a modification of the model that we discussed in Section 11.3 to provide patient-specific decision support about the evaluation and management of pulmonary nodules. The decision support system, a prototype that is not in clinical use, was developed by Gillian Sanders at Duke University, Michael Gould at Southern California

Kaiser-Permanente, and colleagues (see the paper by Sanders *et al.* (2000) for a description of an earlier prototype for this system). The system has a Web-based interface that enables clinicians to enter information about a specific patient. This information is transmitted to a computer that runs the decision model using as model inputs the patient-specific information entered by the clinician.

The clinician first enters information that helps estimate the pre-test probability of cancer, based on a clinical prediction rule (see Swensen *et al.*, 1997). The clinical prediction rule uses the patient's age, size, and location of the nodule, appearance of the nodule, history of extrathoracic malignancy, and history of smoking to estimate the pre-test probability that the nodule is malignant. The clinician can also enter information about her assessment of the risks associated with diagnostic procedures, based on information she knows about the patient. For example, an older patient, or a patient with breathing problems, might be at higher risk for a needle biopsy than are other patients.

The decision support system then analyzes the decision model using the inputs entered by the clinician. The output of the decision support system, transmitted back to the clinician via the Internet, is an analysis of the outcomes and costs associated with different management strategies, based on the patient-specific information. The system generates a patient-specific algorithm, and tables that show health and economic outcomes, and cost-effectiveness, for different management strategies for the clinician's patient. Thus, Alchemist performs a real-time analysis adjusted for the clinical characteristics of the patient. A clinician could then use the model's results to help guide therapy.

Another important aspect of individual decision making is incorporation of the patient's utilities for health outcomes into decisions. Although the Alchemist system, as currently designed, does not allow the user to input patient-specific utilities, inclusion of utilities would be a straightforward extension. To incorporate patient-specific utilities, the clinician could assess a patient's utilities for the relevant outcomes using the techniques such as the standard gamble or the time tradeoff, and then enter the utilities using the Web-based interface to the decision model.

11.4.2 Challenges for individual-patient decision making

A system such as Alchemist provides a mechanism for synthesizing the best available evidence and for incorporating patient-specific information in a formal decision-making framework. Such an approach has the potential to build on a comprehensive body of evidence and on the tools of decision making that you have studied in previous chapters.

However, developers and users face significant challenges in using models for individual decision support. The information available to tailor the probabilities of chance events, such as the mortality from surgery or a diagnostic procedure, may be limited. Fortunately, the analyst or clinician can use sensitivity analysis to decide whether such uncertainties are important. In addition, the representation of a patient's utilities is complex. For problems in which quality of life is an important determinant of the preferred treatment alternative, a patient-specific model would be improved by using the patient's utilities for the relevant health states. Models can alert clinicians to the importance of utilities for a specific problem and identify which outcomes are particularly important in terms of patients' utilities. In addition, few models capture risk preference fully (as discussed in Chapter 7). Finally, for a decision support system that is used in practice, the developers would need a method for keeping the system current and for modifying both the structure and inputs to the model when new information or alternatives become available. Such a process would likely require ongoing funding, another potential challenge, especially if the decision support system is not proprietary.

The methodologic challenges are active areas of research. We note that even if we can meet these challenges, generally a model cannot capture all of the factors of a decision that are relevant for a specific patient. However, such systems are meant to be aids to judgment, not a substitute for it. Thus, the appropriate question is not whether a model can capture every relevant consideration, but whether the patient and clinician can make more informed decisions with the aid of a model-based analysis than without one. We believe that decision models have substantial potential to help make better informed decisions.

Summary

In this chapter, we discussed how to choose among advanced modeling techniques, how to use a model to develop screening policy, how to analyze a complicated diagnostic problem, and how a model might be used as an aid for individual decision making. The main goal of the chapter was to illustrate how analysts apply the concepts you learned in earlier chapters to real-world problems. Decision models are now used in the development of clinical guidelines, as the basis for cost-effectiveness analyses and as the basis for analyses of complex screening, diagnostic, and therapeutic decisions.

Decision models are particularly useful for:
- Integrating evidence about alternatives, probabilities, and preferences.
- Illuminating tradeoffs between length of life, quality of life, risk, and costs.
- Describing the tradeoffs between harms and benefits in a formal framework that takes into account their probabilities and the patient's utilities for them.

- Identifying the factors that are key determinants of the effectiveness and cost-effectiveness of alternatives.

Although most clinicians will not be involved in the development of models like those in this chapter, they can apply the underlying concepts in daily clinical practice. These concepts can help clinicians understand when to order tests, how to interpret them, how to weigh harms and benefits, how to understand chance events and probability, and how to understand the role of patients' preferences (utilities) in decisions. As should be evident from the many examples in the book, good decisions do not always lead to good outcomes, and bad decisions do not always lead to bad outcomes. The play of chance is an inevitable part of medical decision making. But clinicians who understand the concepts covered in this book have a powerful framework for helping patients make decisions that increase the likelihood that they will have the outcomes that are most consistent with their preferences.

Bibliography

Bendavid, E., Young, S.D., Bayoumi, A.M. *et al.* (2008) Cost effectiveness of HIV monitoring strategies in resource-limited settings – a Southern African analysis. *Archives of Internal Medicine*, **168**, 1910–18.

This study uses a microsimulation model to evaluate cost-effectiveness of management strategies for HIV.

Briggs, A., Weinstein, M., Fenwick, E. *et al.* (2012) Model Parameter Estimation and Uncertainty Analysis: A Report of the ISPOR-SMDM Modeling Good Research Practices Task Force-6. *Medical Decision Making*, **32**(5), 722–32.

This paper provides best practices for parameter estimation and uncertainty analysis.

Caro, J., Briggs, A., Siebert, U., and Kuntz, K. (2012) Modeling Good Research Practices – Overview: A Report of the ISPOR-SMDM Modeling Good Research Practices Task Force-1. *Medical Decision Making*, **32**(5), 667–77.

This paper provides an overview of a series of papers that describe best practices in modeling, developed by a joint task force of the International Society for Pharmacoeconomics and Outcomes Research (ISPOR) and the Society for Medical Decision Making (SMDM).

Felli, J.C. and Hazen, G.B. (1998) Sensitivity analysis and the expected value of perfect information. *Medical Decision Making*, **18**, 95–109.

This article introduces the concept of expected value of information, an important, advanced topic, not covered in the chapter.

Gould, M.K., Sanders, G.D., Barnett, P.G. *et al.* (2003) Cost effectiveness of alternative management strategies for patients with solitary pulmonary nodules. *Annals of Internal Medicine*, **138**, 724–35.

This study is the basis of the example in Section 11.3 of the chapter.

Joyce, V.R., Barnett, P.G., Bayoumi, A.M. *et al.* (2009) Health-related quality of life in a randomized trial of antiretroviral therapy for advanced HIV disease. *Journal of the Acquired Immunodeficiency Syndrome*, **50**, 27–36.

This study uses the time tradeoff, standard gamble, EQ-5D, and the health utilities index version 3 to assess the quality of life with HIV infection.

Karnon, J., Stahl, J., Alan, B. *et al.* (2012) Modeling using Discrete Event Simulation: A Report of the ISPOR-SMDM Modeling Good Research Practices Task Force-4. *Medical Decision Making*, **32**(5), 701–11.

This paper provides best practices for developing and analyzing discrete-event simulation models.

Long, E.F., Brandeau, M.L., and Owens, D.K. (2010) The cost effectiveness and population outcomes of expanded HIV screening and antiretroviral treatment in the United States. *Annals of Internal Medicine*, **153**, 778–89.

This study uses a dynamic compartmental model to assess population health and economic outcomes of expanded HIV screening and treatment.

Owens, D.K. and Nease, R.F. (1997) A normative analytic framework for development of practice guidelines for specific clinical populations. *Medical Decision Making*, **17**, 409–26.

This article demonstrates a method for tailoring guidelines to specific populations using expected value of information.

Paltiel, A.D., Weinstein, M.C., Kimmel, A.D. *et al.* (2005) Expanded screening for HIV in the United States – an analysis of cost effectiveness. *New England Journal of Medicine*, **352**, 586–95.

This study evaluates HIV screening using a microsimulation model.

Pitman, R., Fisman, D., Zaric, G.S. *et al.* (2012) Dynamic Transmission Modeling: A Report of the ISPOR-SMDM Modeling Good Research Practices Task Force-5. *Medical Decision Making*, **32**(5), 712–21.

This paper provides best practices for developing and analyzing dynamic transmission models.

Roberts, M., Russell, L., Paltiel, A.D. *et al.* (2012) Conceptualizing a Model: A Report of the ISPOR-SMDM Modeling Good Research Practices Task Force Working Group-2. *Medical Decision Making*, **32**(5), 678–89.

This paper describes a conceptual framework for modeling and how to choose a modeling approach.

Sanders, G.D., Nease, R.F., and Owens, D.K. (2000) Design and pilot evaluation of a system to develop computer-based site-specific practice guidelines from decision models. *Medical Decision Making*, **20**, 145–59.

This paper describes an early version of the Alchemist decision support system.

Sanders, G.D., Bayoumi, A.M., Sundaram, V. *et al.* (2005) Cost effectiveness of screening for HIV in the era of highly active antiretroviral therapy. *New England Journal of Medicine*, **352**, 570–85.

This study is the basis of the example in Section 11.2 of the chapter.

Siebert, U., Alagoz, O., Bayoumi, A.M. *et al.* (2012) State-Transition Modeling: A Report of the ISPOR-SMDM Modeling Good Research Practices Task Force-3. *Medical Decision Making*, **32**(5), 690–700.

This paper provides recommendations for the development, analysis, and reporting of state-transition models.

Swensen, S.J., Silverstein, M.D., Ilstrup, D.M., Schleck, C.D., and Edell, E.S. (1997) The probability of malignancy in solitary pulmonary nodules. *Application to small radiologically indeterminate nodules. Archives of Internal Medicine*, **157**, 849–55.

This paper describes a clinical prediction rule to predict the probability of cancer in solitary pulmonary nodules.

Index

(Note: Page numbers in *italics* refer to Figures; those in **bold** to Tables.)

Medical Decision Making, Second Edition. Harold C. Sox, Michael C. Higgins and Douglas K. Owens.
© 2013 John Wiley & Sons, Ltd. Published 2013 by John Wiley & Sons, Ltd.